The laboratory revolution in medicine

Modern medicine is based on the laboratory. It is in the laboratory that diagnostic tests are performed, that diseases are identified, that therapies are tested, and new scientific knowledge is produced. It is this basis in the laboratory which is seen to provide the power and authority of modern medicine.

Laboratory medicine developed in the nineteenth century, principally in Germany, France, Britain and the United States of America. While a number of scholars have studied various aspects of laboratory medicine in the nineteenth century, no attempts have hitherto been made to synthesise such work and to present a view of the whole subject.

This book brings together leading researchers on the history of laboratory medicine in Europe and America. Each brings their special expertise to bear on the general subject of the nature and genesis of laboratory medicine. Together, they provide a much needed account of how medicine in western industrial societies acquired its distinctive power and authority through association with the laboratory. These historical studies are followed by a short concluding section of 'Reflexions' by scholars from the fields of laboratory studies, philosophy of science, and gender studies.

This collection forms a companion volume to *The medical renaissance of the sixteenth century* (1985, edited by Andrew Wear, Roger French and I. M. Lonie), *The medical revolution of the seventeenth century* (1989, edited by Roger French and Andrew Wear) and *The medical enlightenment of the eighteenth century* (1990, edited by Andrew Cunningham and Roger French).

The laboratory revolution in medicine

Edited by
ANDREW CUNNINGHAM
and
PERRY WILLIAMS
Wellcome Unit for the History of Medicine, University of Cambridge

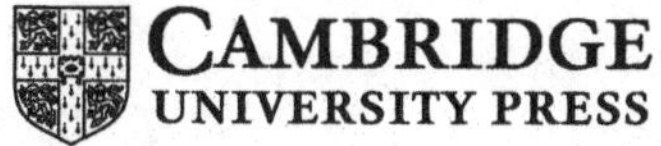

PUBLISHED BY THE PRESS SYNDICATE OF THE UNIVERSITY OF CAMBRIDGE
The Pitt Building, Trumpington Street, Cambridge, United Kingdom

CAMBRIDGE UNIVERSITY PRESS
The Edinburgh Building, Cambridge CB2 2RU, UK
40 West 20th Street, New York NY 10011–4211, USA
477 Williamstown Road, Port Melbourne, VIC 3207, Australia
Ruiz de Alarcón 13, 28014 Madrid, Spain
Dock House, The Waterfront, Cape Town 8001, South Africa

http://www.cambridge.org

First published 1992
First paperback edition 2002

A catalogue record for this book is available from the British Library

Library of Congress Cataloguing in Publication data
The laboratory revolution in medicine / edited by Andrew Cunningham
and Perry Williams.
p. cm.
Companion v. to: The medical renaissance of the sixteenth century
/ edited by A. Wear, R. K. French. and I. M. Lonie. 1985; The medical
revolution of the seventeenth century / edited by Roger French and
Andrew Wear. 1989; and The medical enlightenment of the eighteenth
century / edited by Andrew Cunningham and Roger French. 1990.
ISBN 0 521 40484 3 (hardback)
1. Diagnosis. Laboratory – History – 19th century. 2. Medicine –
Research – History – 19th century. I. Cunningham, Andrew, Dr.
II. Williams, J. P., Dr. III. Medical renaissance of the
sixteenth century. IV. Medical revolution of the seventeenth
century. V. Medical enlightenment of the eighteenth century.
[DNLM: I. History of Medicine, 19th Cent. – Europe. 2. History of
Medicine, 19th Cent. – United States. 3. Laboratories – history –
Europe. 4. Laboratories – history – United States. WZ 60 L123]
RB37.L2755 1992
616.07'56'09034–dc20 91-36254 CIP
DNLM/DLC
for Library of Congress

ISBN 0 521 40484 3 hardback
ISBN 0 521 52450 4 paperback

Contents

Illustrations

Contributors

Wai Chen	26 Belsize Park, London NW3 4DU
Andrew Cunningham	Wellcome Unit for the History of Medicine, University of Cambridge
Nicholas Jardine	Department of the History and Philosophy of Science, University of Cambridge
Richard L. Kremer	Department of History, Dartmouth College, Hanover, New Hampshire
Bruno Latour	Centre de Sociologie de l'Innovation, Ecole Nationale Supérieure des Mines, Paris
Timothy Lenoir	Program in the History of Science, Stanford University
Michael A. Osborne	History Department, University of California, Santa Barbara
Stewart Richards	Wye College, University of London
Hilary Rose	Department of Applied Social Studies, University of Bradford
John Harley Warner	Section of the History of Medicine, Yale University School of Medicine
Paul Weindling	Wellcome Unit for the History of Medicine, University of Oxford
Perry Williams	Wellcome Unit for the History of Medicine, University of Cambridge

Acknowledgements

We are most grateful to the Wellcome Trust for their generous support of the Cambridge Wellcome Unit conference from which this volume took its origin.

We would also like to thank those who contributed papers at the conference which are not published here: Bill Bynum, John Pickstone, Stella Butler, Harry Paul, and most especially Merriley Borell.

Harmke Kamminga and Thomas Schlich helped with checking the text, and Don Manning made most of the photographs: our thanks to all three.

Introduction

ANDREW CUNNINGHAM AND PERRY WILLIAMS

If you feel unwell and go to see a doctor or are admitted to hospital, the chances are that the physicians will take a sample of your body – generally blood, tissue or urine – and send it away to another place for testing; in such cases the decision as to whether you are ill or not, and if you are, what disease you have, will be primarily taken not by you and not by your doctor but by a laboratory test. If you require treatment, this will probably involve the administration of medicinal substances prepared not by you nor by your doctor but in a highly specialised factory-like laboratory. If you decide to become a doctor yourself, your formal professional training will begin not with general practice, nor with hospital work, but with study of the medical sciences, in lecture rooms, libraries and laboratories. If you have already qualified as a doctor and are trying to decide which field of medicine to enter, you will find that the highest professional prestige is attached not to saving large numbers of lives through preventative medicine in the Third World, not to providing service to the community through general practice, nor even to hospital consultancy, but to medical research in scientific laboratories.

Why should the laboratory have become so dominant in modern medicine?

It has taken historians a long time to begin addressing this question. A start was made, one might think, over twenty years ago, when Erwin Ackerknecht posited a threefold distinction between the 'bedside medicine' which held sway in Western Europe from the Middle Ages to the eighteenth century, the 'hospital medicine' especially associated with Paris between 1794 and 1848, and the 'laboratory medicine' which predominated thereafter, right up to our own time.[1]

In fact, of these three categories, neither 'bedside medicine' nor 'laboratory medicine' were much taken up at first by historians.[2] Rather it was 'hospital medicine' that was studied, largely because of its suitability for making comment – complimentary or critical – on certain features of modern medicine, of which it was seen as marking the origin. There was certainly plenty of justification for this view. For as is now generally accepted, following the work of Ackerknecht, Foucault and others, the rise of 'hospital medicine' involved a dramatic transformation in both the *location* of medicine and its *content*. The hospital became the centre of medical teaching and research and the arbiter of medical knowledge. Teaching at the bedside of hospital patients became the norm – an essential part of a medical education, and not just an optional extra if one had the time and the money. The patients became a resource for medical research – something only made possible by the increased power of doctors within hospitals. In the realm of medical knowledge, humoral pathology was replaced by anatomical pathology, in which disease was primarily identified with lesions. As a result, post-mortem examinations became routine, in order to identify pathological changes after death, and distinctive diagnostic techniques (such as percussion, palpation and auscultation) were developed for identifying the same changes before death – techniques which were pointless to anyone not within the clinical system of thought.[3] All of

[1] Erwin H. Ackerknecht, *Medicine at the Paris Hospital 1794–1848* (Baltimore, 1967), pp. vii and xi. 'Hospital medicine' is sometimes also referred to as 'clinical medicine', following Foucault's terminology (see note 3) and the modern practice of referring to the hospital part of medical education as 'clinical'. This can be confusing; originally the term 'clinical' meant no more than 'at the bedside', so that there would have been no distinction with 'bedside medicine'. It was only after the rise of hospital medicine that 'clinical' was identified with 'hospital', so that for us an 'out-patient clinic' is not a self-contradiction.

[2] One notable use of 'bedside medicine' is N. D. Jewson, 'The disappearance of the sick-man from medical cosmology, 1770–1870', *Sociology*, 10 (1978), pp. 225–44.

[3] The classic works on this subject are Ackerknecht, *Medicine at the Paris Hospital*; and Michel Foucault, *The Birth of the Clinic: An Archaeology of Medical Perception*, trans. A. M. Sheridan (London, 1976; original French edn, 1963). Different perspectives are provided by David M. Vess, *Medical Revolution in France 1789–1796* (Gainsville, Fla., 1975), who emphasises the role of army surgeons; Toby Gelfand, *Professionalizing Modern Medicine: Paris Surgeons and Medical Science and Institutions in the 18th Century* (Westport, Conn., 1980), who emphasises the role of pre-revolutionary surgeon reformers; Russell C. Maulitz, *Morbid Appearances: The Anatomy of Pathology in the Early Nineteenth Century* (Cambridge, 1987), who concentrates on the development of pathological anatomy; and Robert Kilpatrick, 'Nature's schools: the Hunterian revolution in London hospital medicine 1780–1825', unpublished Ph.D. thesis (University of Cambridge, 1989), who argues that hospital medicine developed independently in London.

these features of early nineteenth-century 'hospital medicine' are of course fundamental to the medicine of our own culture.

By thus identifying modern medicine's origin with the rise of hospital medicine, historians have inadvertently minimised and obscured from view the later change from hospital medicine to laboratory medicine; it was as though the rise of the laboratory was simply the addition of another resource, the possibility of doing the same thing better. What we are now appreciating is that the claim that medicine should be based on the laboratory actually involved demoting the importance of the hospital. Claude Bernard's famous statement of the claim in 1865 makes this clear:

> I consider hospitals only as the entrance to scientific medicine: they are the first field of observation which a physician enters; but the true sanctuary of medical science is a laboratory; only there can he seek explanations of life in the normal and pathological states by means of experimental analysis. I shall not concern myself here with the clinical side of medicine; I assume it as known or as still being perfected in hospitals by the new methods of diagnosis which physics and chemistry are constantly giving to symptomatology. In my opinion, medicine does not end in hospitals, as is often believed, but merely begins there. In leaving the hospital, a physician, jealous of the title in its scientific sense, must go into his laboratory; and there, by experiments on animals, he will seek to account for what he has observed in his patients, whether about the action of drugs or about the origin of morbid lesions in organs or tissues. There, in a word, he will achieve true medical science.[4]

From a perspective in which the primary site of medical teaching, medical research and medical knowledge and authority was the *hospital*, Bernard's claim that to be a true physician one had to pass through the *laboratory* was a staggering one. What this suggests is that the transition to laboratory medicine was a revolution at least as great as the transition to hospital medicine which preceded it.

In the English-speaking world, we are now beginning to get a picture of that revolution as a result of work in a number of different traditions. Historians of the medical sciences are examining the creation in the nineteenth century of new disciplines such as bacteriology, and identifying fundamental changes in old disciplines such as physiology – which only in the time of Magendie and Müller went from being a study concerned with *organs* and other parts serving the animal soul, a discipline closely associated with anatomy, to a study of the *processes* of living bodies.[5] Historians of the

[4] Claude Bernard, *Introduction to the Study of Experimental Medicine*, trans. Henry Copley Greene (New York, 1957; original French edn, 1865), pp. 146–7.

[5] **Physiology**: Frederic Lawrence Holmes, *Claude Bernard and Animal Chemistry: The Emergence of a Scientist* (Cambridge, Mass., 1974); W. R. Albury, 'Experiment and explanation in the physiology of Bichat and Magendie', *Studies in the History of Biology*,

antivivisection movements are reminding us that one consequence of this new concern with living processes and experimental control was that most of the new life sciences were based to a quite unprecedented extent on experiments on living animals.[6] Historians of scientific institutions, interested in the social organisation of science, are charting the rise of the laboratory from the private chemical workrooms of the start of the century to the university-based research schools of mid-century to the huge state-funded institutes of the end of the century.[7] Historians of medical education and the medical profession are studying the rise of the elementary teaching laboratory in the middle of the century, and the increasingly dominant role of laboratory science in medical practice.[8] Historians of epidemiology

1 (1977), pp. 47–131; Gerald L. Geison, *Michael Foster and the Cambridge School of Physiology* (Princeton, 1978); John V. Pickstone, 'Bureaucracy, liberalism and the body in post-Revolutionary France: Bichat's physiology and the Paris School of Medicine', *History of Science*, 19 (1981), pp. 115–42; Timothy Lenoir, *The Strategy of Life: Teleology and Mechanism in Nineteenth-Century German Biology* (Dordrecht, 1982; reprinted Chicago, 1989); John Lesch, *Science and Medicine in France: The Emergence of Experimental Physiology 1790–1855* (Cambridge, Mass., 1984); W. Bruce Fye, *The Development of American Physiology: Scientific Medicine in the Nineteenth Century* (Baltimore, 1987); Gerald L. Geison (ed.), *Physiology in the American Context 1850–1940* (Bethesda, Md, 1987); L. S. Jacyna, 'Medical science and moral science: the cultural relations of physiology in Restoration France', *History of Science*, 25 (1987), pp. 111–46; William Coleman and Frederic L. Holmes (eds), *The Investigative Enterprise: Experimental Physiology in Nineteenth-Century Medicine* (Berkeley, 1988); Stephen Jacyna (ed.), *A Tale of Three Cities: The Correspondence of William Sharpey and Allen Thomson* (London, 1989). **Pathology**: Russell C. Maulitz, 'Rudolf Virchow, Julius Cohnheim and the program of pathology', *Bulletin of the History of Medicine*, 52 (1978), pp. 162–82; L. S. Jacyna, 'The laboratory and the clinic: the impact of pathology on surgical diagnosis in the Glasgow Western Infirmary, 1875–1910', *Bulletin of the History of Medicine*, 62 (1988), pp. 384–406. **Bacteriology**: K. Codell Carter, 'The Koch–Pasteur dispute on establishing the cause of anthrax', *Bulletin of the History of Medicine*, 62 (1988), pp. 42–57; Thomas D. Brock, *Robert Koch: A Life in Medicine and Bacteriology* (Madison, Wis., 1988); Bruno Latour, *The Pasteurization of France*, trans. Alan Sheridan and John Law (Cambridge, Mass., 1988; original French edn, 1984).

[6] Richard D. French, *Antivivisection and Medical Science in Victorian Society* (Princeton, 1975); Coral Lansbury, *The Old Brown Dog: Women, Workers, and Vivisection in Edwardian England* (Madison, Wis., 1985); Nicolaas A. Rupke (ed.), *Vivisection in Historical Perspective* (London, 1987); E. M. Tansey, 'The Wellcome Physiological Research Laboratories 1894–1904: the Home Office, pharmaceutical firms, and animal experiments', *Medical History*, 33 (1989), pp. 1–41.

[7] The classic study of the social organisation of scientific work is Joseph Ben-David, *The Scientist's Role in Society: A Comparative Study* (Englewood Cliffs, 1971). Major recent works include: Robert Fox and George Weisz, *The Organization of Science and Technology in France, 1808–1914* (Cambridge, 1980); David Cahan, *An Institute for an Empire: The Physikalisch-Technische Reichsanstalt 1871–1918* (Cambridge, 1989); Jeffrey Allan Johnson, *The Kaiser's Chemists: Science and Modernization in Imperial Germany* (Chapel Hill, 1990).

[8] Arleen M. Tuchman, 'Science, medicine and the state: the institutionalization of scientific medicine at the University of Heidelberg', unpublished Ph.D. thesis (University of Wisconsin, 1988); 'Experimental physiology, medical reform, and the politics of education

and public health are pointing to the importance of the laboratory-based germ theory of disease in establishing the basis of disease-management in the colonies of the European imperial powers at the end of the nineteenth century, and in shaping modern attitudes to cleanliness and hygiene.[9] Historians of instruments are studying the rapid development of new investigative techniques, especially in microscopy and in the graphic recording of changing physiological quantities, and the increasing application of such research instruments to clinical use.[10] Historians of business are drawing attention to the increasing industrial role of the laboratory, especially in the drug

at the University of Heidelberg: a case study', *Bulletin of the History of Medicine*, 61 (1987), pp. 203–15; 'From the lecture to the laboratory: the institutionalization of scientific medicine at the University of Heidelberg' in Coleman and Holmes (eds), *The Investigation Enterprise*, pp. 65–99; S. V. F. Butler, 'Science and the education of doctors in the 19th century: a study of British medical schools with particular reference to the development and uses of physiology', unpublished Ph.D. thesis (Manchester University, 1982); 'A transformation in training: the formation of university medical faculties in Manchester, Leeds and Liverpool, 1830–1884', *Medical History*, 30 (1986), pp. 115–32; Russell C. Maulitz, '"Physician versus bacteriologist": the ideology of science in clinical medicine' in Morris J. Vogel and Charles E. Rosenberg (eds), *The Therapeutic Revolution: Essays in the Social History of American Medicine* (Philadelphia, 1979), pp. 91–107.

9 Michael Warboys, 'The emergence of tropical medicine: a study in the establishment of a scientific speciality' in G. Lemaine *et al.* (eds), *Perspectives on the Emergence of Scientific Disciplines* (The Hague, 1976); Charles E. Rosenberg, 'Florence Nightingale on contagion: the hospital as moral universe', in his (ed.), *Healing and History: Essays for George Rosen* (London, 1979); William Coleman, *Death is a Social Disease: Public Health and Political Economy in Early Industrial France* (Madison, Wis., 1982); C. E. Gordon Smith and Mary F. Gibson, 'Yellow fever in South Wales, 1865', *Medical History*, 30 (1985), pp. 322–40; James Trostle, 'Early work in anthropology and epidemiology: from social medicine to the germ theory, 1840 to 1920', in Craig R. Jones (ed.), *Anthropology and Epidemiology: Interdisciplinary Approaches to the Study of Health and Disease* (Dordrecht, 1986), pp. 35–57; William Coleman, *Yellow Fever in the North: The Methods of Early Epidemiology* (Madison, Wis., 1987); Richard J. Evans, *Death in Hamburg: Society and Politics in the Cholera Years 1830–1910* (Oxford, 1987); Roy MacLeod and Milton Lewis (eds), *Disease, Medicine and Empire: Perspectives on Western Medicine and the Experience of European Expansion* (London, 1988); Paul Weindling, *Health, Race and German Politics Between National Unification and Nazism, 1870–1945* (Cambridge, 1989).

10 Merriley Borell, 'Extending the senses: the graphic method', *Medical Heritage*, 2 (1986), pp. 114–21; 'Instrumentation and the rise of modern physiology', *Science and Technology Studies*, 5 (1987), pp. 53–62; 'Instruments and an independent physiology: the Harvard Physiological Laboratory, 1871–1906', in Geison (ed.), *Physiology in the American Context*, pp. 293–321; 'Marey and d'Arsonval: the exact sciences in late 19th-century French medicine', in J. L. Berggren and B. R. Goldstein (eds), *From Ancient Omens to Statistical Mechanics: Essays on the Exact Sciences Presented to Asger Aabae* (Copenhagen, 1987), pp. 225–37; Robert G. Frank, Jr, 'The telltale heart: physiological instruments, graphic methods, and clinical hopes, 1854–1914' in Coleman and Holmes, *The Investigative Enterprise*, pp. 211–90; Stella Butler, R. H. Buttall and Olivia Brown, *The Social History of the Microscope* (Cambridge, n.d.); Brian Bracegirdle, *A History of Micro-Technique: The Evolution of the Microtome and the Development of Tissue Preparation* (London, 1978).

industry.[11] Finally, sociologists and anthropologists are offering a new perspective from which to study laboratories, by examining their role in the construction of knowledge and technology through the building of social alliances.[12]

To bring these different perspectives together for an examination of the whole subject of the origins and nature of the laboratory revolution in medicine we organised a conference on 'Medicine and the Laboratory'. This book contains revised versions of some of the papers given there, together with others. Rather than focusing on the personalities and work of a few celebrated laboratory scientists such as Bernard, Pasteur and Koch, to which discussion of the laboratory in medicine has conventionally been limited, we have tried to cover issues of more general importance about the bringing into existence of laboratories in medicine, about the power they came to wield, and about what precisely goes on inside them. Our aim has been to open up a wider discussion of 'the laboratory revolution in medicine'.

Thus Timothy Lenoir raises the questions: why did teaching and research laboratories, especially those for experimental physiology, become institutionalised in German medical education before their benefits to the practice of medicine were visible? It was not a simple matter of growth, he argues, but was closely related to a shift in ideology: what he calls the 'discourse of practical interest'. This new discourse provided the ideological foundations for the second wave of institute building, which brought regular education in experimental physiology to the mass of doctors. He traces the connections of this ideology with the concept of Progress and with the material improvement and the industrialisation of Germany. The promotion

[11] Jonathan Liebenau, *Medical Science and Medical Industry: The Formation of the American Pharmaceutical Industry* (Basingstoke, 1987); 'Paul Ehrlich as a commercial scientist and research administrator', *Medical History*, 34 (1990), pp. 65–78.

[12] H. M. Collins and T. J. Pinch, *Frames of Meaning: The Social Construction of Extraordinary Science* (London, 1982); G. Nigel Gilbert and Michael Mulkay, *Opening Pandora's Box: A Sociological Analysis of Scientists' Discourse* (Cambridge, 1984); H. M. Collins, *Changing Order: Replication and Induction in Scientific Practice* (London, 1985); Michael Lynch, *Art and Artifact in Laboratory Science: A Study of Shop Work and Shop Talk in a Research Laboratory* (London, 1985); David Gooding, '"In Nature's School": Faraday as an experimentalist' in David Gooding and Frank A. J. L. James (eds), *Faraday Rediscovered: Essays on the Life and Work of Michael Faraday, 1791–1867* (Basingstoke, 1985), pp. 105–35; Steven Shapin and Simon Schaffer, *Leviathan and the Air-Pump: Hobbes, Boyle, and the Experimental Life* (Princeton, 1985); Bruno Latour and Steve Woolgar, *Laboratory Life: The Construction of Scientific Facts*, 2nd edn (Princeton, 1986); Peter Galison, *How Experiments End* (Chicago, 1987); Bruno Latour, *Science in Action: How to Follow Scientists and Engineers Through Society* (Milton Keynes, 1987); David Gooding, Trevor Pinch and Simon Schaffer (eds), *The Uses of Experiment: Studies in the Natural Sciences* (Cambridge, 1989).

of the practical (as opposed to *Wissenschaft*, knowledge for its own sake) was part and parcel of this movement, he argues, and hence laboratories, which now taught the practical, were made central to the training of doctors. 'Physicalism' too was part of this movement, and he examines the rise of physicalism in German physiology with a study of the early careers of Emil du Bois-Reymond and Hermann Helmholtz and their associates in the 1840s, through to their involvement in the Berlin Physical Society and the training offered by Magnus in the 1850s and '60s, in which physiology was treated as a branch of physics and as an essential practical science.

The laboratories themselves are the focus of the chapters by Richard Kremer and Paul Weindling. Kremer discusses three attempts to set up physiological institutes in Prussia in the early period, with a detailed analysis of the negotiation process involved in persuading (or failing to persuade) the state officials that such facilities needed to be built and funded: that future physicians need an experimental and experiential education in physiology was still not yet accepted as obvious. Weindling compares the funding, location and internal organisation of two of the great institutes of the late nineteenth century, the Pasteur Institute in Paris, more pluralist in its organisation and flexible in its relations, and Robert Koch's more centralist and hierarchical Institute for Infectious Diseases in Berlin. These two institutes were the germ theory put into bricks and mortar, and with their different structures and emphases they provided the great centres for the dissemination of the germ theory and of belief in the centrality of the laboratory to medicine, through their training of an international corps of researchers and teachers.

The chapters by John Harley Warner, Michael Osborne and Stewart Richards serve to illustrate the long process which was necessary to convince ordinary practitioners and members of the public to accept the authority of the laboratory. Warner describes how American physicians before the Civil War had become committed to the Parisian model of medical science in which authority was based on clinical experience, so that laboratory medical science was initially resisted as a theoretical, mystifying and elitist form of knowledge; the eventual acceptance of the claims of the laboratory towards the end of the century, he argues, thus involved a change in the form of knowledge supposed to carry authority. Osborne explores the considerable resistance to Pasteurian views on disease causation put up by Louis-Félix-Achille Kelsch, a French military physician and epidemiologist at the Val-de-Grâce hospital who, though knowledgeable about and interested in bacteriology, consistently minimised its significance for military medicine; even while admitting the aetiological role of germs, he maintained that environmental factors were crucial for their virulence, and they were therefore not sufficient to account for the outbreak of epidemics. A concern with disease causation was not enough, in itself, to convert one to Pasteurian views, for Kelsch was very concerned with disease causation; but his view of what this involved was wider than that of the bacteriologists. As a believer in medical geography, Kelsch preferred 'that great laboratory of nature' (as he called it) to the laboratory of the microbiologists.

The existence and practice of the medical laboratory, particularly the experimental physiological laboratory but also the microbiological and pharmaceutical laboratories, depend crucially on the experimental use of animals. When these laboratories became more common, both for teaching and research, more and more animals were regularly (to use the technical term) 'sacrificed' in them in the cause of science. This vastly extended use of experimental animals necessitated a profound change in sensibility on the part of the practitioners of laboratory medicine. The live animal had to be transformed into, and be perceived as, simply a neutral object of scientific investigation and not as a perceptive pain-feeling fellow-creature being put to the torture.[13] There were loud objections to this attempted transformation in perception and sensibility, especially in Britain, and the medical laboratory was thus the site of struggle between the antivivisectionists and the advocates of experimental research. Stewart Richards discusses these disputes about the regulation of vivisection in late nineteenth-century Britain and makes an important distinction between ethical and aesthetic objections to the physiological laboratory, observing that while the use of anaesthetics to relieve the suffering of the animal greatly weakened the ethical argument against vivisection, yet the aesthetic objection was left untouched: attitudes for or against vivisection, he concludes, depended as much on feeling (aesthetics), in particular that of revulsion, as they did in the scientific argument that the animals were safely anaesthetised and therefore free from suffering.

Two chapters deal with the role of the laboratory in the actual construction of medical knowledge, and how it determines the form

[13] On this transformation see Michael E. Lynch, 'Sacrifice and the transformation of the animal body into a scientific object: laboratory culture and ritual practice in the neurosciences', *Social Studies of Science* 18 (1988), pp. 265–89.

and authority of such knowledge. Andrew Cunningham studies the case of plague to examine how concepts of infectious disease were transformed by the laboratory, showing how a disease which was formerly identified by symptoms was turned into a disease which could only be identified in a laboratory through determining there the presence or absence of a specific micro-organism or pathogen. Wai Chen examines the Inoculation Unit at St Mary's Hospital, London, founded by Sir Almroth Wright, and argues that its entire programme of medical research was shaped by the laboratory's role as a commercial vaccine factory; he argues that even the most famous product of that laboratory – penicillin (which was not a vaccine, of course) – was given an identity constructed by the requirements of the laboratory's vaccine programme.

In the final section of the book, three scholars with different theoretical perspectives offer their reflexions on the subject of laboratory medicine. Bruno Latour, whose work has done so much to suggest new perspectives on the historical investigation of the role and importance of laboratories in medicine, writes from the perspective of the anthropology of science. In a revised version of the talk which he gave in the final session of the original conference, he encourages us to move away from sociological concepts like professionalisation and institutionalisation when trying to understand the origin and power of the laboratory in medicine, and instead to look at the opposition to the laboratory and how it was overcome; to pursue the analogy between the laboratory and the factory, and the simultaneous production of both goods (or facts) and a market for them; and to revive Foucault's notion of 'discipline' as applying both to what happens inside the laboratory, say to microbes or experimental animals, and outside the laboratory, to professional colleagues. From the perspective of the philosophy of science, Nicholas Jardine observes that the traditional presentist historiography of the laboratory was created by the nineteenth-century laboratory-propagandists to legitimate their own enterprise, and he looks towards the creation of a new historiography which would combine the insights of the historiographies of texts and discourses, of networks, and of social interests, while supporting a commonsense ontology and engaging with the content of science through the investigation of specific laboratory practices. From the perspective of gender studies, Hilary Rose calls for us to ask how far the laboratory vision, the particular manual and mental skills taught by the teaching laboratory, was the product not merely of a specific class but of a specific gender within that class.

Reflecting on how the original conference (and indeed this book) not only suffered from a gender imbalance in its participants, but scarcely touched on gender issues at all – the significant exception being the session devoted to Stewart Richards's chapter on vivisection, where feelings and sensibility for the first time were discussed – she speculates on how a conference in a feminist utopia might see the laboratory revolution of the nineteenth century and patriarchal studies of it, such as (for the most part) this book.

Taking all these contributions together, we can see certain common themes. One is that the claims made on behalf of the laboratory – both the cognitive claims of representing nature more accurately and authentically and in an unmediated way, and the practical claims of delivering clinical benefits – were not in themselves self-evident or naturally compelling. Admittedly, these claims were propounded with enormous confidence. For example, it was frequently stated and assumed by advocates of the medical laboratory that the new techniques and instruments of the laboratory had had the human element totally removed, so that they were completely objective, and in the laboratory Nature was most herself and spoke clearly in her own voice. Thus Robert Koch said that by the use of photographic techniques in the laboratory 'the microscopical object copies itself', and there could therefore be no doubt as to what Nature was saying; an editor of the *Lancet* wrote that with the invention of the sphygmograph 'the pulse ... writes its own diagram, and registers its own characters', and Almroth Wright said that his laboratory techniques of the capillary pipette 'evolved themselves'.[14] Those who made claims for the practical benefits of the laboratory were no less assertive. Famously, Claude Bernard looked forward to a time when experimental physiology would have made the aetiology of every disease as well-known as that of scabies (caused by a mite), and the cure of every disease no less certain: 'we cure it *always* without any exception, when we place ourselves in the known experimental conditions for reaching this goal'.[15] Nevertheless, the conclusion of our contributors is that such claims had little justification. The new techniques and tests were not obviously objective; for example, Almroth Wright's sophisticated, much-used and supposedly 'self-

[14] R. Koch, 'On the investigation of pathogenic organisms', trans. Victor Horsley, in W. Watson Cheyne (ed.), *Recent Essays by Various Authors on Bacteria in Relation to Disease* (London, 1886), pp. 1–64, at p. 20; *Lancet* editorial, quoted in Frank, 'The telltale heart', p. 211; A. E. Wright, *Handbook of the Technique of the Teat and Capillary Glass Tube: And its Applications in Medicine and Bacteriology* (London, 1912), p. v.

[15] Bernard, *Introduction to the Study of Experimental Medicine*, p.214.

evolved' laboratory procedures for the measurement of the 'opsonic index' were not objective to those who did not believe in the existence of opsonin (which would nowadays include all of us). The therapeutic spin-offs of laboratory science were virtually non-existent until the end of the century; though microscopy and analytical chemistry had early applications in the area of *diagnosis*, these were initially techniques that were brought to the bedside, and were therefore more an extension of the clinical approach than laboratory medicine. In general, our contributors consider that the plausibility of these claims about the importance of the laboratory made by the advocates of laboratory medicine in the nineteenth century is not something to be assumed; rather it is one of the things to be explained.

As a consequence of this, many of our contributors explicitly represent the laboratory revolution not as a self-evident piece of progress, a change which needed no justification, but as the outcome of a group struggle: the victory of advocates of the laboratory over others. Hospital physicians, the most powerful and most crucial group of those sceptical of the necessity, the usefulness or even the relevance of laboratories, were still maintaining fierce opposition in the early twentieth century. Of the other main opponents to the laboratory, the less powerful and less strategically important general practitioners of medicine were won over only to a limited degree, and antivivisectionists have of course never been persuaded by the claims of the laboratory. Recovering the perspective of the opponents, as some of our authors have done, is a very effective way of revealing the contingency of the values and interests associated with laboratories, seeing them as the creation of groups with very particular situations in society.

Taken together, the chapters of this book point the way to a more comprehensive picture of 'the laboratory revolution in medicine', similar to the one currently being developed for the laboratory revolution in the physical sciences:[16] a perspective which integrates, firstly, the activity which went on inside the laboratories – not just the creation of theories but more fundamentally the choice of objects of study and the development of instruments and techniques to prove particular theories; secondly, the relationship between laboratory researchers or advocates and other groups in society; and thirdly, the nature of the society in which these changes took place. Several of the chapters link the rise of the laboratory first to the rise of the

[16] Frank A. J. L. James (ed.), *The Development of the Laboratory: Essays on the Place of Experiment in Industrial Civilisation* (Basingstoke, 1989).

professions – not merely professionalisation, the reorganisation of groups to increase their status, but the reorganisation of *society* in the nineteenth century which gave a leading role to a new professional class laying claim to expert knowledge and certain values such as freedom, truth and objectivity; and second to the rise of industry, which placed a new premium on deterministic causal laws in the realm of theory and on technical control in the realm of practice. In general, the laboratory revolution can be set alongside the political, industrial and philosophical revolutions of the nineteenth century as one aspect of the transformation from a society dominated by Church and aristocracy to one dominated by the industrial, commercial and professional classes.

One confirmation of this view comes from noting in which countries it was that laboratory medicine originated. Although laboratory science and laboratory medicine are now universal, it is remarkable that they have come within a mere hundred and fifty years to dominate the many other forms of knowledge and medicine which formerly flourished all over the world. The distinctive feature of the countries where laboratory medicine originated – Western Europe, particularly the German states, France and Britain, and the United States of America – was that for the most part they had industrial and commercial interests which led to the acquisition of overseas colonies, and it was through these that their culture, including their medicine, was exported. Seen from a global perspective, therefore, 'the laboratory revolution in medicine' was a development in the native medicine of modern Western Europe; this medicine was then made universal by exportation – an act which was, as Weindling puts it, 'the assertion of cultural supremacy through medical science'.[17]

Indeed it was one of the greatest supporters of the expansionist Second Empire in France, Louis Pasteur, who made one of the most passionate claims for the importance of the laboratory:

> if the conquests useful for humanity touch your heart, if you are astounded by the surprising effects of electrical telegraphy, daguerreotype, anaesthesia and so many other admirable discoveries, if you are jealous of the part your country may boast in the development of these marvels, then – I implore you – take an interest in these sacred dwellings, so expressively called *laboratories*. Ask for them to be multiplied and ornamented. They are the temples of the future, of wealth and well-being.[18]

[17] See Chapter 5 below. On the exporting of laboratory institutions, see Ilana Löwy, 'Yellow fever in Rio de Janeiro and the Pasteur Institute mission (1901–1905): the transfer of science to the periphery', *Medical History*, 34 (1990), pp. 144–63.

[18] Pasteur, 'Le budget de la science', first published 1868; reprinted in *Oeuvres de Pasteur*, ed. Pasteur Vallery-Radot, 7 vols. (Paris, 1922–39), vol. VII, pp. 199–204, at p. 200; as translated

The laboratory revolution called for by Pasteur and Bernard was accomplished: laboratories indeed became 'sacred dwellings'. Laboratory culture is so closely entwined with the society that gave it birth that in the present state of social organisation we are practically compelled, in Bruno Latour's phrase, to make a 'detour through the laboratory'.

in René Vallery-Radot, *The Life of Pasteur*, trans. Mrs R. L. Devonshire (London, 1937; original edition, 1901), p. 152, with modifications; emphasis as in original French.

1

Laboratories, medicine and public life in Germany 1830–1849

Ideological roots of the institutional revolution

TIMOTHY LENOIR

Introduction

The most celebrated aspect of medical education in German-speaking lands during the nineteenth century is the introduction of organised training in experimental methods and the use of a variety of scientific instruments and diagnostic aids as a standard part of the medical curriculum. Understanding the factors driving these institutional developments in Germany has been the focus of much research, but it has always been a field mined with paradox. For it is not at all evident why teaching and research laboratories should have become institutionalised within German medical faculties in institutes for anatomy and physiology at such an early date, well in advance of any demonstrable benefits of the laboratory to medical practice.[1]

One resource for addressing these issues has been the institutional dynamics of the German academic system. The works of Joseph Ben-David and Awraham Zloczower, R. Steven Turner and Charles McClelland have amply documented the workings of a bureaucratic rationale oriented in terms of the ideology of the Humboldt reforms supporting *Lehr-und-Lernfreiheit*, and *Wissenschaft um ihrer selbst willen*.[2] In their treatment of the practical workings of the academic

[1] The institutionalisation of medical specialities in Germany is catalogued in Hans-Heinz Eulner, *Die Entwicklung der medizinischen Spezialfächer an den Universitäten des deutschen Sprachgebietes* (Stuttgart, 1970).

[2] See in particular: Awraham Zloczower, *Career Opportunities and the Growth of Scientific Discovery in Nineteenth-Century Germany, with Special Reference to Physiology* (New York, 1981); Joseph Ben-David and Awraham Zloczower, 'Universities and academic systems in modern societies', *European Journal of Sociology*, 3 (1962), pp. 45–84; Joseph Ben-David, 'Scientific growth: a sociological view', *Minerva*, 2 (1963), pp. 455–76; R. Steven Turner, 'The growth of professorial research in Prussia, 1818 to 1848 – causes and context', *Historical Studies in the Physical Sciences*, 3 (1972), pp. 137–82; Charles McClelland, *State, Society and University in Germany, 1700–1914* (Cambridge 1980);

system these authors have drawn special attention to the institutional structures controlling career advancement, particularly the role exercised by high standards of qualification for academic appointments, which were administered by autonomous state ministries in an open, competitive market.

In a recent article I have suggested that this institutional model requires some significant modification. In particular, by focusing on the institutional dynamics of the 'star system', it does not distinguish between the fundamentally different character and orientation of the institutes constructed in the period from the late 1860s to about 1880 and their predecessors constructed in the period between the 1820s and the 1840s. These new institutes dwarfed their first-wave predecessors by several orders of magnitude in physical plant and budget, as well as in the numbers of students who received laboratory training in them. The model developed by Ben-David and others, however, treats this second wave of institutes as a natural outgrowth of the institutional dynamics of the academic system established in the early period; the old institutes simply got larger as the demands for laboratory space and equipment required for the growth of knowledge became more complex. In contrast to this, in a case study exploring the foundation of Ludwig's institute in Leipzig, which was the first of the second-wave physiological institutes, and du Bois-Reymond's institute in Berlin, which was one of the last, I have argued that the new institutes registered a major shift in ideology and in the intended clientele of physiological institutes, a shift which brought about an integrated approach to physiology and oriented the field towards medical and clinical research. Whereas the earlier institutes were primarily intended to bring into close personal contact with a man of scientific genius an elite corps of students destined to advance the frontiers of knowledge, the new institutes were designed to impart laboratory training to the man of average talent intended for a career in routine medical practice.[3] My study confirms for the medical

Steven Turner, Edward Kerwin and David Woolwine, 'Careers and creativity in nineteenth-century physiology: Zloczower redux', *Isis*, 75 (1984), pp. 523–9.

[3] Emil du Bois-Reymond gave expression to the new policy orientation behind the formation of what he referred to as the 'new temples of science' in the inaugural lecture dedicating his new institute in 1877: '[It] is not on account of the geniuses (may there be many among you) that this institute is here; geniuses have always succeeded in making their way even without such institutes. Rather to impart sound physiological intuition and rigorous inductive training as light and armor in the insecure half-darkness of medicine to the person of average intelligence, indeed to the person of lesser ability; that is the reason for the existence of this institute, and if it achieves this purpose, the sacrifices for it will not have been too great.' See Emil du Bois-Reymond, 'Der physiologische Unterricht sonst und jetzt' in *Reden* (Leipzig, 1912), vol. 1, p. 651.

sciences a thesis developed by David Cahan for the physical sciences; namely, that there was an institutional revolution in the organisation of science in the German states as science was self-consciously harnessed to the needs of a nascent, industrialising, capitalist economy.[4] In light of this new ideological imperative, natural science and rigorous methodical thinking, once regarded as the proper mental equipment for the elite intellectual leadership of the nation, was now regarded as essential for rank-and-file professionals, the 'Durchschnittsköpfe' as du Bois-Reymond referred to them.

These results suggest all the more strongly that we take another look at what was going on in the first phase of institution-building. Many features of the institutional model are certainly correct, but its focus was upon explaining how the norms governing teaching, research and publication were assembled into a coherent institutionalised role, a problem focus which is rather too strongly presentist in orientation and insufficiently sensitive to complexities of interest, context and contingency within the perspectives of the actors themselves. One difficulty with this approach, for example, is that it treats the building of the early institutes as completely imposed from above by enlightened state ministries of education and culture. But were these noble and high-minded objectives the only interests of the state ministries? Were the sorts of efforts to exercise social and political control through medical and educational institutions to which we have been alerted by historians such as Michel Foucault absent in Germany, in states otherwise famous for their obsession with control? No less missing from this account is any sense of institutions as structures mediating multiple objectives of the various groups in whose interests the institutions are constructed and maintained, including those persons recruited to make careers within their walls. More directly related to the point of this chapter, if the thesis concerning the 'institutional revolution' can be sustained, are the roots of the shift in ideological commitments that made the new institutional mission possible, the sources of its legitimating narrative.

Recently a number of historians have addressed the sorts of questions raised above by exploring how academically trained physicians attempted to acquire a monopoly over the provision of

[4] See David Cahan, 'The institutional revolution in German physics', *Historical Studies in the Physical Sciences*, 15 (1984), pp. 1–65; Timothy Lenoir, 'Science for the clinic: science policy and the formation of Carl Ludwig's institute in Leipzig' in William Coleman and Frederic L. Holmes (eds), *The Investigative Enterprise* (Berkeley, 1988), pp. 139–78.

health care between the mid-1820s and early 1850s, and how these efforts affected the development of medical institutions. In two well-documented studies, Claudia Huerkamp and Ute Frevert argue that interests in securing discipline and state authority motivated the state to support the professionalisation strategies of physicians.[5] They argue that academically trained physicians, particularly the *Wundärzte* and *Kreisphysici*, were used as agents of state control in the rural communities by giving them power of decision in matters of public hygiene, especially in administering smallpox vaccinations, registering births and deaths, and treating mental illness, as well as in settling disputes concerning the legitimacy of local healers to practise, and other local health matters. Other studies have suggested that by making an activist scientific medicine the intellectual core of their efforts and by linking it with the instrumental armamentarium of microscopes and the new diagnostic tools, the professionalising efforts of academic physicians created an environment conducive to the support of laboratory medicine.[6]

My concern in the present chapter is to consider the place of the laboratory within the social and cultural context of the early nineteenth century, particularly in the period of the late 1830s and 1840s. During this period the necessity of including the laboratory as an essential component in a professionalisation project was largely unproven. My purpose here is to show that discussion about the power of diagnostic tools, laboratories, scientific medicine and rational therapeutics should rather be seen as an important ideological element in a narrative legitimating a moderate liberal vision of social and political progress and as part of a social process linked with the formation of a distinctive German middle class. Recent work by German social historians provides helpful orientation. The new German social history has argued that along with the dissolution of feudal corporate forms of social organisation, one of the major developments of the *Vormärz* period was the emergence of a bourgeois middle class with its own values, self-image and culture. In place of the splintered multitude of groups of *Honoratioren*, *Bildungsbürger*, bankers, business people, military officers, state officials, etc., making

[5] Claudia Huerkamp, *Der Aufstieg der Ärzte im 19. Jahrhundert* (Göttingen, 1985). Ute Frevert, *Krankheit als politisches Problem* (Göttingen, 1983).

[6] See Timothy Lenoir, 'Social interests and the organic physics of 1847' in Edna Ullmann-Margalit (ed.), *Science in Reflection* (Boston, 1988), pp. 169–91; Arleen Tuchman, 'Science, medicine, and the state: the institutionalization of scientific medicine at the University of Heidelberg', unpublished Ph.D. dissertation (University of Wisconsin, 1985).

up the traditional *Bürgertum* a new homogeneous class was born.[7] In their work on the emergence of the middle class, Hans-Ulrich Wehler, Jürgen Kocka and Rheinhart Koselleck have focused primarily on the structural factors of population growth: the demographic, economic and political changes conditioning these developments. Without minimising the power of these structural conditions as constraints on action, I am rather concerned about the self-conscious efforts of various groups of individuals to actively *construct* a new bourgeois culture and, with it, a narrative legitimating the interests of the new middle class in Germany. My aim in this chapter is to show that discourse about the natural sciences and laboratories participated in this process in two ways. First, those interested in forging a bourgeois culture emphasised the importance of shaping what they called a national public life.[8] In the literature devoted to this project, science was seen as a model of public life. Second, discussions about laboratories as model forms of social organisation and the positive prospects of contributions from the laboratory toward material progress in industry and medicine were important elements of a narrative in which this image of a new German bourgeoisie as the progressive class of the future was constructed and legitimated. Rather than studying the establishment of a particular social role or the place of experimental science in professionalisation strategies, I am interested in laboratories as elements of a bourgeois *mentalité*.[9]

In order to depict laboratories as forms of life in which this *mentalité* was nourished, I will follow some of the actors – namely, du Bois-Reymond, Helmholtz, Ludwig and occasional others – who began their careers in the early laboratories and later participated in the second wave of institution building. I will depict their goals and

[7] See the extremely impressive synthesis and evaluation of these studies in Hans-Ulrich Wehler, *Deutsche Gesellschaftsgeschichte*, vol. II: *Von der Reformära bis zur industriellen und politischen 'Deutschen Doppelrevolution', 1815–1845/49* (Munich, 1987), especially pp. 185–210.

[8] One of the strongest statements of this issue was given by Jakob Burckhardt in a lengthy review article he wrote on the Berlin exhibition of 1842. Two historical paintings by Belgian painters, Louis Gallait's *Abdication of Charles V* and Charles de Bieve's *Signing the Compromise of 1566*, had created a sensation for their powerful realism. Burckhardt asserted that no German painter could paint such a historical work and offered as an explanation that 'in order to be able to create painting of historical realism it is not sufficient simply to have had a history; more important it is necessary to have participated in a public life [ein öffentliches Leben]'. See Jakob Burckhardt, 'Bericht über die Kunstausstellung zu Berlin im Herbst 1842', *Kunstblatt*, 24 (1843), no. 1, pp. 1–2, no. 2, pp. 5–7, no. 3, pp. 9–12, no. 4, pp. 13–15. The quotation is from p. 15.

[9] The most useful discussion on the different senses of ideology and its relation to a form of life is Raymond Geuss, *The Idea of Critical Theory: Habermas and the Frankfurt School* (Cambridge, 1981).

their visions of what it was possible to achieve, in light of the constellation of beliefs and attitudes they held about the society in which they wanted to live, and I will link these ideological components to the practical actions of these individuals and others whom they knew. Using a variety of sources I will reconstruct a field of interacting discourses which represents 'the politics of practical interest'. Clustered around the concern with practical interest in various forms are subjects which the actors in my study took to be crucial to their lives: these include economic growth, industrialisation and the ways to ameliorate poverty engendered by new social changes, as well as views about the constitution both of society and of disease; about the relation of the state to the medical profession and the state's role in the organisation of trade; and about realism, materialism and practical interests in philosophy and politics. My aim is to illustrate the ways in which the discourses within this web were mutually supporting. These contingent and interlocking fields of discourse enabled certain representations to authorise and organise domains of practice.

Wehler points out – and he does not claim to be the first to do so – that class formation involves a complex of factors such as occupational background, family politics, socialisation experiences, social and geographical mobility, and minority traditions. No less crucial is conflict with opposed forces, particularly political conflict.[10] The laboratory and its place in the new culture of industrial society was defined by conflict. For the process I am describing, the revolutions of 1848–9 were a watershed, on the far side of which an agenda was formulated and the elements of an ideology coalesced which legitimated the institutional revolution of the 1860s. During the late 1840s and early 1850s the actors who created the laboratories of the institutional revolution and defined their cultural role encountered resistances to achieving their purposes. They experienced constraints on their actions, constraints provided by the walls, both visible and invisible, of the institutions in which they lived and negotiated their future.

Born from this encounter with constraints was a project for remaking the world. To illustrate these formative processes I will focus on the early stages of the careers of du Bois-Reymond, Helmholtz and Ludwig, in which they all turned from idealism to 'practical interest' in various areas of intellectual and political life. The discourse of practical interest generated enthusiasm for

[10] Wehler, *Deutsche Gesellschaftsgeschichte*, vol. II, p. 197.

materialism and for an instrumentalised link between medical theory and practice, providing the ideological foundations of the second wave of institution building.

The discourse of practical interest

The values and images, the projected reforms of economy and politics, the vision of the future and the appreciation of certain features of the present articulated by the discourse of practical interest expressed important elements of the common culture of the students working in Johannes Müller's laboratory. A partial portrait of this culture, from an actor's perspective, emerges from the published correspondence of Helmholtz and the correspondence between du Bois-Reymond and his father during his student years and the early stages of his attempt to carve out a career for himself in Berlin. Additional letters between du Bois-Reymond and other friends, including Helmholtz, Brücke, Ludwig and Eduard Hallmann, as well as the correspondence between Helmholtz and his father, fill out the picture.

The letters of du Bois-Reymond and Helmholtz to their parents reveal both similarities and differences in the values and outlook of the two generations. The political and economic circumstances of the late 1840s made the differences become tensions. By the standards of the 1830s and 1840s both the fathers, Felix du Bois-Reymond and Ferdinand Helmholtz, were basically 'liberal', Helmholtz's liberalism being of a more idealist cast. But both men were more conservative than their sons, particularly with regard to religion. Although the Revolution of 1848 made both generations more conservative, the idealism of the older generation was shown to be a bankrupt illusion, while the moderate liberalism of the younger generation emerged as the basis of a realist approach to the future.

Ferdinand Helmholtz had been a *Landstürmer*, a volunteer in the wars to free Prussia from Napoleonic imperialism, and his burning passion was the formation of a united German state, a dream he shared with most members of his generation who had engaged in the struggle against Napoleon and who had passed through the first phase of the new humanistic *Gymnasium* and research seminars. They believed this idealism of the spirit would eventually produce material results. Helmholtz frequently expressed such views in the circle of his family and close friends, and on several occasions he even made public professions of such views in his classes at the Potsdam *Gymnasium*, where he was responsible for the programme of German language instruction.[11] In the late 1840s, on the eve of the Revolution of 1848, Ferdinand Helmholtz was censured for such outbursts and for his participation in a local organisation called the *Treubund*, expressing strong religious conservatism and criticising the policies of the regime. Bitterly disappointed by the outcome of the Revolution, Ferdinand Helmholtz would in later life seek refuge in subjective idealism.

The letters between Hermann Helmholtz and his father depict an ongoing discussion, which frequently assumed the proportions of a struggle, over epistemological issues. The father, Ferdinand Helmholtz, had been a student of Johann Gottlieb Fichte, and in the letters he advocates Fichte's subjective idealism. Ferdinand Helmholtz's closest friend was Immanuel Hermann Fichte, the son of the famous philosopher and a well-known idealist philosopher-theologian in his own right. I. H. Fichte was Hermann Helmholtz's godfather. In his letters Ferdinand Helmholtz explicitly announced his agreement with Fichte's religious and political views. These letters illuminate the conservative liberalism of the head of the Helmholtz family.

From the late 1830s I. H. Fichte was one of the leading philosophers opposing the Hegelians. He expressed his opposition in numerous books and articles, but his most influential forum was the journal which he co-edited with Christian Hermann Weiße, the *Zeitschrift für Philosophie und spekulative Theologie*. Fichte and Weiße's programme was 'speculative theism'. As a propaedeutic to their ultimate theological aims, they needed to develop an epistemology and a theory of science [*Wissenschaftslehre*] resting on a different concept of knowledge than the one Hegel presupposed. Rather than treating the knowing subject and the object of knowledge as different aspects of the same identity, namely as the temporalised self-revelation of the Absolute, as Hegel had advocated, Fichte wanted to reintroduce an objective empirical moment independent of the subject. For Fichte, there certainly is a subjective element in experience, but thought is not just a subjective game. The necessity of thought, he wrote, immediately presupposes the necessity of being or reality. Emphasis on the objectivity of empirical experience could reverse the splintering of philosophers into hostile camps which the terrorism of the 'identity philosophy' had produced. 'Philosophy needs to recognise the objective system of things in the world', wrote Fichte. 'This system is the foundation of true community among philosophers and at the

[11] See Leo Koenigsberger, *Hermann von Helmholtz*, 3 vols. (Brunswick, 1902), vol. 1, pp. 4–6.

same time that which brings philosophy into continuous reciprocal contact with the other sciences.' To encourage this ecumenicism, Fichte dropped the blatant programmatic mission of his journal by renaming it the *Zeitschrift für Philosophie und philosophische Kritik*. In the first issue of the new series, he proposed a general philosophical congress to take place in September 1847 in Gotha.

At the risk of jumping ahead of our story to events of the late 1840s, it is useful to characterise Fichte's (and Ferdinand Helmholtz's) 'Gotha Programme'; for it provides useful orientation within the discourse between the generations in the 1840s, a discourse which erupted into a full-fledged confrontation in Johannes Müller's laboratory:

> As certain as the heart and soul of *Wissenschaft* is free research, it is also certain that she cannot make her pure claims of legitimacy dependent upon practical needs. Because for *Wissenschaft* practical interests do not exist; her only concern is with objects of research... To *Wissenschaft* as such it is irrelevant whether this or that form of government, or this or that church of religious viewpoint is dominant. For her, state and church, politics and religion, are not real objects, rather they are ideas, ideal objects of her investigation... And therefore every proper investigation of such practical questions is truly and in the deepest sense conservative; for the ideas of the state, of freedom and of religion are the only permanent supports of the existing order [*alles Bestehenden*], the powers capable of saving humanity from error and destruction.[12]

On the eve of the Revolution, Fichte sought to unite the splintered factions of philosophical schools and bring them together in support of the state. At the Gotha congress he advocated adopting a republican constitution within the community of academic philosophers and preserving peace by turning away from practical interests. Unfortunately, this meant excluding – temporarily – outspoken materialists from the government of the philosophical republic:

> Only one direction in philosophy should be put aside in its present stage of development – and certainly not silenced for all time; that is materialism. In consideration of the general social conditions which have presently become the concern of civilised humanity, this direction of philosophy more than any other single cause has contributed to the diminished reputation of philosophy among the German people; for it [materialism] has dissolved the calm of the spirit which philosophy requires.[13]

[12] Immanuel Hermann Fichte and Hermann Ulrici, 'Ankündigung der vom Jahre 1847 an erscheinenden Zeitschrift für Philosophie und philosophische Kritik, als Fortsetzung der Fichteschen Zeitschrift für Philosophie und speculative Theologie', *Zeitschrift für Philosophie und philosophische Kritik*, 17 (1847), p. 4.

[13] *Zeitschrift für Philosophie*, 18 (1847), pp. 309–21, at 310–11. These were the words of the representative of the Duke of Gotha who opened the congress, and endorsed by Fichte in his presentation of the proceedings. The same attitude was expressed by Hermann Ulrici, Fichte's co-editor in the new *Zeitschrift*; see his 'Die wissenschaftlichen Tendenzen im Verhältniß zu den praktischen Interessen', *Zeitschrift für Philosophie*, 17 (1847), pp. 25–37.

This same liberalism, constrained by fears of the effects of materialism and the pursuit of practical interests on the moral order, permeated the household of the young Emil du Bois-Reymond. In 1838 as the nineteen-year-old du Bois-Reymond began his university study in Bonn, he faced the problem that confronted many young Bürger of choosing a career appropriate to his talents and commensurate with his social station. Like his comrades and cohorts, he brought with him a fairly well-formed set of self-expectations, a sense of where he 'belonged' in society and what his prospects might be for realising his aspirations. Like many a young nineteenth-century Bürger, he also carried a heavy responsibility for advancing the station of his family. His father's letters constantly reminded him of that fact. In frequent passages, the father, Felix du Bois-Reymond, extolled the opportunities open to Emil which had been unavailable to the 'poor beggar from Neûchatel.'[14]

A man with a simple education, Felix du Bois-Reymond had worked himself into a position of respectability as a Prussian bureaucrat, and as a mid-ranking member of the privileged educated class, he wished for his son to achieve the highest status within the Bildungsbürgertum. Like Ferdinand Helmholtz, Felix du Bois-Reymond was an idealist of the old school. In a letter to Eduard Hallmann, Emil du Bois-Reymond characterised his father's philosophical views and his own difficulties with them:

> It is impossible for me to get along with my father, a totally committed Kantian and therefore one of the slyest dialecticians in the world. Reference to the immediate facts of consciousness is never allowed; rather after the insufficiency of human capacity to grasp the interconnections of the universe is demonstrated, only the dry *tabula rasa* of scepticism remains possible, from which one can *ad libitum* either take the path according to Hegel's expression *sicut canis redire ad vomitum* or throw oneself in the arms of the tradition of revelation and the dualist ideas of good and evil. That a third path other than this Kantian standpoint of self-destruction might be possible – the path of healthy human understanding which takes the world as it is – is dismissed as crass Lockeanism, and so forth.[15]

After attending the philosophical and anthropological lectures of Immanuel Fichte[16] and immersing himself in Schelling, Goethe and a

[14] These letters are in the du Bois-Reymond papers at the Staatsbibliothek Preussischer Kulturbesitz in Berlin, Depositum Runge-du Bois-Reymond, K 10, III, 3.

[15] *Jugendbriefe von Emil du Bois-Reymond an Eduard Hallmann*, edited by Estelle du Bois-Reymond (Berlin, 1918), p. 52.

[16] Du Bois-Reymond discusses these courses with his father in his letters during the year 1838–9 which he spent in Bonn. The lectures of Fichte are among those beside which he placed an asterisk indicating their special appeal to him. The letters are in the du Bois-Reymond papers at the Staatsbibliothek Preussischer Kulturbesitz in Berlin, Depositum Runge-du Bois-Reymond, K 10, III, 3.

variety of *Naturphilosophen*, Emil du Bois-Reymond rejected that idealist world-view and the old-style Kantianism of his father.

Apart from revealing typical parental hopes, the letters between du Bois-Reymond and his father provide important clues to reconstructing the image of the society in which those hopes could be realised. Occasionally in his letters, Felix du Bois-Reymond suggested useful and important reading for his son, particularly articles in *Lexikons*, compendia discussing philosophical, social and especially economic issues. The references are not haphazard, for during the period of the correspondence Felix du Bois-Reymond was busy completing a four-volume work on social problems in Germany[17] (which he published under the quasi-pseudonym of Bodz Reymond, perhaps in order not to draw the criticism of his superiors in the Prussian ministry), and on the problems of poor relief created by industrialisation. The letters indicate these problems were discussed with regularity and intensity at home.

In Felix du Bois-Reymond's view, the main threat industrialisation presented to the social order was the manner in which economic competition disrupted solidarity and undermined religious values. As the solution, he proposed preserving older guild structures and preventing the displacement of crafts and trades by the concentration of capital in large factories. His suggestion did not go unnoticed. It was discussed, among other places, in the liberal *Conversations-Lexikon der Gegenwart* published by F. A. Brockhaus (4 vols., Leipzig, 1838–41). The author of the articles on pauperism and free trade called Felix du Bois-Reymond's book important but dissented from the conclusions of this 'otherwise liberal and politically unmotivated [*politisch unbefangenen*] man'.[18]

Having characterised the views of the father, I now want to consider the views of the son. The voluminous material preserved from du Bois-Reymond's period of youthful *Sturm und Drang* provides a vista of considerable proportions. In correspondence and in reading notes, du Bois-Reymond refers both to the content of the Brockhaus volumes and to other literature of a social and political

[17] Bodz Reymond, *Staatswesen und Menschenbildung* (Berlin, 1837–9).

[18] 'Gewerbefreiheit' in *Conversations-Lexikon der Gegenwart*, vol. II, pp. 413–21, especially p. 414. Also see 'Pauperismus', vol. IV, part I pp. 65–74, especially p. 68. The *Conversations-Lexikon* was related to a much larger, thirteen-volume encyclopaedic work published by F. A. Brockhaus, *Conversations-Lexikon: Allgemeine deutsche Real-Encyklopädie für die gebildeten Stände*, 8th edn (Leipzig, 1833–7). In constructing this portrait, I draw upon these works and upon the 9th edition of Brockhaus, a fifteen-volume work published in Leipzig between 1843 and 1848. Henceforth, I will refer to the editions of the larger work as *Real-Encyklopädie* (8th edn) and *Real-Encyklopädie* (9th edn), respectively.

nature. From these materials, we can reconstruct fairly clearly the image du Bois-Reymond had of his career chances as well as of the society that would make that career realisable.

Among the most highly praised sources in Emil du Bois-Reymond's letters are articles appearing in the Brockhaus *Lexikon* and in the *Deutsche Vierteljahresschrift*, a quarterly journal for politics, science, medicine and religion, published by Cotta in Stuttgart, the first issue of which appeared in 1837. The principal themes in these sources provide a framework within which many of Helmholtz's and du Bois-Reymond's practical decisions in their early careers become intelligible, for the two men shared the general orientation to politics, society and culture expressed in this literature.

One of the major objectives of editors of lexicons and journals of politics and culture during the 1830s and 1840s in German states was to awaken an appreciation among the middle classes of their own culture. They sought to build a self-confident image of the Bürgertum as the truly progressive class in contemporary society, in politics as well as in cultural production. The article 'Conversation' in the 1833 *Real-Encyklopädie* explains that in polite circles it was no longer acceptable to discuss simply topics related to the fine arts, music, art and theatre.[19] A person from the educated Bürgerstand was expected to have a general knowledge of *Lebensphilosophie*, natural history and anthropology, geography and geology, and political and cultural history: topics of relevance to contemporary active life in politics and the world. The well-bred Bürger, so the article instructed, should strive to achieve a sense of 'guter Ton' in conversation, a well-balanced sense of important themes, clearly presented without embellishment or pedantry. One should assist in making every person present feel an active participant in and contributor to the *Gesellschaft*.

Gesellschaft, cooperation and group solidarity are prominent themes in much of this literature. For example, one of the opening articles in Brockhaus's *Conversations-Lexikon*, entitled 'Adel und Bürgerstand der neuesten Zeit',[20] focuses on resolving the growing tensions between a small but increasingly important *Geldaristokratie* and the nobility. These social tensions were presented as the main obstacle to the realisation of the political and economic aims of the Bürgerstand. Unlike England, where cooperation had been achieved between the upper classes, the article observed, the German nobility was closing its ranks more self-consciously than at any time in the

19 'Conversation' in *Real-Encyklopädie* (8th edn), vol. II, p. 856.

20 *Conversations-Lexikon*, vol. I, pp. 50–5.

past. Indeed, the article went on to note, it was not surprising that the nobility had taken exclusive measures to preserve its social position, for in a state where education had become a necessary prerequisite to achieving a position in any branch of the civil service or military, a tendency of the two classes to mingle socially had been unavoidable and intermarriages were frequent. Moreover an increasingly large number of noble landed estates, *Rittergüter*, were passing into the hands of wealthy Bürger. If these trends continued, the article noted, the nobility would have no real basis for asserting its privileged status at all.[21]

Committed to non-revolutionary courses of action, the authors assembled by Brockhaus and Cotta pinned their hopes for political change on loosening the barriers between the upper classes of German society; in their social calculus the educated middle class was the key element. But there was also a distinct danger: that the middle class, whether educated or not, did not 'know how to value and preserve its own distinctive honour'.[22] The progressive changes the middle class hoped to bring about could all be undermined if the intellectual leadership did not cultivate and preserve distinctive middle class values. If instead the leadership allowed itself to be co-opted by the current ruling elites through assimilating aristocratic culture and values, the hopes for any real change in German society would be dashed. A theme closely connected with this was the notion that it was also necessary to break down the barriers within the Bürgerstand between the educated elite and the uneducated or non-academically trained middle classes. This was believed to be particularly critical for the future of German industry; for German industry could not survive if it were forced to develop in the helter-skelter pattern of English industrialisation. Germany had to set its course for industrialisation according to a different compass.[23] Only through the regular and concerted application of science for technological progress could German industry expect to catch up and compete with England. To this end it was necessary that academically trained scientists be brought into the faculties of the schools of trade and industry and that closer contact be established between these two groups.[24]

Closely associated with these themes of social and cultural solidarity among the middle classes were discussions of political

[21] *Ibid.*, p. 53. [22] *Ibid.*, p. 53.

[23] On this subject see the important work of Ilja Mieck, *Preußische Gewerbepolitik in Berlin 1806–1844* (Berlin, 1972); and Friedrich Zunkel, *Der Rheinisch-Westfälische Unternehmer 1834–1879* (Cologne, 1962).

[24] 'Gewerbewesen' in *Conversations-Lexikon*, vol. II, pp. 421–8.

organisation. One of the most frequently mentioned themes was the impetus to progress in the 1830s imparted by new collective forms of organisation among the Bürger classes. In an extensive discussion of clubs, societies and other types of cooperative organisations, the *Deutsche Vierteljahresschrift* concentrated on societies among natural scientists as models for rational reform which would encourage rational cooperation and avoid the dangers of revolution.[25] Organisations such as Lorenz Oken's *Verein deutscher Naturforscher und Aerzte* were praised as forerunners of German national unity and as models for nationally oriented reform-minded groups in other countries such as the British Association for the Advancement of Science in Britain. Similar appreciation of societies for promoting scientific knowledge was expressed in Brockhaus's *Real-Encyklopädie*,[26] and the *Conversations-Lexikon* devoted an extensive article to the Göttinger Magnetischer Verein organised by Carl Friedrich Gauss, Wilhelm Weber and Alexander von Humboldt. International cooperation on scientific projects such as that promoted by the Magnetischer Verein would not only indirectly assist German unification by regularising communication and contact between German states but through its leadership role would also enhance the recognition of 'German Science'.[27] The authors argued that if 'German Science' were recognised by foreign scientific groups as a distinct national orientation, this would further the cause of uniting Germany from within.

The most important of the new cooperative forms of organisation were economic, especially the German Customs Union (Zollverein). The literature most discussed in the circle of Johannes Müller's students expressed a self-conscious moderate liberalism; its central thread was the advocacy of German national unity. But unity was not to be achieved by political struggle or revolution. Rather it was to emerge from economic reform and the pursuit of material interest.[28]

[25] Mone, 'Über das deutsche Vereinswesen' *Deutsche Vierteljahresschrift* (1839), no. 3, pp. 205–34. The article 'Berliner Vereine', in *Grenzboten*, 5 (1846), no. 1, pp. 178–84, assured its readers that there was no need to fear Vereins as a source for spreading communist and socialist doctrine, which in any case were modern forms of humanism (p. 181).

[26] 'Naturforschervereine' in *Real-Encyklopädie* (8th edn), vol X, pp. 169–70.

[27] 'Magnetischer Verein' in *Conversations-Lexikon*, vol. III, pp. 436–40.

[28] See, for instance, Friedrich Nebenius, 'Über die Wirkung des Großen deutschen Zollvereins', *Deutsche Vierteljahresschrift* (1840), no. 2, pp. 253–314. Nebenius argued that commercial unity leads to the gradual interlocking of other interests, including, ultimately, legal reforms (pp. 255–6); the multiplication of all forms of communication and contact between different groups (p. 271); improvements in the conditions of the workers resulting from higher demand for labour and resultant wage increase, rising rents, and profits on capital (p. 280);

The best interest of the state was an economic policy supporting the material well-being of its citizens.[29] This was best accomplished through construction of the Zollverein, encouragement of industry, and free trade within the economic boundaries of the German states. Far from being opposed to large landed wealth, this literature saw a strong Germany arising from a balance between the interests of *Großgrundbesitz* and nascent industry, particularly the core industries surrounding the development of the railroads.

With respect to the realisation of political reform and the unification of Germany, the authors of these articles harboured no idealist illusions. They did not expect, nor did they advocate, political revolution.[30] The lengthy article 'Constitutionen als Tendenz der Zeit' in Brockhaus[31] argued, for example, that the only protection against revolution was reform.[32] But what they had in mind were not democratic legal and political reforms; their engine of change was to be gradual reform generated by improved material circumstances. Changes in the material basis of society would ultimately force changes in the legal and political superstructure. The article 'Constitutionelles Leben' in the *Conversations-Lexikon* and various articles on trade and industry resounded with the message that the unification of Germany would be effected through the expansion of industry, particularly the railways. The interlinking of material interests throughout Germany would generate the need for regulating transport, furthering credit and creating legal safeguards for the growth of industry. These developments would gradually force the laws in all the German states to approach the same form; and from there it would be a short step to a stable constitution in a nation united through and grounded in its material interests.

increase in population (p. 282); and growth in cultural goods, particularly education in technical and scientific subjects (p. 283). Gustav Höfken, 'Erweiterung des deutschen Handels und Einflusses durch Gesellschaften, Verträge und Ansiedlung', *Deutsche Vierteljahresschrift* (1842), no. 2, pp. 172–218, argued for unity through economic expansion. Also, see Ignaz Kuranda, '1845–1846' in *Grenzboten*, 5 (1846), no. 1, pp. 1–12, especially pp. 3–4.

29 See 'Materielle Interessen' in *Conversations-Lexikon*, vol. III, pp. 557–64.

30 For an especially clear statement, see Kuranda, '1845–1846', p. 12: 'Of course those who smell revolution and spot communists in the woodwork will raise their cries against us and lay all the nonsense of their denunciatory phantasies at our feet. But we can observe them with calm, because we are not revolutionaries. We do not hope for violent upheavals in the future. The German people, which is so late in coming to the great table [*Arterstafel* (*sic*)] of self-determination at which other peoples have long been seated, the German people who are much more mature and prepared as they stand at the gates of freedom than all the other nations were who passed through them, this Germany will not find it necessary to tread a bloody path. Her path is less steep and more secure.'

31 *Real-Encyklopädie* (8th edn), vol. II, pp. 818–38.

32 *Ibid.*, p. 823.

The moderate liberals assembled by Brockhaus and Cotta, then, foresaw a constitutional monarchy as the natural outgrowth of the evolution of material interest. 'Constitutionen als Tendenz der Zeit'[33] argued against a society organised around the unfettered pursuit of private, individual interest and defended instead Friedrich Schlegel's notion of the collective beliefs (*Gesammtüberzeugung*) and the constitution of the local community (*Gemeindeverfassung*) as the basis for public law and individual freedom. A constitutional monarchy would preserve these principles and conform best, so the article argued, with the natural moral character of the German nation. A popular representative government based on democratic principles would not protect the state from the excesses of the French Revolution, for it would not be an expression of true higher moral interests of the people. The parliament of a true representative government would be an expression of the 'present average moral development of the people' (*mittlern Geistesbildung des Volkes*) rather than a collection of agents acting on behalf of individual material interests.

While the authors assembled by Brockhaus and Cotta ardently advocated industrialisation as the cure to all problems, they did not defend free trade. They argued for free trade within the Zollverein but believed that during the take-off phase of German industry tariff barriers should be erected in order to foster the accumulation of capital necessary to compete successfully with England.[34] These barriers might be removed once German industry had reached maturity. Just what counted as 'maturity', however, was variously interpreted. One appropriate option was tucked away nicely in the article entitled 'Handelsfreiheit', which defended the notion that no country ever has enough capital to develop all branches of its industry to fullest potential.[35] The state should actively encourage domestic consumption and promote the accumulation of capital in a variety of industries, not just those oriented towards export. Furthermore, the state should support industrial growth through the construction of railways, improved roads and waterways, and improvements in communication, such as telegraphs, postal systems and newspapers.

While they adopted a limited free-trade doctrine and welcomed government support for industry, moderate liberals did not look kindly upon state intervention in the labour market. And if societies,

[33] *Ibid.*, pp. 818–38.
[34] See the article 'Industrie' in *Real-Encyklopädie* (9th edn), vol. VII, pp. 431–4.
[35] Handelsfreiheit' in *Real-Encyklopädie* (9th edn), vol. VI, pp. 620–1.

clubs and other cooperative forms of organisation promoted middle-class interests, they had exactly the opposite effect for workers. In the labouring classes doctrines of free trade should be enforced without hesitation. Precisely this issue had concerned Felix du Bois-Reymond, prompting his four-volume work on the causes of pauperism, *Staatswesen und Menschenbildung* (Berlin, 1837–9). While the elder du Bois-Reymond had sought a remedy in state support of guilds and worker self-help organisations, the article 'Gewerbefreiheit' argued that all restrictions on choice of work and freedom of mobility should be removed.[36] Du Bois-Reymond's work had identified the concentration of capital in the new industries as the cause of working-class material and moral depravity. Against this position, the Brockhaus article argued that in Prussia, where guilds were allowed to continue in the old trades, the material condition of the workers was not worse in the new factories where restrictions on the labour market were removed.[37] The Brockhaus volumes and the Cotta *Vierteljahresschrift* argued that the new factories were in fact the sources of increased material welfare for workers. Allowing workers to organise unions and permitting them to strike had evil consequences. Factory owners had the financial resources to hold out longer than workers; and during the period when the plant was shut down by a strike, they would take advantage of the opportunity to introduce improvements in machinery, which would further reduce wages when the defeated workers returned.[38] On the other hand, new machinery actually increased productivity and improved working conditions. In no way were the new factories the sources of pauperism or other social ills; those causes had to be sought in other more 'general conditions of society'.[39] Overall the Brockhaus and Cotta position was that only by furthering material interests would the social and political changes desired by most Germans come about. The best way to ensure that future was to protect industry and remove any obstacles to the full development of the capacities of the 'productive middle classes', the agents of historical change.

The centrality of economic reform to the moderate liberal programme made representing the preferred course of action tricky: it needed to be distinct from a path of rampant individualism and unfettered material interest, identifiable instead as a way oriented towards gradual material improvement guided by political and moral responsibility. Crucial to this plan were the modes of representation

[36] 'Gewerbefreiheit' in *Conversations-Lexikon*, vol. II, pp. 413–21.
[37] *Ibid.*, p. 414.
[38] 'Fabriken' in *Real-Encyklopädie* (9th edn), vol. V, pp. 171–4.
[39] *Ibid.*, p. 174.

and images for the production of knowledge that would authorise and legitimate its truth.[40]

The philosophical component of these new modes and images was captured for moderate liberals in an anonymous article in the *Deutsche Vierteljahresschrift* in the early 1840s. The strong reaction to the artificial idealism of German philosophy indicated the need to return to common-sense realism. The time was past when one believed reality could be grasped through an *a priori* deductive construction. 'What is being demanded now', the article observed,

> in the realm of the spirit as well as in nature is a more positive type of research into reality and a more substantial spiritual nourishment than the delightful play with ideas can provide... Even philosophy must begin with facts and experience, whether they be internal or external. Furthermore even the German no longer wants to be just a thinking being but also a being of action, and he is increasingly less satisfied with dead and fruitless knowledge which preaches its own powerlessness in life, and which may be capable of explaining things but which in practice can neither control nor command things and is incapable of doing anything in the real world.[41]

But the solution was not to be found in an escape to a crass French materialism either. The sound path to the future lay in uniting the best features of idealism and materialism in a common-sense realism.[42] Dogmatic and extremist positions were to be replaced by an eclecticism which drew together all parties.

Nearly every domain of public discourse was permeated by this deep concern to avoid vulgar (French) materialism on the one hand and (English) utilitarianism driven solely by private interest on the other. One of its most turbulent manifestations was in discussions of painting, for here, as might be expected, the issue of choice of subject matter and manner of representation appropriate to the values and goals of society was brought sharply into focus. In painting, the preferred strategy was to mark out a particular German style of realism which united materialism and idealism.

This effort was echoed in other domains as well. Articles on 'Materielle Interessen'[43] and 'Zeitgeist'[44] are miniature portraits of

[40] On 'images of knowledge' as structures for authorising knowledge production, see Yehuda Elkana, *Anthropologie der Erkenntnis: Die Entwicklung des Wissens als episches Theater einer listigen Vernunft* (Frankfurt-on-Main, 1986), especially pp. 46–58.

[41] Anon., 'Streit des Diesseits und des Jenseits in der deutschen Philosophie', *Deutsche Vierteljahresscrift* (1843), no. 2, pp. 1–73, at p. 61.

[42] *Ibid.*, pp. 62–3.

[43] 'Materielle Interessen'.

[44] 'Zeitgeist' in *Real-Encyklopädie* (9th edn), vol. xv, p. 500. 'In today's *Zeitgeist* lies a tendency toward civic and religious freedom, a noble sympathy for humane forms of organisation, and a lively sense of material progress. Whether or not an over-estimation of material interests is a sickness [*Krankheit*] of the time... is a much disputed issue.'

the Brockhaus attempt to strike a balance between materialism and idealism. The growth of material interests was taken to be a prerequisite for the pursuit of higher intellectual goals. Material and immaterial interests reinforced one another and had to be pursued together. None the less, the pursuit of material interests depended on according a certain priority to higher intellectual goals; for

> immaterial interests are the guarantor for the flowering of the material interests. However energetically material interests are pursued, as soon as immaterial interests are neglected, all efforts to achieve material well-being become fruitless. A people that stands tall spiritually and morally, will not and cannot be in need and does not have to be concerned for its well-being or for its freedom. In spite of the most favourable natural circumstances, an intellectually dull and morally corrupt people can never achieve material growth, and even the material well-being it has already achieved stands in danger of decline with the decay of its intellectual and spiritual base.[45]

The central strategy in the moderate liberal position was to represent a turn towards industry; securing the foundation of the state in shared material interests was viewed as the only reasonable means to bring about progress through cooperation of different classes. There were few mixed messages in this literature concerning the identity of the most valuable members of society, upon whom Germany's future depended. At the head of the list were two groups, the rising industrialists and what the Brockhaus article on universities called the 'new breed' of academicians.[46] On the side of the industrialists were men like David Hansemann and Friedrich Harkortt, men of outstanding ability motivated by deep patriotic feelings. They were important not only because their factories were generating wealth and creating new jobs for a growing population, but also because they were models of what individual initiative motivated by a deep patriotic commitment to the fatherland and to the common good in the pursuit of material interests could accomplish for the state. It was Hansemann, for instance, who had established a fire insurance fund, which benefited everyone in his city of Aachen.[47] Moreover, it was through the private enterprise of such individuals that other critical problems confronting the state could be solved. Industry could not only create jobs and absorb the growing excess population on the land. Through organisation of *Aktiengesellschaften* similar to Harkortt's *Unterstützungs-Verein*, it was conceivable that industry could take over the state's responsibility for financing poor

[45] 'Materielle Interessen', p. 562.
[46] 'Universitäten' in *Conversations-Lexikon*, vol. IV, part II, pp. 155–72, especially p. 164.
[47] 'Hansemann' in *Conversations-Lexikon*, vol. II, pp. 733–5.

relief. The persistent theme throughout this literature was that the state needed the entrepreneurial class and must do whatever was necessary to further and accommodate its interests. This positive message was frequently interlaced with a threat, however. The message resounded that the *Geldaristokratie* was not content to stand by and hope for the recognition of their just demands by the ruling classes. Both the Brockhaus article 'Materielle Interessen' and articles in the *Deutsche Vierteljahresschrift* observed that the potentially most politically dangerous class in Germany was the wealthy middle class.[48] Events in France during the 1830s had taught that a course of political action oriented towards improving material welfare and encouraging the development of material interests had to be co-ordinated with political reforms giving the most active members of society a participatory role, or disaster would ensue.

In this discourse of practical interest, science joined industry to form the twin pillars of the state. Moderate liberals, as I have noted, valued science as a model for building cooperative forms of social organisation leading to rational progress and the cultural unity of the German nation. No less important, however, were the contributions of science to technology and improvements in the material conditions of life. The image of the new breed of natural scientist was that of a person uninterested in dogmatic speculative systems. The most progressive scientific fields were chemistry and physics, particularly mechanics, electricity and magnetism. The educated person as well as the simple farmer, noted the Brockhaus article on 'Naturwissenschaften', could not look at the trains and steamships upon which German industry was finding its way into the world without recognising that the path to progress in the future was the command of natural forces through the application of science to technology. It was in fact the promise of this union of science and technology that made physics the leading field in the sciences; and within physics the premier speciality was work in electromagnetism. The telegraph line constructed by Gauss and Weber for their magnetic researches was just one example of the path to the promised land.[49] The leaders in other fields such as medicine and physiology were making progress by breaking with philosophical orientations and linking their theories and methods more closely to chemistry and physics.[50] Thus, Justus

[48] 'Materielle Interessen' pp. 561–2.

[49] See the articles 'Eisenbahnen' and 'Electromagnetismus' in *Real-Encyklopädie* (9th edn), vol. I, pp. 1115–36 and 1140–4, respectively.

[50] See 'Medicin und Chirurgie' in *Conversations-Lexikon*, vol. III, pp. 583–7, especially p. 584.

Liebig was praised for creating the model laboratory in Giessen which was now being reproduced in other German universities such as Göttingen and Leipzig. Liebig, the article admitted, had offended lots of people, but he would be remembered by future historians as one of the truly great scientists. Through Liebig's 'scientific mission'[51] chemistry was becoming a 'German' subject. While he was important as a theorist of chemistry, Liebig's main contribution was in developing simple techniques which could be applied broadly; his work on chemical processes of fermentation was likely to transform completely agriculture and medicine.[52]

Johannes Müller was similarly praised for having broken with the speculative approach to nature he had taken up as an enthusiastic student of Hegel and for having adopted instead 'a thorough interpenetration of theoretical and empirical research' which had opened up a new era in medicine.[53] The article on physiology noted that together with Charles Bell, Müller's comparative anatomical and experimental work on nerve function had laid the foundations for the field of neurophysiology. 'No branch of physiology', the Brockhaus author claimed, 'has had such a fruitful effect on practical medicine as the new theories of nerve function, and the important surgical advances of operative orthopaedics made by Stromeyer and Dieffenbach trace their origins to the application of the new physiological principles'.[54] Like Liebig, Müller was a model of *bürgerliche Intelligenz*. He had achieved worldwide renown through his scientific achievements in physiology, making the subject virtually dependent, so the article argued, on German advances. He organised his work not in the form of a grand system but rather in the form of a useful compendium. But Müller was also the type of independent, self-motivated new breed of academician who mixed private initiative and public concern, as evidenced, the article noted, by his efforts to build a school which would make a major impact, by his extensive publishing activities and efforts to present his views to larger audiences, and through his recent successful business ventures in Berlin.[55] Within the educated elite Müller and Liebig were of the same

51 'Liebig' in *Real-Encyklopädie* (9th edn), vol. VIII, pp. 746–7.

52 One of the longest articles in the *Deutsche Vierteljahresschrift* in the first decade of its existence was Justus Liebig, 'Das Verhältniß der Physiologie und Pathologie zur Chemie und Physik, und die Methode der Forschung in diesen Wissenschaften', *Deutsche Vierteljahresschrift* (1846), no. 3, pp. 169–243.

53 See 'Müller' in *Real-Encyklopädie* (9th edn), vol. X, p. 26; 'Müller' in *Conversations-Lexikon*, vol. III, pp. 757–8.

54 'Physiologie' in *Conversations-Lexikon*, vol. IV, part I, p. 209.

55 What these were precisely, I have been unable to ascertain.

stamp as Hansemann and Harkortt among the civic-minded entrepreneurs. These men personified the values of the new *Mittelstand* that would bring about German national unity.

Departures from this ideal personal profile were criticised, even among persons who were acknowledged to be making important contributions towards the establishment of the moderate liberal vision of progressive society. Dieffenbach, for example, was described as the greatest surgeon of all time. He had improved old techniques and introduced a variety of pathbreaking new procedures for correcting strabism and stammer. His new methods in facial plastic surgery were miraculous. On the other hand, 'Dieffenbach's effectiveness as a teacher is more than slightly limited by his exclusively practical orientation, which stands in the way of a more rigorous scientific orientation.'[56] Johann Lukas Schönlein was the object of similar damning praise. Schönlein's contributions were equally significant for science and for humanity:

> Distinguished at the bedside by his deep practical insight and his brilliant understanding of the individual case, [Schönlein] is captivating in the lecture hall through his wonderful vision of medicine in general. His main objective is to connect the principles of medicine, especially nosology, to natural history; and thus he is the creator of a nosological system for classifying diseases in a manner similar to natural history into classes, families, groups [*sic*], and species. By means of this system characteristic symptoms are united to diagnoses and individual diseases are either related to one another or separated from one another with the deep penetrating glance of an outstanding observer employing all the technical means science has to offer.[57]

The problem with Schönlein was not limitation of vision or failure to unite theory and practice, but rather unwillingness to publish his ideas and make them accessible to a larger audience. His work was actually the model of progress, but only his innermost circle of students knew and understood it. Schönlein seemed to lack the deep sense of civic responsibility and the cooperative commitment to the future needed to conform to the ideal image of a German scientist.

The image of medicine presented in this literature was that of a field at the dawn of a new era of progress led by an embattled camp of scientists. Medicine in the eighteenth and early nineteenth century had been dominated by 'systems'. By contrast, no single system dominated the current medical agenda. Medicine was in a building period in which it was attempting to understand better the facts of medical

[56] 'Dieffenbach' in *Real-Encyklopädie* (9th edn), vol. IV, pp. 344–5, at p. 345.
[57] 'Schönlein' in *Real-Encyklopädie* (9th edn), vol. XII, pp. 742–3, at p. 743.

experience with new methods and apparatus adapted from other empirical sciences, particularly physics, chemistry and physiology:

From physics we are borrowing the laws of acoustics in order to shed light on respiratory diseases, diseases of the heart, and the abdomen through auscultation and percussion...; from chemistry we are borrowing reagents with which we are researching the normal and pathological excretions of the body; and where the unarmed eye is incapable of determining normal from pathological tissues, just like the physiologists, we use the microscope, an instrument which is becoming a symbol of the new medicine.[58]

The author of the article on microscopical discoveries explained that progress in pathology and practical medicine would depend on more advanced microscopical investigation of normal tissues; but the kinds of important advances to be expected from introducing the microscope into practical medicine could already be seen in Rudolf Wagner's work on the contents of blood in pathological processes.[59] The new scientific medicine, particularly 'physiological medicine', was aggressively interventionist and no longer dominated by therapeutic nihilism, the Brockhaus author argued:

A mountain of materials is being assimilated upon which the true art of healing, therapy, will be able to draw. Furthermore, the oft repeated objection voiced by the uninformed that the art of healing lags far behind the art of identifying disease is no longer valid... Numerous diseases whose ravages the physician previously had to stand by helplessly observing with folded arms are no longer considered mortal and incurable by today's medicine; and, just as Caspar has demonstrated statistically that general mortality has declined significantly in our day, so it would be incorrect not to attribute much of this to progress in medicine, however much of the decrease may be attributable to the general progress of civilisation. Medicine owes this genuine improvement, this blessed advance to the direction it has taken in the present, a direction which no system could have guaranteed.[60]

It is important to bear in mind that while the 'image' of society described in this popular literature reflected the concrete circumstances of life in the 1830s and 1840s, it was by no means a simple transparent reporting of situations. The society described in these pages was only in part a society that existed; in even greater measure, it was a society that a group of moderate liberals hoped to construct in part through such discourse. When socio-economic changes were beginning to place noticeable strains on the existing system, the authors of these articles were attempting to persuade others of the correctness of their vision of managing a society. In 1840 they were

[58] 'Medicin und Chirurgie', pp. 584–5.

[59] 'Mikroskopische Entdeckungen' in *Conversations-Lexikon*, vol. III, pp. 646–56, especially p. 655.

[60] 'Medicin und Chirurgie', p. 585.

standing only at the beginning of developments that accelerated over the next two decades. In 1840 the relevant public to which the Brockhaus articles and other liberal journals spoke may have been relatively small and weak.

Indeed, there are indications in some of the literature on medicine that the position they articulated as the standpoint of 'scientific medicine' was an embattled one, that medicine also had its dark side. The Brockhaus author complained of overcrowding in the medical *Stand* and of the consequences it had in preventing physicians from practising their art. To eke out a living, physicians were being driven to pamphleteering and to trading in quack medicine. The author assured his readers that the causes lay much deeper than the medical profession itself, and he expected that the overcrowding of the market would soon 'drive the price of the product down to such a level that the day labourer will be unable to find his wage and be forced to take up some other honourable trade'.[61] Whereas the Brockhaus author saw the cure for overcrowding in the invisible hand of the market, the author of an extensive article in the *Deutsche Vierteljahresschrift* saw the market as precisely the problem.[62] The public did not know how to evaluate properly the ability of a physician but judged simply in terms of the size of the practice. As every good physician knew, a physician with a large practice could not be a good one. He could not devote the time needed to evaluate each case on its merits and to keep abreast of the latest scientific developments necessary for improving his diagnostic and therapeutic skills. Physicians with large practices would be forced to employ simple, routine therapies and frequently, out of expedience, they could slip into employing folk remedies and quack medicine in order to ensure their popularity. Since the public lacked the knowledge to distinguish between routine and difficult cases, physicians with large practices tended to secure their position by taking only cases with well-known courses and therapies. The practitioners of the new scientific medicine, mostly young physicians with small or no practices, were not only disadvantaged; they were imperilled:

> In the last decades a series of great discoveries have given medicine new vigour, but these astonishing advances have been of the sort to make the physician's activities and treatments *more complicated* rather than simpler... What used to be left to the province of rich experience and the physician's tact, and even with this advantage being incapable of offering a sufficient guarantee against possible error, no longer

[61] 'Medicin und Chirurgie' p. 587.

[62] Anon., 'Das gewöhnliche Abschätzen der Aerzte nach ihrer Praxis', *Deutsche Vierteljahresschrift* (1847), no. 3, pp. 235–69.

needs to remain doubtful, unclear, or hidden from the man who is acquainted with a series of investigations and who is sufficiently well-trained in them. Pharmacology [*die Arzneiwissenschaft*] is more exact, more certain than ever before. She owes this exactness to the great refinements enjoyed by the other branches of the natural sciences. Physics, chemistry, anatomy, and especially physiology, microscopy and pathological anatomy now belong to the most important studies of the well-educated physician. It is to these fields that medical science owes the incalculable advantages with which it is throwing off the chains of mysticism and seeking to make the precision of the mathematical sciences its own.[63]

The real training and experience with these new scientific tools began only after completion of university course work and passing the state medical exams. Healing had on this account become more rather than less difficult.

The author of this article really saw no simple solution to the problem – or at least he did not propose a short-term remedy. It had become a conflict between younger physicians with scientific training and older colleagues with outdated education, diagnostic skills and therapies. One possible solution was cooperation. The amount of time required to master the new techniques implied that medicine would benefit from specialised practice. Older physicians and physicians with large practices should consult with their more knowledgeable scientifically-trained colleagues.[64] But the organisation of medical practice and the role played by the public in the medical market undermined cooperation between physicians; 'medical politics' [*ärztliche Politik*] demanded of the physician with a large practice that his diagnosis be certain, his prescription decisive – and his knowledge mysterious. In such a market the practitioner of scientific medicine could never gain a foothold.

Another article in the *Deutsche Vierteljahresschrift* from the same year proposed the obvious solution to the problem; it was, of course, the moderate liberal prescription for guaranteeing rational progress in all areas of the economy, namely, state intervention.[65] If the state was interested in the health of its citizens, and if it was interested in promoting progress in medicine through the advances of science, then the state must regulate the provision of medical services. The author pointed out that the recent furore in medical circles concerning control over homeopathists and water curers had raised the issue of free trade in the medical market. This article proposed that free trade in medicine would lead to disastrous consequences. On the other hand, making all physicians officials of the state would be equally

[63] *Ibid.*, pp. 253–4.
[64] *Ibid.*, p. 257.
[65] Anon., 'Die Heilkunde und der Staat', *Deutsche Vierteljahresschrift* (1847), no. 1, pp. 1–40.

problematic. This would encourage the public to think that the state was favouring a particular class of people and restricting freedom of choice in medical care. Some formal means had to balance these interests.

This author proposed expanding the official duties of the presently existing state medical examiner [*Gerichtsarzt*], giving this official increased jurisdictional and policing powers, and raising the standards for appointment to such positions. To ensure that they represented the interests of the state, the medical examiners should no longer be practising physicians with occasional official responsibilities in the area of public hygiene, but rather paid state officials with no private practice. Hygiene had actually developed to such a degree that it deserved to be considered as a medical speciality in its own right. Medical examiners, according to this proposal, should have a normal university training in medicine; but after passing the medical exams, prospective medical examiners should study intensively experimental chemistry, forensic medicine, public hygiene [*medizinische Polizei*], veterinary science and pharmacy [*pharmaceutische Waarenkunde*].[66] The powers to be accorded to the state medical examiner were extensive, and they could in no way have been interpreted as favouring the interests of physicians without academic and scientific training. In order to assist the state in researching the causes of endemic and epidemic diseases, the state medical examiner was to be empowered to examine all the records of physicians in his district. Because he was no longer a practising physician, this authority was presumed not to cause conflict with the local physicians, who otherwise might fear an attempt to steal away their patients. The medical examiner was to be given authority over apothecaries, homeopathists and midwives. 'Above all the medical examiner must keep a watchful eye on quackery practised by unauthorised persons, all complaints of this sort should come under his purview, and he should be empowered appropriately to deal with them... The medical examiner should not simply appear as a legal consultant to the court, but rather he must be the judge himself and be given police powers'.[67] Furthermore, private vaccination should be eliminated and complete responsibility for vaccination be given over to the medical examiner.

The author of this proposal was all too aware that the power he wished to accord the state medical examiner would be perceived as motivated by special interests:

[66] *Ibid.*, p. 27.

[67] *Ibid.*, p. 24.

> Those who want to see the principle of complete freedom in medical matters established, will probably see too much power and force concentrated in the hands of the state. One thinks of the many uneducated healers, who, no matter what objections we may raise, have often in fact produced cures of which no physician was capable. On the one hand it would be disadvantageous to the public if these options were eliminated, and on the other hand, if the state retained the sole right of instruction and accreditation, the *Stand* of physicians would be threatened by a one-sided education, so that in the final analysis the patient would not enjoy the blessing of a genuinely free medical science but rather experience the doubtful and ambivalent influence of an 'Austrian', or 'Prussian', or 'Bavarian' medicine.[68]

But these objections could be immediately answered, he argued. In order not to create the impression that such measures were intended to limit the choice of medical care and to restrict medical practitioners to those designated or approved by the state medical officials, the author argued that his proposal actually contained a mechanism for protecting the practice of non-orthodox physicians such as homeopathists, herbalists, water curers, chiropractors, and other lay healers. Even these persons would have to admit, it was argued, that if they were genuinely capable of curing, their methods should be capable of standing up to examination. Having passed an examination administered by the medical examiner, their practice would henceforth be authorised and protected by the state. No one, not the state, not the patient, not even the healer benefited from keeping their cures and wonder drugs secret.[69]

Let me summarise the ideological position staked out in this literature designated for the educated public, which I have characterised as the moderate liberal programme. First, progress in achieving the transformation of society that many liberal middle-class Germans hoped for was seen to be effected best through an alliance of the Bildungsbürgertum and entrepreneurial groups. The values essential to this alliance were a commitment to the creation of a unified German state, in which the talent, industry and initiative were protected, rewarded, and recognised as the sources of future well-being of the body politic. Secondly, confident that the future of the state depended on this alliance of *Bildung* and *Besitz*, the group fashioning the moderate liberal programme believed that their interests should be specially encouraged and protected economically, socially and professionally. Weber and Mannheim's descriptions of a 'staatstragende Schicht' in German society of the first decades of the twentieth century could easily apply to the group self-image I am describing. Furthermore, among the natural candidates for intellectual

[68] *Ibid.*, p. 29.

[69] *Ibid.*, p. 30.

leadership of this class-in-the-making were the new breed of academicians representing the most progressive disciplines, particularly political economy and the natural sciences, and, within the natural sciences of the 1840s, the most progressive disciplines of chemistry, physics and physiology.

By virtue of their social and family backgrounds as well as through their own talents and interests, both du Bois-Reymond and Helmholtz found this ideology expressive of their own world-view. It was certainly not, I have attempted to show, an orientation in complete accord with that of their fathers, but there were many common elements. Their exposure to new forces affecting career choices and paths of professional and social development rendered these young persons receptive to moderate liberalism. In du Bois-Reymond's case, the contact with German national unity in the social and political discussions at home joined other dimensions of his local life-world to render him receptive to these viewpoints. Consider, for example, the way he structured his leisure-time activity by participation in a *Turnverein*. Du Bois-Reymond became an active *Turner* in 1828 and continued to be active through his days as a university student and young *Privatdozent*. The *Turnverein* were extremely nationalistic in orientation, dedicated to the principles of 'freedom, independence and the fatherland'.[70] Gymnastics contributed to these ideals not only the development of physical skill and athletic prowess but also the notion of freedom. An article in the *Deutsche Vierteljahresschrift* described the experience of the young *Turner*: 'Here at the gymnasium the boy is in his element, the playground is his state, and to be sure a free state, in which every talent and every force, every tendency and direction is allowed unhindered expression, because here only talent and strength [*Kraft*] count for anything'.[71] Gymnastics, together with the collection of patriotic literature and songs of the *Turnverein*, would strengthen moral independence and lead to the inner formation and development of individualism.

Müller's laboratory

The image of a progressive laboratory science in the service of practical improvements in surgery and medicine constructed by Brockhaus was one thing; as du Bois-Reymond and Helmholtz discovered, its reality was slightly different. The disparity between

[70] F. W. Klumpp, 'Das Turnen', *Deutsche Vierteljahresschrift* (1842), pp. 219–73, at p. 228.
[71] *Ibid.*, p. 248.

what it could be in this image fabricated by the liberal press and the reality of what it was, in fact, served to provide a focus for tensions and build a momentum for change. The dynamics of this process are apparent in the careers of Müller's students during the 1840s and the deep fissures that opened between some factions of the younger generation and their *Doktorvater* (a struggle which mirrored the generational tensions with their own fathers) at the end of the decade.

To illustrate this point I want to consider briefly the actual life of Müller's laboratory. The most salient characteristic of the activities in Müller's laboratory is that while laboratory 'experience' was considered essential to the production of knowledge, laboratory training played an insignificant role for the practitioner. Only those preparing for careers as academic scientists acquired extensive laboratory experience. Moreover, even these advanced students do not seem to have acquired laboratory training *per se*. Rather they were permitted to work in the laboratory of a major professor where they picked up the skills of laboratory science through a limited amount of observation coupled with unsupervised attempts to teach themselves.

Friedrich Bidder, who was himself a student in Müller's lab in 1834, provides a vivid description of the activities there in his 'Lebenserinnerungen'.[72] Müller's exercises in dissection, offered every winter semester, were attended normally by about 150 to 200 medical students. The students were divided up into groups working on twenty different corpses.

> After the group assignments had been made, the students would be left completely to their own designs. Müller would appear at most for a half-hour in the hall in order to cast a quick glance here or there; a rigorous introduction to anatomical preparation was out of the question... Most of the students had not the slightest idea what the parts were they were supposed to prepare. A few of them had a handbook for anatomical preparation.[73]

Bidder, who had already completed a course of medical study in Dorpat with Heinrich Rathke, where the only human dissection he had ever done was on the day of his state medical qualifying examination, attracted Müller's attention on one of the professor's dashes through the anatomical theatre. His skilled hand in dissection earned Müller's praise and the 'electrifying invitation: Herr Doktor, why don't you join me upstairs in my Kabinet. You will be able to work much better there away from all this confusion.'[74] In the two-

[72] Excerpted and published by P. Morawitz in an article titled 'Vor Hundert Jahren im Laboratorium Johannes Müllers, von weil. Prof. Dr Friedrich Bidder, Dorpat' in *Münchener medizinischer Wochenschrift*, 81 (1934), pp. 60–4. [73] *Ibid.*, p. 62.

[74] *Ibid.*, p. 62.

room private laboratory of Johannes Müller, Bidder joined Henle, Schwann and Reichert. He learned the art of anatomical preparation and the leading questions of physiological research at the side of these future scions of Müller's school. Perhaps most revealing of the level of anatomical instruction at that date was the presence of no more than a single microscope in Müller's lab.

The lectures on physiology held every summer term were equally disappointing. Bidder had expected that

> the man who was so deeply concerned to give the doctrines of physiology empirical foundations would have made every effort to give his auditors such experiences and to demonstrate the methods by which they are acquired. That was, however, not the case at all. The students and other auditors had to be satisfied with theoretical discussions. In his lectures encompassing the entire domain of physiology Müller only twice offered the students an occasion to observe something.[75]

At the root of the problem described in these passages by Bidder was a particular conception of the objectives of physiology as a discipline. Physiology for Müller was *Wissenschaft*; and he understood that term precisely in the sense of the Prussian educational reformers. What he sought was a unified science of life, the pillars of which were comparative anatomy, particularly embryological investigations, and experiment. Both in his inaugural address as a professor in Bonn and in the introduction to his monumental *Handbuch der Physiologie des Menschen*, Müller, declaring himself to be the heir of the biological tradition expounded in the writings of Kant and Goethe, explicitly stated that observation and experiment were instruments leading to a synthetic philosophical understanding of the nature of life. To construct this *verständige Physiologie* was Müller's announced purpose. The operative control over nature was not necessarily consonant with this disciplinary objective.

In his many dealings with the *Kultusministerium* Müller always stressed his programme of constructing a unified science of life. It was a programme that appealed to ministers for whom the support of *Wissenschaft um ihrer selbst willen* was part of a plan for providing the values and the spiritual elite needed to disseminate them to the youth of the nation. Such thinking was not only behind the call of Müller to Berlin but also behind his appointment in both the philosophical and medical faculties.[76] Through Müller's activities the ministers hoped to enrich the empirical, technician-like orientation of

[75] *Ibid.*, p. 63.

[76] See Manfred Stürzbecher, 'Zur Berufung Johannes Müllers an die Berliner Universität', *Jahrbuch für die Geschichte Mittel- und Ostdeutschlands*, 21 (1972), 184–226, especially p. 192.

the medical curriculum with the spirit emanating from the research seminars of the reformed philosophical faculty, the spiritual bulwark of the nation.

The attitudes I have attributed to Müller were by no means confined to him alone among the naturalist scientists in the Prussian professoriate. R. Steven Turner has shown similar attitudes in the memoranda prepared by chemists for the *Kultusministerium* in response to Liebig's scathing critique of the condition of the natural sciences in Prussia in 1840.[77] According to these memos, Liebig's factory-like laboratory in which young men worked from morning until late evening was much too utilitarian in its orientation. Prussia had its technical schools and *Realschulen* to attend to the practical needs of the state. The medical faculty, in particular, criticised Liebig's claims for chemistry for not growing out of an appreciation of the unity of learning. Moreover, Liebig's laboratory was based upon exploiting a set of techniques and apparatus he had developed for performing organic analysis. While valuable, such methods, which could be taught even to ordinary minds, did not yet qualify as *Wissenschaft*. Chemistry of the sort taught by Liebig had not progressed beyond the stage of describing and classifying. It was not yet a theoretical science aimed at finding the causes of phenomena.

Institutes designed in light of the principle of *Wissenschaft um ihrer selbst willen* were extremely individualistic in their orientation towards research. This was in keeping with one of the fundamental concepts behind the Humboldt reforms: namely, to produce creative minds freed from the oppressive regimentation of the Frederician state. The effects of this science policy are illustrated once again in the work of Johannes Müller. In contrast to Liebig, for example, Müller's research did not pursue a single objective. He moved from work in experimental physiology utilising vivisectional techniques in the early 1830s to work in sensory physiology. In the late 1830s came a period of work (with Schwann) on digestion utilising chemical methods. This was followed by research on cellular development (particularly in its application to pathology). Interspersed throughout these researches was extensive work in comparative anatomy and embryology, and, finally, research on alternating generations. As Müller's interests shifted, so too shifted the orientation and fields of research of the inner circle of his assistants and students. The result was successive waves of student-clusters entering the academic market with different

[77] R. Steven Turner, 'Justus Liebig versus Prussian chemistry: reflections on early institute-building in Germany', *Historical Studies in the Physical Sciences*, 13 (1982), pp. 133–9.

sorts of research objectives and frequently different sorts of disciplinary aims. Because of the various orientations he gave his students, Müller has been credited with contributing to the foundation in Germany of several different research fields in the biological and medical sciences, including experimental physiology, cellular pathology, embryology and zoology. If there was a common disciplinary thread in these researches, it was oriented around physiology from a zoological or zootomical perspective. This conception of the discipline was not fundamentally medical in orientation but rather aimed at a more generalised science of vital phenomena.

This approach did not sustain concentrated effort upon the development of research skills, techniques and instrumentation in a particular area such as physiology; nor did it refine them through laboratory training so that they would enter the repertoire of standard practice. Indeed, between 1835 and 1858, the average amount spent in Müller's institute on materials and experimental animals for instruction in physiology was only 18 thaler.[78] This was hardly the sort of investment needed to transform the practice of medicine by infusing it with results obtained at the research front. But this, of course, was precisely the genius of Liebig's institutional reform proposals. In 1840 they went strongly against the grain of the reigning ideology of *Wissenschaft*.

New directions: science for the clinic

A new wind began to stir just a few years later, its direction determined by developments which enhanced the promise of contributions to medical practice from laboratory training. Its conditions lay as well in the efforts of a growing rank of reform-minded academically trained physicians who saw in these technical changes a rationale for freeing themselves from state control and establishing medicine as a free profession. They wanted to replace state control by autonomous associations of self-policing physicians and to establish a unified educational standard for all practising physicians. Carrying this plan through meant strengthening the qualifications of physicians by introducing laboratory training into the medical curriculum, a

[78] From records in the Zentrales Staatsarchiv Merseburg, Historische Abteilung II, Generalia Universitäts-Sachen, Acta 'Die ordentlichen jährlichen Ausgaben für die naturwissenschaftlichen und medizinischen Institute der deutschen und österreichischen Universitäten' betreffend, Rep. 76va Sekt. 1, Tit. xv, Nr 17, Bd 1. Quoted from Axel Genz, 'Die Emanzipation der naturwissenschaftlichen Physiologie in Berlin' unpublished Dipl. med. dissertation (Magdeburg, 1976), pp. 33 and 7.

move which in turn implied restructuring existing institutions. This movement must be seen as consistent with the programme, outlined by Brockhaus intellectuals for instance, to create a bourgeois state.

The problem confronting the medical reform movement was that they were in the position, rife with contradictions, of attempting to reverse the role the state had played in the professionalisation of medicine. In Prussia this was an effort aimed at continuing and expanding the advantages secured for academically trained physicians by the ministerial edict of 1825 while removing the state controls which had brought about those changes. The edict of 1825 had nullified the earlier ministerial introduction of free trade into medicine in 1818.[79] The new system designated three classes of physicians: namely, physicians and two classes of surgeons. Medical personnel designated as 'physician' were henceforth required to complete a four-year course of academic studies at a university with written and practical examinations. This course of study qualified them to practise internal medicine. Most physicians went on to pass a further set of examinations in surgery which provided certification as a general practitioner.

Different classes of surgeons were designated according to academic qualification. Class-1 surgeons (*Wundärzte 1. Klasse*) were required to complete three years of study at one of the provincial medical colleges in Münster, Magdeburg, Greifswald and Breslau. The entrance requirement for this course of study was two years' attendance at a gymnasium (*Sekundareife*). From the beginning this lower status designation proved to be relatively unattractive; in 1826, one year after the new edict, the numbers of persons registered as physicians and class-1 surgeons were 1,906 and 323.[80] By 1837 this designation was made even less attractive by the introduction of residence restrictions preventing class-1 surgeons from settling in a community where a general practitioner was already in residence. Thus in 1843, 821 persons qualified as class-1 surgeons whereas 3,037 achieved certification as physicians. The edict of 1825 defined much lower qualifications for class-2 surgeons (*Wundärzte 2. Klasse*) of whom 2,102 were certified in 1826, and required that they could only practise in rural areas outside of towns and villages. The result of this decision was that in rural areas lay healers and non-certified medical personnel played a greater role than before.

The next two decades witnessed strong growth in the demand for

[79] See Huerkamp, *Der Aufstieg der Aerzte*; Frevert, *Krankheit*.
[80] Wehler, *Deutsche Gesellschaftsgeschichte*, vol. II, pp. 232–6.

general practitioners outside of positions in state service. In the 1840s alone the number of graduating medical students exceeded the number of available state and academic positions for academically trained physicians by 80 per cent. Rather than signalling a situation of overcrowding, these numbers reflected increased demand for general practitioners both in cities and in rural areas. Whereas 49 per cent of all physicians were in state service in 1826, by 1843 the proportion had fallen to 36 per cent. Moreover, even physicians in state service received the major proportion of their income from private practice. Corresponding with this development was a steady decrease in the attractiveness of the designation as surgeon. The number of persons registered as class-2 surgeon, for example, decreased from 2,102 in 1826 to 1,353 in 1843.

The reform movement of the 1840s, led by physicians such as Rudolf Virchow, sought the abolition of the three-class designation and the introduction of a standardised professional training, namely that of the general practitioner. These efforts were successful. Between 1849 and 1852 the provincial medical colleges for training surgeons were closed, and university training became standard for all physicians. All other medical personnel, such as midwives, were placed under the authority of academically trained physicians. Hence, by 1852 academically trained physicians gained complete monopoly (with the support of the state, to be sure) of the provision of health care.

Closely associated with these developments were efforts to reform clinical medicine by linking diagnostic procedures to causal theories based in physiology and pathology. Johann Lukas Schönlein, who accepted a call to Berlin in 1840, was one of the leaders in this movement.[81] But he was not alone. At exactly the same time in Tübingen Karl Wunderlich was generating enthusiasm for the construction of a rational medicine. They were soon to be joined by others in this endeavour, most notably Virchow, Henle and Pfeufer. The programmes of these individuals differed in the emphasis they placed on key elements of the reform package, and while these differences in emphasis were not without consequence for the theory and organisation of clinical practice, there was essential agreement on the core of their proposed scientific medicine. For my purposes Wunderlich's 'physiological medicine' is most significant, because it was in large part responsible for shaping the local institutional

[81] Johanna Bleker, *Die naturhistorische Schule 1825–1845: Ein Beitrag zur Geschichte der klinischen Medizin in Deutschland* (Stuttgart, 1981).

linkages between physiology and medicine which affected the work of Ludwig, Helmholtz and du Bois-Reymond.

The basis of Wunderlich's physiological medicine was a reconstitution of disease: the notion that illness and disease is the result of a disturbance in the normal functioning of an organ or system of organs. In his journal, the *Archiv für physiologische Heilkunde*, Wunderlich waged holy war against the defenders of specific disease entities. He also opposed the view that pathological anatomy provided the sole source of scientific medicine. Rather, he advocated the investigation through experimental physiology of the laws of normal organ function. Grounded in physiology, scientific medicine would investigate the causes of pathological lesions and the relationship between lesions and symptoms of disease. Wunderlich's central objective was to trace changes in organ function back to chemical and physical changes taking place at their anatomical locus. In his programme, therefore, pathology was only a tool to be employed in tracing the pathways of disturbed organ function. In a similar way he argued that scientific medicine must use the microscope and chemical investigations both as research tools and as diagnostic aids. But their relevance as diagnostic tools depended upon establishing a causal relationship with the physical and chemical basis of normal organ function.[82]

This interest in medical reform was reflected in gradual changes in the course offerings in medical faculties. The University of Berlin, which had the largest number of medical students during the period, is a representative locus of difficulties encountered by the reformers. The first of the new generation of courses which offered laboratory training to the general medical student was Henle's two-hour course in general microscopic anatomy in the summer semester of 1839.[83] Considering that Müller's cabinet possessed only one microscope, Henle's course could not have attracted large numbers of students. For the most part, interested students would have had to share Henle's microscope or supply their own, a possibility for the first time in the late 1830s with the introduction of the inexpensive achromatic microscopes produced by Plössel in Vienna and by Pistor and Scheick in Berlin.[84] That there was indeed growing student interest in the new

[82] Karl Wunderlich, 'Das Verhältniss der physiologischen Medicin zur ärtzlichen Praxis', *Archiv für physiologische Heilkunde*, 4 (1845), pp. 1–13. The various programmes for scientific medicine which proliferated during the 1840s are discussed in Bleker, *Die naturhistorische Schule*, pp. 114–26.

[83] *Vorlesungsverzeichniss* of the University of Berlin, 1839.

[84] See Tuchman, 'Science, medicine, and the state', especially chapter 3.

scientific medicine, and in the microscope as a potential diagnostic tool, is indicated by the fact that after Henle's departure Ehrenberg began to offer exercises in the use of the microscope for physiology.[85]

Following the arrival of Schönlein in 1840, one small private course in the new diagnostic techniques of auscultation and percussion was offered. By 1843 the interest in diagnostic methods had expanded to include offerings on the chemical analysis of blood, urine and other secretions. In the winter semester of 1843, Simons, a future founding member of the Berlin Physical Society, offered two courses in pathological and physiological chemistry, accompanied by demonstrations with chemical and microscopic experiments.[86]

The turning point in the perceived importance of such practical courses, emphasising training in the use of the microscope and in the new diagnostic methods, seems to have occurred in Berlin about 1845. In the summer semester of that year Ernst Brücke offered a course on the theory of the microscope and its use in the examination of healthy and diseased tissues. This course joined Ehrenberg's exercises in the use of the microscope for physiology; Simon's (now four-hour) course on pathology and therapeutics with demonstrations with the microscope; Heintz's course on physiological chemistry with experimental demonstrations; and Ebert's practical exercises in auscultation and percussion – at least five course offerings in which medical students were initiated into the technical methods of the emerging scientific medicine. From 1847 onward the number of such courses offering practical experience in microscopy, experiment and the use of chemical and physical diagnostic methods increased to seven; in 1848, eight such courses were offered; fifteen in the tumultuous summer semester of 1849 amidst the fighting on the barricades; and by 1856, there was an ongoing average of eleven courses offering practical exercises in experimental technique and diagnostic procedures to medical students. By the late 1850s scientific medicine was fully recognised as the organising principle of the medical faculty. In 1861,

[85] This course appears in the *Verzeichniss* for the first time in the summer semester of 1842. Ehrenberg continued to offer it every year thereafter. Du Bois-Reymond mentioned in a letter to his friend Hallmann the difficulties in trying to persuade people like his father that 'the instrument has virtually become a tool of medical diagnosis, especially in the field of practical pathology where it has already produced such astonishing results that its rapid disappearance as a temporarily popular scientific industry is scarcely imaginable'. Quoted from *Jugendbriefe*, p. 66, letter of 19 August 1840. Du Bois-Reymond reports having bought a stethoscope and practiced auscultation and percussion during his semester break in the spring of 1841. See *Jugendbriefe*, pp. 88–9, letter of 25 May 1841.

[86] These courses were announced in the listings under the natural sciences in the philosophical faculty.

Virchow, du Bois-Reymond and Langenbeck engineered the demise of the old examination, the *Tentamen philosophicum* and replaced it with the *Tentamen physicum*. Where technical subjects had previously been absent from the examinations, the *physicum* examined over six areas related to experimental physiology, pathological anatomy and physiological chemistry.[87] By this time the shift was completed from a general medical science with a comparative anatomical and morphological approach as its conceptual core to a conception of the discipline rooted in an activist, experimental physiological and chemical approach.

Reshaping the discipline: du Bois-Reymond and physical physiology

Keeping in mind this overview of the orientation and objectives of Müller's laboratory and the structure of the environment in which it was functioning, I want to return to the inside of the laboratory itself. This site offers a profile of the tensions within a local context manifesting themselves as a split along generational as well as ideological lines. The careers of Helmholtz, Brücke, Ludwig and, most richly, du Bois-Reymond, exhibit similar trajectories. The sort of conservative orientation evident in the views of their fathers was shared by Johannes Müller, the *Doktorvater* of all but Ludwig. In spite of the description of him in Brockhaus as a model progressive, Müller actually exemplifies the Bildungsbürger: uninterested in participating in the construction of a homogeneous bourgeois culture of the sort depicted in the moderate liberal press. In another context I have argued that the rejection of Müller's *Lebenskraft* and the orientation towards physical reductionism evident in Helmholtz's and du Bois-Reymond's early writings mirrored their reactions to the idealism and religious conservatism of their fathers.[88] Here I am more concerned with the ways in which these young men began to link their own interests with other like-minded individuals in founding the Berlin Physical Society. Particularly in the aftermath of the Revolution of 1848, they came to see that their intellectual efforts and the collective work of the Berlin Physical Society required the sort of legitimation offered by the politics of practical interest, and they quite

[87] See Theodor Billroth, *Über das Lehren und Lernen der medicinischen Wissenschaften an den Universitäten der deutschen Nation nebst allgemeinen Bemerkungen über Universitäten: Eine culturhistorische Studie* (Vienna, 1876), pp. 208–13.

[88] See my paper 'Social interests and the organic physics of 1847'.

consciously acknowledged the importance for their own work of making the society it envisioned more than a utopian dream.

The letters from du Bois-Reymond to Hallmann, which span the period September 1839 to November 1850, lend insight into the relationships among Johannes Müller and his students. They provide information as well concerning some of the events leading to the founding of the Berlin Physical Society. Of special interest in this regard is the account in these letters of du Bois-Reymond's choice of a dissertation topic.

Both Helmholtz and du Bois-Reymond began their advanced research as microscopical anatomists.[89] In fact, far from rejecting the type of developmental and morphological studies that had been Müller's great contribution to physiology, du Bois-Reymond initially wanted to pursue the same line of comparative embryology. Work in microscopical anatomy seemed at first glance to offer the solution to the personal doubts and deep depression that had befallen him in the autumn of 1840. In a letter to Hallmann he included an excerpt from his diary which expressed his turmoil:

> Cleft between philosophy and the study of scientific details; between life as it is described in novels and autobiographies of famous men and reality that lies before me. Impossibility of raising myself from being the receptive onlooker, which has been my nature up to now, and getting myself together [*mich zusammenraffen*] for independent research activity... Connected with this the inability to enjoy the moment as it is, rather always seeing it as a formative moment for a future lying completely in the blue. The inability furthermore, not to think of myself in this future as a contemplative, busy, famous and admired man, but rather as it should be, as a useful person sacrificing his personal interests and purposes for the common good... and added to this being held in high esteem in social circles and by persons, whose hopes one never feels certain of being able to fulfil.[90]

Five months later du Bois-Reymond was able to report that he had begun to see his way through this personal crisis. His deep relationship with Karl Reichert seems to have helped. To Hallmann he noted, 'I only know one person to whom I owe more for progress in worldly wisdom than him, and that person is you.'[91]

Reichert was at the time Müller's prosector, a microscopical anatomist with a Midas touch,[92] as he was depicted by du Bois-Reymond; his special experience was in applying the cell theory to problems of development. As one of two topics in which du Bois-Reymond might earn his spurs as an independent researcher, Müller had proposed that he work under Reichert's direction in applying the

[89] Helmholtz's dissertation was a comparative microscopical investigation of the origins of nerve fibres: 'De Fabrica Systematis Nervosi Evertebratorum', 1842.

[90] *Jugendbriefe*, pp. 75–6. [91] *Ibid.*, p. 84. [92] *Ibid.*, p. 81.

cell theory to the cleavage of the frog's egg.[93] With great enthusiasm du Bois-Reymond set himself to the task, only to be sorely disappointed. The paper that reported his results, he explained, was filled with rich observations, and while he thought he had overcome all the difficulties through an elegant application of mathematics, which deserved to be in Müller's *Archiv*, his hopes were disappointed. 'Reichert demonstrated irrefutably to me how little I understood how to think in the spirit of nature [*im Geist der Natur zu denken*].'[94]

Du Bois-Reymond wrote that he did not take this rebuff from his prosector personally, but it is hard to believe that the experience did not leave its marks. For someone striving to become an independent researcher the inability to think 'im Geist der Natur' was evidence of incompetence. Among Müller's students it was a phrase with a special significance, for it recalled directly the famous phrase of Müller's inaugural lecture in Bonn in which he had ushered in a new era in physiology. Du Bois-Reymond did not yet have the right stuff.

This touches directly upon vitalism, a question at the heart of the enterprise of physiology in the early 1840s. As I have argued elsewhere, Müller and others of his generation defended a form of biological holism.[95] Müller maintained that there was a special force, the *Lebenskraft* associated with biological organisation that was incapable of being reduced to or generated from elementary physico-chemical forces. The *Lebenskraft* was a force *sui generis*. For Müller, Karl Ernst von Baer, Rudolf Wagner and others, experimental intervention into the life of the organism would yield at best questionable results concerning organ function. They preferred instead to allow detailed comparative anatomies and above all embryology to provide insight into the workings of the *Lebenskraft*. Since in the present state of the art direct experimentation was not deemed admissible, a special kind of speculative inference was required of the researcher to turn the data of his anatomical preparations into a dynamic physiological process. As Müller described it, this was truly a *denkende Naturauffassung*. While 'intuition' into the processes of nature has always been the mark of a truly great scientist, it is easy to imagine that, since the acquisition of the ability to think 'im Geist der Natur' is not easily transmissible through a prescribed set of methods or learnable procedures, the approach advocated here could easily become an elitist tool for

[93] *Ibid.*, p. 85.
[94] *Ibid.*, p. 89, letter of 25 May 1841.
[95] Timothy Lenoir, *The Strategy of Life: Teleology and Mechanics in Nineteenth Century German Biology* (Dordrecht, 1982; reprinted Chicago, 1989).

preserving control over a research area, or at least perceived as such by those who were having difficulty gaining admission to the inner sanctuary of science. As du Bois-Reymond had learned, mastery of a battery of microscopical techniques was not sufficient to enter the exclusive club of physiologists.

Given the extent of the various pressures – from home, from himself and from the enormous competition for virtually non-existent positions – it is not surprising that du Bois-Reymond wrote on 25 May 1841, after the failure of his attempt at embryology, 'in my present status quo an independent work is the absolute most important thing.'[96] It was in this situation that Müller's second proposal began to absorb his whole attention. And indeed, the second problem Müller proposed to du Bois-Reymond turned out to be more fortunate. He suggested that, given du Bois-Reymond's background in physics and mathematics, he was perfectly suited to do research in nerve physiology. An appropriate study seemed to be a re-examination and continuation of Matteucci's experiments on the relationship of electricity to the 'nervous principle'. Du Bois-Reymond found a number of positive aspects that recommended this problem. First, it was an important research area that had not been investigated in light of the latest findings in electricity and magnetism:

> Apparently everyone who has examined the problem up to now (except old Humboldt, who has long since lost sight of the problem since the discovery of electromagnetism and induction) has understood either nothing about physics or nothing about physiology. Thus it has come about that no one has yet been able to grasp the subject from the standpoint from which I am going to attack it. The few persons to whom I have spoken about my ideas on this matter have filled me with the boldest hopes.[97]

Immediately after receiving from Müller the suggestion of following up Matteucci's work, du Bois-Reymond's letters and notebooks record that he set about constructing a sensitive galvanometer and that he founded a youthful *Naturforscher-Verein*, consisting of five members, which met every fourteen days. Formed in 1841 this group was later to evolve into the Berlin Physical Society. In its early stages the organisation did not have a 'programme'. Its initial purpose was rather to discuss the latest scientific literature, which would be of mutual assistance in their fledgling scientific projects.

After settling on a topic and forming his student *Verein*, du Bois-Reymond began for the first time to question seriously the assumptions and approach of the older generation. The letters henceforth

[96] *Jugendbriefe*, p. 89. [97] *Ibid.*, p. 89.

ceased to mention Reichert as a confidant and advisor. Ernst Brücke took his place: 'In Brücke I have once again everything that one human being can have from another. And thus, this summer through all sorts of influences which are difficult to describe accurately without being able to specify precisely the points of advance, I have come a good way further in life, or rather, in the art of life.'

At this point the letter (9 August 1841) moves into a line of thought that was to occupy du Bois-Reymond in one form or another for the rest of his life:

Reichert had a little girl as first born and is behaving like a worthy papa. This brings me to a subject, which to be sure belongs out of the category of miscellany but which must be treated. I would like to know your opinion concerning the (latent) dispute between Henle, Stilling and Schwann on the one side and Reichert on the other side with respect to the physical relationships of organisms. I am gradually coming around to Dutrochet's view: the more one advances in the understanding of physiology, the more motives one has to cease believing that the phenomena of life are essentially different from the phenomena of physics.[98]

Du Bois-Reymond continued by reiterating the basis of the disputes between these men. Reichert, he pointed out, was of the opinion that while the attempt should be made to reduce as many aspects of the phenomena of life as possible to physico-chemical causes, this could not explain everything connected with biological organisation. In criticising this teleomechanist position, which Reichert had taken over from Müller, du Bois-Reymond pointed out that

for him the cell theory brings no further advantage other than that of an internal view of organic substance; other than that he simply translates to the cell as element all the problems that one has sought to solve for the entire organism unsuccessfully for such a long time... Meanwhile it became clear to me with time that so pitifully little can be gained in this way and that without question a rich treasure of explanation and reduction is yet to be gained by application of physics and chemistry.[99]

Having discussed the professional grounds of the dispute, du Bois-Reymond reintroduced the personal factors that had heightened the tensions within Müller's household:

After I had been brought completely back to the field of physics by Müller the wounds [*die Wunde*] split open and I found myself with Reichert in my hair without end and without victory. For from both sides one can only argue *a priori*, and as long as no *a posteriori* moment is given to decide the argument, everything remains an inextricable antinomy... I was reminded of this story by Reichert's fatherhood insofar as I can no longer hide from myself that if early on he was very productive, he has also taken early refuge in these views in a manner disappointing for a person of his age; he is thoroughly fossilised therein; and therefore in all dimensions finished very young.[100]

[98] *Ibid.*, pp. 97–8. [99] *Ibid.*, p. 98. [100] *Ibid.*, pp. 98–9.

This harsh judgement of a man who did indeed continue to be a productive researcher, who ultimately ascended to occupy the chair of anatomy at the University of Berlin, and who was elected to fill Müller's place in the Academy, leaves room to conjecture that the disagreement was as much in their personal relationship as it was over scientific principles. Apart from this, however, there are other aspects of this statement which provide insight into the full complex of factors motivating du Bois-Reymond. First it is important to note that du Bois-Reymond felt that the issue of whether to pursue a reductionist or teleomechanist approach was, at least for the present, incapable of being settled empirically. Thus the basis for making a commitment to one framework or the other – and we have seen above that du Bois-Reymond was consciously seeking a philosophical framework that would harmonise with his interests in scientific details – could not be rendered simply by the falsification of one of them. The preference was, we see in the passage quoted above, given to the approach which seemed on the side of progress (*Fortschritt*): a term that entered du Bois-Reymond's vocabulary at this point and remained throughout his career as the sufficient justification for supporting the physiology he professed. Reichert, 'the worthy papa', was a fossilised morphologist. His work was not allied with the forces of progress. In order to secure himself a position he had, as du Bois-Reymond viewed it, given up the search for truth at a far too early age and joined the forces of reaction: forces which du Bois-Reymond and his friends saw represented by Johannes Müller. Whereas Müller had earlier been an inspiration to du Bois-Reymond, he, too, began to represent everything to which they were opposed. 'Müller,' du Bois-Reymond announced to Hallmann, 'you probably do not know that he is extremely right wing both politically and religiously.'[101]

In the autumn of 1841, describing himself as the incipient Faraday of physiology, du Bois-Reymond began to fill several notebooks with his readings of Matteucci and details for constructing a galvanometer sensitive enough to register small bioelectric currents; in the spring of 1842, he recorded his first serious experimental researches on the '*Froschstrom*', induced current in frogs. At the same time he noted in a letter to Hallmann that he and Brücke had taken the oath:

> To defend the truth that in the organism no other forces are active except the common physical-chemical forces; that where for the present these do not suffice for an explanation, either the manner of their action must be worked out for the concrete

[101] *Ibid.*, p. 114, letter of March 1843.

case by means of the physical-mathematical method, or new forces must be assumed which, being of the same dignity as the physical-chemical, are inherent in matter and are always only to be reduced to repulsive and attractive components.[102]

Organic physics was to be their lever in redefining the discipline of physiology in such a manner as to exclude Müller and the other practitioners of the morphological approach:

In physiology things are uncommonly quiet. People are beginning to see that this direction is exhausted and that new yeast must come into the batter or else the atoms will stop vibrating... There are only anatomists here now, but considerable progress has already been made in that morphology on the one side and organic physics and chemistry on the other side have begun to separate more strongly than before. It must eventually come about that physiology as such represents a mere empty framework from which the content has been stolen and transformed.[103]

The 'fiery sword of physics'[104] was to be their weapon in this struggle. Leaving the electrophysiological investigations[105] intended to 'create respect for physiology among the physicists',[106] I will focus on the organisation that grew out of du Bois-Reymond's *Naturforscher-Verein*, namely the Berlin Physical Society. It was through this and similar organisations that the personal aspirations, cognitive interests and images of society held by similarly situated individuals were transformed into a spring of collective action.

The Berlin Physical Society and the articulation of practical interests

Their need of expertise in experimental physics led the young organic physicists to Gustav Magnus.[107] An introduction was not necessary, for four members of du Bois-Reymond's and Brücke's *Naturforscher-Verein* – namely, Gustav Karsten, Wilhelm Heintz, Karl Hermann Knoblauch and Wilhelm Beetz – were all students of Magnus. Magnus had a library and laboratory as well as an extensive collection of

[102] *Ibid.*, p. 108. [103] *Ibid.*, p. 127, letter of 17 June 1846.

[104] The description was a recollection of Ludwig. See Ludwig to du Bois-Reymond, 3 September 1855, in Estelle du Bois-Reymond (ed.), *Zwei grosse Naturforscher des 19. Jahrhunderts: Briefwechsel zwischen Emil du Bois-Reymond und Carl Ludwig* (Leipzig, 1927), translated by Sabine Lichtner-Ayed and edited by Paul F. Cranefield (Baltimore, 1982), p. 88.

[105] For a discussion of du Bois-Reymond's work in neurobiology, see my study, 'Models and instruments in the development of electrophysiology, 1845–1912' *Historical Studies in the Physical and Biological Sciences*, 17 (1986), part 1, pp. 1–54.

[106] *Jugendbriefe*, p. 108.

[107] For biographical details on Gustav Magnus, see Max Lenz, *Geschichte der königlichen Friedrich-Wilhelms-Universität zu Berlin* (Halle, 1910–18), vol. III, pp. 278–82; Hermann Helmholtz, 'Zum Gedächtniss an Gustav Magnus' in *Vorträge und Reden* (Brunswick, 1896), vol. II, pp. 33–51. The article on Magnus in the *Allgemeine deutsche Biographie* is excellent.

industrial models and physical and electrical apparatus in his home.[108] He generously encouraged his students, as well as mechanics from Berlin, such as Halske, and engineers from the technical branch of the military, such as Siemens, to make use of these resources. Du Bois-Reymond's group soon joined forces with Magnus and his circle of physics and technology enthusiasts, eventually formally constituting themselves on 14 January 1845 as the Berlin Physical Society.

The reasons for Magnus's encouragement of the young researchers are no less interesting than their reasons for seeking him out. Magnus's career was characteristic of the problems confronting academics in the reactionary 1830s and 1840s. Certainly no one in Berlin appreciated the importance of Liebig's proposal for improving the support and status of laboratory training more than Magnus.[109] Having studied technology, physics and chemistry with Hermstaedt and Gmelin in Berlin, Magnus had, like Liebig, continued his studies by spending several months with Berzelius in Stockholm and then a year with Dulong, Thenard and Gay-Lussac in Paris. When he returned to Berlin he had hoped to make his habilitation in technology, with the eventual prospect of replacing the old Hermstaedt. There had been a long-standing argument against this field since the era of the Humboldt reforms, for technical studies did not fit the mould of abstract science for its own sake that had been the hallmark of the plans for reorganising the university. Magnus was forced to make a second habilitation, this time in physics, which then enabled him to receive a position as 'extra-ordinary' (*außerordentlicher*) Professor.

This was only the beginning of a long struggle for advancement, however. The situation of the *Extraordinarien* in this period was particularly grim, and most affected were the *Extraordinarien* in the natural sciences. Gustav Rose, for example, manned his post on occasion without pay and waited seventeen years for advancement to *Ordinarius*.[110] Magnus's salary as *Extraordinarius* was insufficient to keep body and soul together, and so, like most of his colleagues, he held a variety of posts. He taught chemistry at the Berlin Technical School, from 1832 to 1840 physics at the artillery and engineering school, and from 1850 to 1856 chemical technology at the new

[108] See, for example, Magnus's letter to the *Kultusminister*, von Altenstein, of 1 April 1834 in which he discusses the difficulties of not having his own teaching laboratory at the university. Sammlung Darmstaedter, F2d 1835, 1912.236 in the Staatsbibliothek Preussischer Kulturbesitz in Berlin.

[109] Magnus and Liebig were close personal and professional friends. See the correspondence between Magnus and Liebig in Liebigiana 58, Bayerische Staatsbibliothek, Munich.

[110] See Lenz, *Universität Berlin*, vol. II, pp. 227, 416, and especially 485.

Technical Institute, which was modelled on the Paris Ecole Polytechnique.[111] Although the author of numerous outstanding papers in chemistry, physics and physiology, Magnus had to wait eleven years before being promoted to *Ordinarius* in 1845. In light of his own experiences it is not surprising that, although himself secure in his position, Magnus was one of the leaders of the university reform movement in 1848 which attempted to improve the situation of the *Extraordinarien* and *Privatdozenten* in the university corporation.[112] Magnus's involvement in liberal projects extended beyond the university. As the son of a prosperous businessman and teacher in the various schools constructed by the liberal finance minister Wilhelm Beuth,[113] Magnus was deeply sensitive to the interests of the fledgling industrialists. For many years he was a member of the physics section of the *Verein für die Beförderung des Gewerbefleißes*, which was central in spreading the gospel of liberal economics. He participated in the organisation of the industrial exhibition in Berlin in 1844, and was the Prussian representative at the exhibitions in London and Paris of 1851, 1855, 1862 and 1867. He was also instrumental in carrying through the reform of the Technical School in 1850 which reorganised the school along the lines of the Ecole Polytechnique by introducing science as a basis for improving technical education.

Magnus used his contacts as the teacher and associate of many Berlin industrialists to enrich his lectures in technology. A believer in the 'hands-on' method of learning things, Magnus arranged field trips to factories and workshops in order to demonstrate the principles of technology. Like many *Extraordinarien*, Magnus held lectures in his home, where he had constructed a physical-chemical laboratory, modest at first but eventually expanding into the most complete collection of physics instruments at the time in Berlin. This collection was later purchased by the state and transferred to the university. Helmholtz's experiments on fermentation were conducted in Magnus's laboratory under his careful three-month supervision in 1845. During the summer semester of 1843, finding himself surrounded by a group of extremely talented young physics enthusiasts, Magnus suggested the formation of a private colloquium which would meet weekly in his house. Among the members of this group were du Bois-Reymond's *Naturforscher-Verein*, i.e., du Bois-Reymond, Brücke,

[111] See Karl Wilhelm Gallenkamp, *Die Friedrich-Werderische Gewerbeschule in Berlin nach ihrer prinzipiellen Stellung in ihrer geschichtlichen Entwicklung* (Berlin, 1874).

[112] Discussed by Lenz, *Universität Berlin*, vol. II, pp. 257–63.

[113] See Ilja Mieck, *Preussische Gewerbepolitik in Berlin, 1806–1844* (Berlin, 1965).

Karsten, Beetz and Heintz. They were joined by six others, including Rudolf Clausius. With the exception of Clausius, who left to study in Halle, this was the group from which the Berlin Physical Society evolved two years later.[114]

It is worth exploring the interests Magnus had in establishing the Society. Although there are no surviving materials for Magnus which could address the issue directly, a number of aspects of Magnus's biography invite speculation. Of special interest is Magnus's 'practical' orientation toward physics, adopted during his university education and his period of study with Berzelius and Gay-Lussac at the Ecole Polytechnique. In Berlin, he found his efforts to develop that perspective hampered by institutional arrangements. This was further complicated by the fact that while the image of the natural sciences was improving as a result of Humboldt's and Müller's activities, these disciplines had by no means yet arrived at a position of power within the university. Furthermore, Magnus himself was frustrated in his efforts to promote his own special view of physics by the fact that he was unable to rise above the status of *Extraordinarius* for eleven years. Since the *Ordinarien* and the faculty senate had the power of determining disciplinary orientations through their control of the examinations and large lecture courses, Magnus had little influence on disciplinary orientations within the university.

This helps us perhaps to understand Magnus's political activities within the university, particularly his active role in the reform movement of the 1840s. One of the principal objectives of the reforms was to gain active participation in faculty deliberations, seats in the faculty senate and voting rights for all *Extraordinarien* and *Privatdozenten*. Had this come about, it would, of course, have greatly increased the power of men like Magnus. By attracting bright young students who could gain the *venia legendi* and become *Privatdozenten*, an 'oppressed' research orientation could ultimately gain strength and power. That this was in fact the real agenda of the day was acknowledged by Johannes Müller in the statement he fashioned rejecting the reform demands as Rector of the university and President of the Faculty Senate in 1848.[115]

The various memorial addresses for Magnus all mention that he was a man who sacrificed his own personal interests for the good of the community and that his unsparing efforts were directed on the one

114 See 'Bericht über die Feier des 50 jährigen Bestehens der physikalischen Gesellschaft am 4 Januar 1896', *Verhandlungen der deutschen physikalischen Gesellschaft*, 15 (1896), no. 1, pp. 15ff.

115 See Lenz, *Universität Berlin*, vol. II, pp. 267–70, discussed below.

hand towards improving the lot of his fellow human beings and on the other to the advancement of *Wissenschaft*. But it is also of interest to the present discussion that Magnus had a quite different view of his own branch of *Wissenschaft*, namely physics. In his memorial address, Helmholtz states that Magnus, having suffered the reign of *Naturphilosophie* in Berlin, was determinedly against any sort of speculation in physics. This judgement included mathematical physics. He wanted to separate strictly mathematical and experimental physics. To be sure, Magnus was not a trained mathematical physicist, but this was not the reason for his insistence, according to Helmholtz. As his own works amply demonstrate, Magnus was in his element whenever the problem at hand called for quantitative results arrived at through applied mathematics. According to Helmholtz, what Magnus opposed was the practice of most mathematical physicists of assuming without empirical evidence the existence of hypothetical entities and then making them the foundations of physics. Examples were the assumed existence of atoms by most physicists in order to explain the properties of bodies, or the assumption that heat is a material fluid. Magnus wanted to base physics not on arbitrary axioms, but rather on measurable quantities.

In this programme of eliminating all speculative elements from physics, Magnus made common cause with J. C. Poggendorff and the coterie of 'measurement physicists' whose works were featured in Poggendorff's *Annalen der Physik und der Chemie*. Like Magnus, Poggendorff was not opposed to the use of mathematics in physics: far from it. Rather, Poggendorff was committed to the notion that physics was the study of what one could measure with instruments.[116] He emphasised over and over again in discussions of electricity and magnetism, for example, that theories about the causes or origins of electricity were rather useless. Theories should be about the phenomena detected by electrometers. To locate the laws of electricity, as revealed by instruments in experimental researches, focussed on number and measure: that was the task of physics in Poggendorff's eyes.[117]

[116] See Christa Jungnickle and Russell McCormmack, *The Intellectual Mastery of Nature: Theoretical Physics from Ohm to Einstein*, vol. 1, *The Torch of Mathematics, 1800–1870* (Chicago, 1986) pp. 122–6. The shift from 'concretising' to 'abstractifying' approaches in German physics has been discussed by Kenneth L. Caneva, 'From galvanism to electrodynamics: the transformation of German physics and its social context', *Historical Studies in the Physical Sciences*, 9 (1978), pp. 63–159.

[117] This was also the task of physics in Magnus's eyes. In the several letters of recommendation for young physicists in the Darmstaedter Sammlung in the Staatsbibliothek Preussischer Kulturbesitz in Berlin (see, for example, Sammlung Darmstaedter, F2d 1835, 1917.427, letter

The co-founders of the Physical Society, therefore, placed a variety of hopes in their common enterprise. For du Bois-Reymond and Brücke it was a means of sharing ideas and information useful to their programme of reforming physiology and of gaining respect for it from the physicists. For Magnus the Society was not only a means for furthering the education of talented young scientists but also a way to spread his own programme of experimental physics. Men like Werner Siemens, who were not concerned about academic politics, brought another set of interests to the Society. As a military man from the technical branch, Siemens was unable to attend courses at the university. A man who had always aspired to be a member of the educated class, according to his own account, Siemens derived a certain sense of legitimation from participating in meetings with the scientific elite. He also acquired knowledge critical for his fledgling electrotechnical enterprise.

In the first issue of its journal, *Die Fortschritte der Physik*, the Berlin Physical Society quietly announced its programme of placing experimental physics at the centre of scientific progress. The aim of the journal, wrote its editor, Gustav Karsten, was to speed the flow of information about the most important advances in physics each year. Whereas other disciplines such as chemistry and physiology had their own *Jahresberichte*, such an organ was completely lacking for the rapidly expanding domain of physics.

The initial question, of course, was how to define and arrange the 'most important advances in physics'. The Society did not attempt such a definition. 'How far we have extended the concept of physics', wrote Karsten, 'can best be gathered from the reports themselves; but by the close interconnection of the different branches of science, it is understandable that disciplines which "appear" to lie far apart from one another are actually united in the same branch'.[118] Indeed the reader would soon discover what that pregnant formulation contained; for experimental physics appeared to unite work in atomic theory, heat, electricity and magnetism as well as physiology. Physiology was simply defined in this journal as a branch of applied

of recommendation for Knoblauch), Magnus always applauds the man who knows how to develop a consistent chain of reasoning based on experiments which elaborate some central or core experiment. In none of the extant letters does he praise a theoretical talent. In his memorial address for Gustav Magnus ('Zum Gedächtniss', especially pp. 44–7), Helmholtz criticised Magnus's reaction to mathematical physics and his conflation of it with speculative nature philosophy. Helmholtz mentions that his own work grew up outside the tradition favoured by Magnus (p. 47).

118 Gustav Karsten, 'Vorbericht', *Die Fortschritte der Physik*, 1 (1845), printed in 1847, pp. viii–ix.

physics. Moreover, the subjects covered were not limited to theoretical advances. In fact theory received relatively little attention in comparison to techniques and instrumentation. 'Mechanical technology', which included practical subjects, especially galvano-plating, was a major feature of the early volumes of *Die Fortschritte der Physik*. The papers read by members of the Society in its bi-weekly meetings emphasised the 'practical' turn they were giving to scientific questions. The tone of the Society was set by papers such as du Bois-Reymond's discussion of his galvanometer (1847), Ludwig's paper on the measurement of pressure in arteries, Knoblauch's papers on techniques for measuring effects of radiant heat, Brücke's paper on methods for making the motions of a vibrating string visible, or Siemens's papers on the construction of an electric spark-timer for measuring velocities (1845) and on the measurement of resistances in electromagnets (1847). The crowning achievement and paradigmatic example of the orientation of the young Society was offered on 23 July 1847. In Helmholtz's paper 'Die Erhaltung der Kraft', the message that measurement is the source of theoretical advance in science was unmistakable. Through the discovery of the principle of the conservation of energy Nature herself seemed to bless the enterprise of the Physical Society of uniting disciplines as disparate as physiology, mechanics and technology through experimental physics.

Imperialistic disciplinary aims were not the only novel features of the Berlin Physical Society that would have struck the readers of *Die Fortschritte der Physik*. The composition of the Society, proudly, perhaps even defiantly, displayed in the journal's foreword, was a cross-section of the rising 'party of progress' in Berlin. Among the fifty-four members of the Society listed in the first volume, twenty-two were *Privatdozenten* in the medical and philosophical faculties, six, including Siemens, were lieutenants from various technical branches of the military, six were listed as *mechanicus*, including Halske and Leonhardt, and several of the members, such as Ludwig Böhm, the stepson of the Kultusminister Johannes Schultze, were students who had not yet completed their doctoral studies. Gustav Magnus was the only professor officially listed as a member of the organisation, although the physicist Heinrich Dove is mentioned as an occasional participant in the proceedings. *Privatdozenten* who were seeking to reform the university and to redefine its disciplinary boundaries, instrument makers and mechanics whose ranks supplied the first generation of Berlin industrial entrepreneurs, in short, men who were also among the most vocal supporters of a variety of legal and political reforms, were united in a common endeavour to promote progress in and through physics. The organisation served as the meeting ground for a number of young men who found themselves forced by circumstances to set out on new paths in order to gain entry into the academic establishment, and the programme they fashioned significantly altered the course of modern science. The Berlin Physical Society served multiple functions, not the least important of which was that it brought together aspiring young scientists and enterprising technologists who were experiencing similar difficulties in different aspects of the social-cultural milieu of Berlin in the 1840s. It was their mutual interests in science, particularly physics, and technology that initially brought them together; but once together, their different perspectives on society, its problems and the changes in it necessary to accommodate their interests began to form into a common bond. Having embarked upon new courses in their careers, these men gained from the Berlin Physical Society a sense of solidarity: they were not alone in their enterprise. Moreover, in the case of its core members, the Society nourished a conviction that they were fighting a kind of holy war against the established authorities, a war in which victory would lead to a more powerful unified Germany.

Revolution and repentance from idealism: an ideology for the new era

Like much of the middle class, the members of the Berlin Physical Society initially welcomed the Revolution of March 1848 with open arms. Some, such as Rudolf Virchow and the mathematician Eisenstein, even participated in the fighting on the barricades on 18–19 March. These were exceptions, however. For the most part these individuals were sympathisers with the cause of the revolution, but they feared to involve themselves in the actual fighting. The struggles on the barricades and in the streets took place primarily between workers and artisans and the military. While the students sympathised with the workers, for the most part they joined their professors on the sidelines. Students and most professors wanted to see legal and political reforms of a republican character as well as the construction of a national constitutional state. They in no way hoped for a radical democratic or communist solution to the political and social problems of the day. When the revolution threatened to go too far, the students organised themselves into squadrons to restore order. Indeed, in order to prevent the more radical students from becoming the core of an armed popular army, Gustav Magnus took command of the student regiments.[119] In spite of these qualifications, we should not infer that the members of the Berlin Physical Society adopted an apolitical stance and did not participate in other significant political events surrounding the Revolution. Several Society members were active in advocating liberal reforms of the universities and academies. The university reforms were seen by the students and their leadership as models for the reform of other institutions.[120]

I have already mentioned Gustav Magnus's active role as one of the speakers of the group of professors and students advocating reforms of the University of Berlin. The group included August Twesten, Moriz Haupt, Friedrich Trendelenburg and Rudolf Virchow. Among the reforms they proposed were the replacement of the state-appointed trustee of the university by a board of trustees, which together with the Faculty Senate and Rector would have complete responsibility for running the affairs of the university rather than merely an advisory function as previously; an open administration and participation of the entire faculty in determining the budget; the right to set salaries according to number of years of teaching; binding authority in matters of appointment and promotion; the introduction of an assembly consisting not only of all the professors but also of the assistant professors and *Privatdozenten* as well, from which committees responsible for conducting the business of the university were to be appointed in free elections – perhaps the most problematic demand; reform of legal jurisdiction in academic affairs; student participation in the election of judges and their right to attend sessions in which judgements were being discussed and handed down; free choice of council from among the university community; right of free association for all students; discontinuation of compulsory lecture courses; publication of examinations; inclusion of the professors on the state examining commission; and an increase in the status of a university degree.[121]

Karl Ludwig became deeply involved in the Revolution in Nassau-Hesse. Having already been hauled before the authorities as a student for assisting another student radical from Göttingen, named Wilhelmi, before his arrest in Marburg, Ludwig continued to work for liberal causes as a young assistant. In Marburg, Ludwig's close friends

[119] Adolf Rüger *et al.*, *Humboldt-Universität zu Berlin: Überblick 1810–1985* (Berlin, DDR, 1985), pp. 32–3. Also see Lenz, *Universität Berlin*, vol. II, pp. 267–70.

[120] See Heide Thielbeer, *Universität und Politik in der deutschen Revolution von 1848* (Bonn, 1983), especially pp. 125–221.

[121] Lenz, *Universität Berlin*, vol. III, p. 264.

were Robert Bunsen and Ludwig Fick, both of whom were politically active. Fick, who was the director of the institute for anatomy and three years older than Ludwig, was one of the leaders of the liberal reform movement in Marburg,[122] defending the 'moderate liberalism' I have discussed above. During the Revolution Fick took part in forming the government, serving on the *Volksrat*. Ludwig joined Bunsen and the historian, Heinrich Sybel, in the leadership of the *Vaterlandsverein*, an organisation which advocated German unification through the formation of a constitutional monarchy under Prussian leadership. Ludwig edited a newspaper, *Der neue Verfassungsfreund*, which advocated the views of the *Vaterlandsverein* in charting a new course. Ludwig, like Magnus and du Bois-Reymond and other members of the Berlin Physical Society, also presented proposals for university reform of the sort advocated by the students at the Wartburg Fest and Jena Congress. But Ludwig joined to his proposals the need to recognise the importance of support for the natural sciences as crucial to the new German nation state. In this respect he embarked upon a course advocated by other members of the Berlin Physical Society, such as Gustav Karsten, who wrote a treatise entitled *Von der Stellung der Naturwissenschaften, besonders der physikalischen, an unseren Universitäten* (Kiel, 1849), intended to influence the deliberations of the committees formed at the Jena Congress on university reform, in which he called for a reconsideration of the issues raised by Liebig in his earlier indictment of the lack of support for laboratory science in Prussia.[123] Ludwig was in personal contact with Liebig during his early years in Marburg, and he, too, was convinced that Liebig's proposals held the formula for progress. The liberal Eberhard ministry, which came into power as a result of the March upheavals, was equally convinced of the importance of science, and Ludwig, Bunsen and Sybel were authorised to begin searching to fill new faculty appointments in physics, botany and mineralogy. Ludwig proposed du Bois-Reymond for the position in physics.

[122] See Christina Vanja, 'Philipps-Universität und Stadt Marburg in der deutschen Revolution von 1848 – Bruno Hildebrand und Karl Theodor Bayerhoffer' in Dietrich Kramer and Christina Vanja (eds), *Universität und demokratische Bewegung* (Marburg, 1977), pp. 73–95.

[123] Concern for the spread of materialism among the students and faculty, as well as for its potential use for reform agitation, led university authorities to confiscate copies of Liebig's *Chemische Briefen* and place it on a list of proscribed books and literature along with Engels' *Lage der arbeitenden Klassen*, all the writings of Feuerbach, articles on proposals for a Prussian constitution, and the republican newspaper *Westphälisches Dampfboot*, three years prior to the Revolution. See Thielbeer, *Universität und Politik*, pp. 76–7.

In a letter dated 12 February 1849, when the air was yet filled with optimism for a liberal victory in which he and du Bois-Reymond might work side by side, Ludwig outlined his view of the political future and the role of the natural sciences in it:

Let us hope that the dwindling funds for our purposes will soon be over; it will soon be recognised that the solution to the revolutionary, i.e. the social issue, is only to be found in the natural sciences; and when this is realised more money will be made available to us. If only we see that happen during our careers, we might then perhaps even have the pleasure of having an assistant or two. It will be up to your Diet. If they force the hand of Manteuffel and his consorts, matters will gaily follow their course, and we will have a free and happy Germany.[124]

Ludwig's enthusiasm during early 1849 continued to grow: 'My heart is so full of Germany,' he wrote, 'but I cannot write much about it to you. I do not see our situation as sadly as you do; the progress that lies in constitutionalism is unmistakable, and its national assembly has given Germany a stability that will develop further.' Ludwig felt it was crucial for his close friend to take an even more active role in the reform movement than he had yet attempted:

You will and must take up a position on free activity in science, and in a few weeks or years, when the cultural seed scattered by these storms starts bearing fruit, your activity will once again be honoured and you will no longer regret walking about as a cowardly murderer of toothless and clawless animals.[125]

[124] Du Bois-Reymond (ed.), *Zwei grosse Naturforscher*, p. 25. Brücke shared Ludwig's views on the 'social question'. In the early phases of the revolution, du Bois-Reymond appears to have adopted a socialist solution to the problems of the working classes, perhaps in opposition to the more conservative proposals of his father. In a letter of 15 July 1848, Brücke wrote: 'Concerning our views on the social situation, it has become clear to me that we differ essentially from one another in that you believe that the question can be solved in a socialist manner through the regulation of the relationships between capitalists and workers, whereas I am of the opinion that such efforts will come to nothing, since in this manner it will never be possible to bring the real value of labour represented by a normal worker into agreement with the prices of his usual food and living requirements. In my view the situation of the workers will only be improved through a change in the legal structure, through a new patent law for all of Germany, through direct taxes and through state protected colonisation and emigration. The primary problem to be resolved remains the customs problem, upon which we always founder because we cannot undo the past. If (so the argument goes) we want to assure our industry a greater value (not simply a higher price because in this way we damage production) and in this manner help the workers, we must raise our customs duties. This helps for the moment, but we put the consumer at a disadvantage and create as a consequence slowly but surely a proletariat just like the English. If we proclaim free trade, our entire artificial industry will collapse at once and the present generation of workers and industrialists are sacrificed to posterity, for the future of Germany lies with free trade and not customs duties. When Trieste and Hamburg, Genoa and Bremen are linked by railways, no German financier will be able to succeed in blockading the two most important European trade routes through customs duties and allowing the traffic to fall to the hands of neighbouring lands.' From Ernst Wilhelm von Brücke, *Briefe an Emil du Bois-Reymond*, part 1, ed. Hans Brücke *et al.* (Graz, 1978), pp. 9–10.

[125] Du Bois-Reymond (ed.), *Zwei grosse Naturforscher*, p. 27.

This exhortation was intended to cheer up his friend, whose own political efforts during the summer of 1848, in the opening months of the Revolution, had fallen flat. Du Bois-Reymond's efforts centred on the Berlin Academy of Science, to whom he presented a petition proposing to open the meetings to the public. In words that must have recalled similar demands made to the French Academy during the Revolution, du Bois-Reymond had written:

Everywhere at this moment the principle of openness is bringing renewal. Everything that senses the life force pulsing through it owes homage to this principle, and the power of public opinion derives its own force from it. Therefore a desire long harboured by many persons has been awakened now more strongly than ever before: the desire that the principle of openness find its place in the domain of science and that the Academy permit the doors of its meeting hall to be opened to anyone who wants to pay honour to the most prestigious representative of German science. To be sure the meetings of the Academy have always been open to anyone who is invited by one of its members. The Academy also holds genuine public sessions from time to time. But in such a constricted form the public is not provided the guarantees through which the trust is developed that a corporation needs in order to be powerful in a constitutional state.[126]

Du Bois-Reymond's concrete proposal was to turn the sessions of the Academy into public events. In addition reports of the sessions were to be published immediately after the meetings rather than months later as was usual practice. Popularised versions of the results were also to be prepared and widely distributed:

Then the liveliest effect of the Academy on the people will begin, and whereas now its existence is scarcely known, or observed with indifference, it will appear as the pride of the nation and an essential component of common life, whose important task it is to take initiative in matters pertaining to science.[127]

The petition was signed by 105 persons, most of whom were members of the Berlin Physical Society, primarily young persons with doctorates or candidates for degrees in philosophy and law. Prominent among the names were Kirchhoff, Remak, Virchow, Wilhelmy, Halske and several persons who identified themselves as 'Mechaniker', such as Schleuter and Langhoff. Du Bois-Reymond explained the rationale behind his proposal in a letter of 6 January 1849 to Hallmann:

I don't need to explain to you the utility and timeliness of the thing. It is clear that in a constitutional state where the budget is approved by chambers, a corporation is powerless unless it has the support of public opinion behind it; that the Academy

[126] Quoted from a petition in the du Bois-Reymond Nachlaß of the Akademie der Wissenschaften der DDR, Akademie-Archiv II: VI a 11. I am grateful to Christa Kirsten and Herbert Hörz for providing me with a copy of the document. See also Friedrich Herneck, 'Emil du Bois-Reymond und die Grenzen der mechanistischen Naturauffassung' in *Forschen und Wirken: Festschrift zur 150-Jahr-Feier der Humboldt-Universität zu Berlin, 1810–1960* (Berlin, 1960), pp. 229–51.

[127] Du Bois-Reymond's petition (note 126), last paragraph.

could not have sunken lower in public opinion than at present; that by guaranteeing the openness of its meetings it would have rendered itself the greatest service; that this reform would bring other equally healthy reforms in its wake; and finally that in an age when art and science appear to have disappeared in the dust of agitated political passions like a coach which has kidnapped one's beloved, an effort aimed at lifting the corporation that represents art and science was well advised.[128]

Indeed, du Bois-Reymond's proposal was praised by the liberal *Vossische Zeitung* as a model for reforming other corporate institutions in Prussia.

All of these individuals were, of course, deeply disappointed by the outcome of the Revolution. The proposals for reform of the University of Berlin made by Magnus and his committee were rejected. In his unenviable position as Rector, Johannes Müller wrote the document rejecting their demands. The proposals would create a majority of one hundred *Privatdozenten* and *Extraordinarien* to fifty-nine full professors, Müller objected. His language revealed that Müller saw the issue as a challenge to authority by the younger generation, and he quickly closed ranks with the full professors in rejecting the demands of youth. There would be nothing to prevent them from using this advantage to appoint young persons to any free position and to protect themselves by allowing academic decisions to be guided by party interests. Müller wrote:

The principle of the majority also rules the organisation and activities of learned organisations. But if the moral worth of this principle is not to be relinquished, acceptance in the faculty as a corporation can only originate from a certain recognition for scientific accomplishments and service, which is properly to be determined by a free test of the person named as professor or of the person being appointed as a teacher. Otherwise it could occur that science which is alien to the principle of the majority is driven as a servant into the background of the business of the faculty and party objectives would come to occupy the foreground of such a corporate body... As soon as the *Privatdozenten* are accorded the same rights as the professors who have either been appointed or called, they cease to be *Privatdozenten* and become professors themselves, the only difference between them and the other professors being that they have acquired those privileges without the scientific accomplishments of the latter.[129]

Müller concluded this stinging rebuff with a plea to the Ministry of Education to consider the suspect motives of the members of the committee who had taken advantage of a moment when the state authorities were paralysed by weakness and confusion in order to make their unreasonable demands. Lenz notes that Müller's reply was not actually delivered until several hours after the liberal Camphausen

[128] *Jugendbriefe*, p. 131.

[129] Quoted by Lenz, *Universität Berlin*, vol. II, part II, pp. 267–9.

ministry had stepped down on 25 June; that is, after the democratic threat had been silenced and an alliance with conservatives was being struck. Lenz notes: 'One sees that our predecessors ... knew how to march in step with the general tendencies of political developments.'[130]

Neither du Bois-Reymond's proposal to reform the Academy nor any of the other proposals made by Ludwig, Bunsen or Karsten fared better. Du Bois-Reymond's petition to open the meetings of the Academy to the public was dismissed on the grounds that it was not permitted by the original statutes and that it was not necessary (fifty select persons were, however, allowed to purchase annual admission tickets).[131] Furthermore, Ludwig was in serious trouble. He had been not only an outspoken proponent of university reforms but also an ardent defender of the liberal Eberhard ministry and the programme for unification with Prussia. With the rejection of a 'German' crown by Friedrich Wilhelm IV and the defeat of Eberhard, Ludwig was in an untenable position. He was forced to resign his position at the University of Marburg and accept a position in Zurich, the haven of German revolutionaries in exile.

In some ways the young men of the Berlin Physical Society learned the same lesson from the Revolution of 1848 that Karl Marx learned. Marx, too, had believed that the class struggle was about to begin. The precondition for this, of course, was that the workers and bourgeoisie existed as classes, and that they were conscious of their interests. Marx came to realise that neither class had reached this stage before the Revolution of 1848, and he repented of his idealism in 'The Eighteenth Brumaire of Louis Bonaparte'. The experience of the Berlin Physical Society members was analogous to Marx's, though their lesson came from the opposite direction. Likewise repenting of their idealism, du Bois-Reymond, Ludwig and their circle of friends became convinced that it had been a mistake to trust in party politics. The literature I have discussed above which advocated the need for a distinctive middle-class consciousness that would value its own culture had turned out to be more programmatic than real. The members of the Berlin Physical Society came to believe they had been carried away with the idealistic illusion that through party politics one could change the organisation of the universities and the place of the natural sciences in the faculties of philosophy and medicine, and ultimately within the state. Du Bois-Reymond's assessment of his own

[130] *Ibid.*, p. 269.

[131] *Jugendbriefe*, p. 132.

predicament and prospects for the future was typical of the other members of the group, even those who had been less directly involved politically:

I cannot reconcile myself to the thought that my future, such as I have dreamed of it for so long (or such as has presented itself to me, to put it in the royal and imperial official style), is now to be destroyed, but I have to reconcile myself to it. And all that shopkeeper rabble that held out such splendid promises so long as it was a question of spurring me on to the most selfless work in the hope of this journey now still gives one good advice on one's way. It would yet be bearable if there were any improvement to be seen in the civilian world. How gladly one would make any personal sacrifice if only 'little Germany' came into being. But all for nothing and less for nothing, only to have the wheels of progress bogged down deeper still, so many hopes dashed, so much human felicity destroyed, such despondency in all hearts! I tell you, we poor ornaments of peace are in a bad way now; happy are those who bear the sword ...[132]

Some months later du Bois-Reymond wrote to Hallmann about the lesson he had learned from the Revolution and about his decision never again to allow himself to be the dupe of political illusions leading him to action in the public arena with no predictable outcome:

The political situation is terrible. I don't want to discuss it ... Here the mood is awful, the ultras of the reaction are now bowing their heads and proving we were right. Where will this end? Where and when will we see each other again? When will I finish my book? In the meanwhile I won't make the mistake of the summer of '48 again and instead I will pursue the path with more sober energy that the skills of science have shown me.[133]

But in another sense the Revolution did bring about much of what the writers of the Brockhaus and *Vierteljahresschrift* articles had been attempting to achieve, for now the course of liberalism for the next decade and a half was set upon rejecting idealism in all its forms and embracing a realism guided by the pursuit of material interest as the path toward solving the political and social questions of Germany. The members of the Berlin Physical Society now clearly saw that the society they envisioned was one in which the ideological elements I have discussed were configured into the moderate liberal narrative legitimating their own 'apolitical' activities. Their day would come, as Ludwig and Brücke had written, when German states recognised that the solution to their social and political problems lay in industrialisation and that German industrialisation required the natural sciences.

No one expressed these sentiments more clearly than Helmholtz in his address as Rector of the University of Heidelberg in 1862. On the

[132] Du Bois-Reymond to Ludwig, 16 February 1849, in Du Bois-Reymond (ed.), *Zwei grosse Naturforscher*, pp. 25–6.

[133] *Jugendbriefe*, p. 134.

eve of the 'institutional revolution' of the late 1860s, Helmholtz wrote: 'Even the proudest and least cooperative absolutist states have had to acknowledge that the power of the state rests upon its wealth, which depends upon command over the forces of nature and their application to agriculture, industry and transportation.'[134] Helmholtz went on to insist that the strength of modern nations lay in unfettering industry and accommodating the political interests of the Bürger classes. Ultimately, he concluded, the key to power lay in expansion of the natural sciences and in their technical application: 'No nation which wants to remain independent and influential can fall behind in this task.'[135]

Helmholtz included in this speech the ringing observation, 'Knowledge is power [*Wissen ist Macht*], and no age has been in a better position to realise it than the present one.' The statement may be taken as the motto of a generation – as long as we understand that by *Wissen* was meant a certain kind of knowledge, useful rather than speculative in orientation, produced by the laboratory rather than the lecture hall, and shaped by the discourse of practical interest in which Helmholtz's speech itself participated.

[134] Hermann Helmholtz, 'Ueber das Verhältniss der Naturwissenschaften zur Gesammtheit der Wissenschaften' in *Vorträge und Reden* (Brunswick, 1903), vol. 1, pp. 180–1.

[135] *Ibid.*, p. 181.

2

Building institutes for physiology in Prussia, 1836–1846

Contexts, interests and rhetoric

RICHARD L. KREMER

Introduction

In 1853, the *Wiener medizinische Wochenschrift* announced: 'Today it is no longer a disputed question whether a physiological institute belongs at a well-organised university, or if one does not exist, whether it should be erected.'[1] Leopold Wittelshöfer, who wrote this report on physiological institutes, could list twelve such institutes which had emerged over the previous twenty years,[2] and could even offer an organisational model for the ideal institute. It would have three divisions, each with its own physical space and apparatus (for physiological chemistry, physiological physics and anatomy/morphology), a room for microscopy, a library, animal stalls and a botanical garden, a large auditorium for lectures, apartments for its director and assistants, stipends for students and a regular budget for salaries and equipment. Wittelshöfer implied that the institutes would offer services for three different clientele: mass lectures for beginning

Acknowledgements: For their criticism and helpful suggestions, I thank R. Steven Turner, Lynn Nyhart, O.-J. Grüsser, Michael Hagner, Yvonne Howell and various participants at the 1988 Cambridge Wellcome Unit's conference on 'Medicine and the Laboratory'. I am grateful to the directors of the Geheimes Staatsarchiv Stiftung Preussischer Kulturbesitz Abteilung Merseburg (henceforth referred to as GStAM), the manuscript section of the Staatsbibliothek Preussischer Kulturbesitz in Berlin (henceforth SPK) and the Universitätsarchiv in Bonn for permission to quote sources from their holdings, and to the staffs of these archives for their friendly assistance. This research has been supported, in part, by the National Science Foundation and a Burke Research Initiation Grant from Dartmouth College.

1 Leopold Wittelshöfer, 'Ueber physiologische Institute', *Wiener medizinische Wochenschrift*, 3 (1853), cols. 606–8, 619–20, 635–6, at col. 607. Wittelshöfer is silently quoting here from Johann Ev. Purkyně, 'Ueber den Begriff der Physiologie ... Rede, gehalten bei der Eröffnung des physiologischen Institutes zu Prag am 6. Oktober 1851', *Vierteljahrschrift für die praktische Heilkunde*, 33 (1852), no. 2, pp. 1–24, at p. 2.

2 Breslau, Rostock, Göttingen, Berne, Jena, Würzburg, Zurich, Berlin, Bonn, Munich, Prague and Vienna.

students, practical exercises for more advanced students, and opportunities for original research by the assistants or students writing dissertations.

At a time, however, when only five German universities had established independent chairs for physiology (at the other universities, physiology and anatomy were combined),[3] Wittelshöfer's account of the institutional strength of the discipline might seem optimistic. Indeed, the so-called 'institutional revolution' for physiology is usually considered to have begun fifteen years later in Leipzig, when Karl Ludwig dedicated his massive new institute which became a model for eleven similar institutes constructed at other German-speaking universities between 1870 and 1890.[4] These 'institutional revolutions' swept the various disciplines of medicine and natural science in the last third of the nineteenth century, and often capped the successful establishment of a new discipline within the university system. Large, new buildings would be constructed, especially equipped for the teaching and research requirements of the discipline, and intended to serve only that discipline. In physics, for example, David Cahan has found that between 1873 and 1915 German states spent over nine million marks to build and equip twenty-three new institutes.[5] No one has yet managed to collect systematically such data for the medical disciplines. But the physiological institutes built after Ludwig's model must have cost nearly as much as did those for physics. These institutional revolutions dramatically changed the nature of laboratory instruction, the scope of scientific research and the scale of state support for science.[6]

Clearly, the early 'institutes', praised so enthusiastically by Wittelshöfer, were not equivalent, at least in scale, to those large-scale *Grossbetriebe* created in physiology's institutional revolution. As Reinhard Riese has noted, university contexts for specialised scientific and medical research, at least in Heidelberg, tended to evolve through phases. Cabinets or collections, often dating from the eighteenth

[3] Hans-Heinz Eulner, *Die Entwicklung der medizinischen Spezialfächer an den Universitäten des deutschen Sprachgebiets* (Stuttgart, 1970), p. 61.

[4] See Heinz Schröer, *Carl Ludwig: Begründer der messenden Experimentalphysiologie, 1816–1895* (Stuttgart, 1967), p. 77; Timothy Lenoir, 'Science for the clinic: science policy and the formation of Carl Ludwig's institute in Leipzig' in William Coleman and Frederic L. Holmes (eds), *The Investigative Enterprise: Experimental Physiology in Nineteenth-Century Medicine* (Berkeley, 1988), pp. 139–78; Eulner, *Die Entwicklung*, p. 63.

[5] David Cahan, 'The institutional revolution in German physics, 1865–1914', *Historical Studies in the Physical Sciences*, 15 (1984), pp. 1–65.

[6] Frank R. Pfetsch, *Zur Entwicklung der Wissenschaftspolitik in Deutschland, 1750–1914* (Berlin, 1974).

century, contained only demonstrative material for lectures or practical exercises and no special locations for experimental research. When such space was created in state-owned buildings, the cabinet often became named an 'institute', to be used by its director and perhaps a few advanced students. As younger students began experimental exercises in the institute, much more space was required and usually either a new construction or extensive remodelling of the existing location followed. Finally for those sciences most successful in capturing state support, a 'large institute' might be built, divided into sections, organised hierarchically, with working places for several hundred students.[7] Riese's final two phases encompass the institutional revolutions. His second phase might best describe the first wave of 'institutes' in physiology chronicled by Wittelshöfer.

Such a typology, however, provides more of a natural history than an ecology of institutional growth in given disciplines.[8] It does not pay attention to the dynamics of institutional change. It does not explore the various interests behind the types of institutions, changing evaluations of research or of pedagogical needs, or possible alternative arrangements for organising teaching and research. Neither does it consider whether the medical disciplines faced peculiar institutional constraints, different from those for disciplines taught in the philosophical faculties. As such, Riese's typology provides little help in resolving what may become a major controversy in understanding the flourishing of natural science at the nineteenth-century German universities.

Over the past thirty years, sociologists Joseph Ben-David and Awraham Zloczower have argued that the decentralised German universities created among themselves a competitive market, competing for students, faculty and reputation. Given the neohumanist ideology of *Wissenschaft* and the 'research imperative' whose origin R. Steven Turner has convincingly tied to Prussian educational reforms enacted early in the century, the system would provide opportunities for scholars as entrepreneurs to create whatever institutions furthered individual goals. States seeking to boost their reputations might be persuaded to construct new facilities or institutes by hard-bargaining candidates for faculty positions. Taking physi-

[7] Reinhard Riese, *Die Hochschule auf dem Wege zum wissenschaftlichen Grossbetrieb: Die Universität Heidelberg und das badische Hochschulwesen, 1860–1914* (Stuttgart, 1977), pp. 215–16.

[8] Charles Rosenberg, 'Toward an ecology of knowledge: on disciplines, context, and history' in A. Oleson and J. Voss (eds), *The Organization of Knowledge in Modern America, 1860–1920* (Baltimore, 1979), pp. 440–55.

ology as a test case, Zloczower tried to correlate variations in research productivity with changes in 'career opportunities' as perceived by young *Privatdozenten*. In these sociological explanations, then, market mechanisms drove the development of German science, especially in the rapid expansion of the universities after 1870. But Ben-David and Zloczower were unable to explain why, at given times, certain disciplines acquired more value in the competitive market than others. Here, they simply fell back on references to the internal, intellectual development of the various disciplines which would provide the raw material for the market economy.[9]

More recently, following the lead of Peter Borscheid and his incisive analysis of the development of chemistry in Baden, scholars have begun to ask whether state interests might have seriously disrupted the free market hypothesised by the sociologists. If the state sought to modernise its economy and society, and if it saw in natural science or medicine potentially useful tools for that task, might it have been willing to violate the 'solitude and freedom' of neohumanist *Wissenschaft* and especially encourage certain sciences in the service of modernisation?[10] This would, of course, restrict the 'currency' available to faculty and university ministries in the free market described by the sociologists. Explanations in terms of state interest in modernisation through science need not, of course, contradict explanations in terms of competitive markets, but rather might offer non-internalist accounts for the mechanisms available to actors in those markets.

Few would deny the major significance of both slowly modernising states and competitive decentralised universities for the rapid development of the scientific enterprise in nineteenth-century Germany.

[9] Joseph Ben-David, 'Scientific productivity and academic organisation in nineteenth century medicine', *American Sociological Review*, 25 (1960), pp. 828–43; Awraham Zloczower, *Career Opportunities and the Growth of Scientific Discovery in 19th Century Germany* (New York, 1981); Joseph Ben-David and Awraham Zloczower, 'Universities and academic systems in modern societies', *European Journal of Sociology*, 3 (1962), pp. 45–84; R. Steven Turner, 'The growth of professorial research in Prussia, 1818 to 1848 – causes and context', *Historical Studies in the Physical Sciences* 3 (1972), pp. 137–82; R. Steven Turner *et al.*, 'Careers and creativity in nineteenth-century physiology: Zloczower redux', *Isis*, 75 (1984), pp. 523–9; H. Schelsky, *Einsamkeit und Freiheit: Idee und Gestalt der deutschen Universitäten und ihrer Reformen* (Reinbek, Hamburg, 1963).

[10] Peter Borscheid, *Naturwissenschaft, Staat und Industrie in Baden, 1848–1914* (Stuttgart, 1976); see essays by William Coleman, Arleen Tuchman and Timothy Lenoir in Coleman and Holmes (eds), *The Investigative Enterprise*, and R. Steven Turner, 'German science, German universities: historiographical perspectives from the 1980s' in Gert Schubring (ed.), *'Einsamkeit und Freiheit' neu besichtigt: Universitätsreformen und Disziplinenbildung in Preußen als Modell für Wissenschaftspolitik im Europa des 19. Jahrhunderts* (Stuttgart, 1991), pp. 24–36.

Still unclear, however, is the timing of both factors, their relative importance for various scientific and medical disciplines, and their relative importance in the various German states. In this chapter, I hope to contribute to this discussion by examining the first attempts to create special institutions for physiology in Prussia. The success of these attempts, although limited, none the less established three of the 'institutes' so lauded by Wittelshöfer in 1853. More important than bricks and mortar, however, are the interests revealed in these episodes, and the rhetorical strategies deployed by various actors seeking to realise these interests. These institutes were among the earliest laboratories at German universities, and thus heralded a new type of patronage from the state and a new social and physical location for university natural science. Only on the basis of such case studies will we be able to refine the macro-theories of modernisation or competition.

Before turning to the proposals for physiological institutes, offered to the Prussian Cultural Ministry between 1836 and 1846, let me make three observations to characterise the unsettled status of physiology at the Prussian universities during the first half of the nineteenth century.

First, within the medical faculties at the six old Prussian universities – Berlin, Bonn, Breslau, Greifswald, Halle and Königsberg – physiology early had established, in part, an institutional autonomy as an independent subject (*Fach*) with its own chair, separate from anatomy. Because of local circumstances in 1811 when the Breslau theological seminary and the old university in Frankfurt-on-Oder were combined into a new university, an *Ordinariat* for physiology was created, the first such independent chair at any nineteenth-century German university. The first holder of this position, however, begged to teach anatomy, where greater student fees would increase his income.[11] Likewise in 1826, again because of local circumstances, the Prussian Cultural Minister, Karl Freiherr von Stein zum Altenstein, divided the chair in Königsberg so that both Karl von Baer and Karl Burdach could be accommodated. At the remaining Prussian universities, however, chairs for anatomy and physiology remained united until well after other German universities had begun to separate them.

[11] August Bartels, hired with the strong support of Karl Rudolphi, professor of anatomy and physiology in Berlin, taught general anatomy, general pathology, anthropology and physiology before returning to Marburg in 1821. See Rudolphi to the Cultural Ministry, 2 October 1811, and the correspondence between Bartels and the ministry in GStAM, Rep. 76va, Sekt. 4, Tit. IV, Nr 1, Bd 1, Bl. 163ff.; Rudolph Heidenhain, 'Purkyně', *Allgemeine deutsche Biographie* (Berlin, 1888), vol. XXVI: pp. 717–31, at p. 717.

Despite its early start, Prussia did not become a leader in granting physiologists independent chairs.

Second, the unsettled institutional status of physiology within Prussian medical faculties was also reflected in the state medical examinations. The famous Prussian medical edict of 1825, which had abolished the separate tracks of surgery and internal medicine for the education of most medical personnel, had not emphasised physiology. For future 'practising physicians', a newly created and controversial *Tentamen philosophicum* was required after the first two years of university study. This examination tried to preserve a fig-leaf of *Bildung* for the increasingly specialised medical students. They would be tested in logic, psychology, physics, chemistry, botany, zoology and mineralogy by professors from the philosophical faculty. For promotion two years later, candidates for the M.D. degree were tested in eight subjects, all from practical medicine except for history of medicine and anatomy and physiology (considered as one *Fach*). The final licensing *Staatsexamen* likewise required little specialised knowledge of physiology.[12]

Third, starting in the late 1830s Prussian medical personnel increasingly began to call for reform of the *Medicinalwesen*, including among other things medical education.[13] This reform movement, which ranged from Virchow's radical social programme to conservative, bureaucratic changes proposed by the Cultural Ministry, peaked by 1848 and then quickly faded as the reaction swept Prussia. Perhaps the most widely read reform essay, written by an official of the Cultural Ministry in 1846, emphasised the importance of physiology as 'the most necessary of all the fundamental sciences'. It advocated adding the subject to all three medical examinations (this would occur in 1856), and urged that physiology be taught via experiment in 'physiological institutes'.[14] The reform authors, however, rarely discussed what type of physiology to teach in the medical faculties. By 1840, at least three distinct approaches to the field had begun to emerge – the anatomical/morphological studies of such as Johannes Müller or Rudolf Wagner, the chemical studies of

[12] Hans Günter Wenig, 'Medizinische Ausbildung im 19. Jahrhundert', Inauguraldissertation (Bonn, 1969); Claudia Huerkamp, *Der Aufstieg der Aerzte im 19. Jahrhundert* (Göttingen, 1985), pp. 45–50.

[13] Kurt Finkenrath, *Die Medizinalreform* (Leipzig, 1929); Erwin H. Ackerknecht, 'Beiträge zur Geschichte der Medizinalreform von 1848', *Sudhoffs Archiv*, 25 (1932), pp. 61–183; Huerkamp, *Der Aufstieg der Aerzte*, pp. 45–50.

[14] Joseph Hermann Schmidt, *Die Reform der Medicinal-Verfassung Preussens*, 2nd unchanged edn (Berlin, 1846), pp. 50 and 77.

physiological processes of such as Friedrich Tiedemann and the physical studies of young scholars like du Bois-Reymond or Eduard Weber. In sum, physiology as a *Fach* in the 1840s was facing a set of unsettled institutional, medical and intellectual conditions in the Prussian universities. The *Fach* appeared to have the potential of becoming a discipline, but the shape such a discipline would take was by no means obvious.

Three Prussian proposals, 1836–1846

Over thirty years before 1869 when Ludwig began the institutional revolution in physiology, the Prussian Ministerium der geistlichen-, Unterrichts-, und Medicinal-Angelegenheiten (the so-called 'Cultural Ministry') received three separate proposals for creating such institutes.[15] Reflecting radically different conceptions of physiology, its status as a *Fach*, its methods of research and its relation to medicine and medical education, these proposals also envisioned different institutional structures and borrowed from various existing models. Before turning to the rhetoric of the proposals and of the responses they engendered, I shall first sketch the proposals and their contexts.

The widely known Breslau physiologist, Jan Purkyně (1787–1869), in 1836 and 1839 sent plans to Berlin for an 'experimental-demonstrative institute'. Opened in 1839 in a building renovated specifically for his purposes, Purkyně's would be the first physiological institute at a German university.[16] In his expansive proposal, Purkyně outlined four goals for the institute: to provide visual demonstrations (*Veranschaulichung*) for his physiological lectures; to enable medical

[15] Note that already in 1829–30, the Cultural Ministry had discussed creating a 'physiologische Experimental-Anstalt' in Berlin, an episode which I have not yet been able to explore. See K. A. S. Schultze to [Altenstein], 12 January 1831, GStAM, Rep. 76va, Sekt. 7, Tit. IV, Nr 9, Bd I, Bl. 69r–70r; K. E. Rothschuh, 'Carl August Sigmund Schultze (1795–1877) und seine Vorlesungen über Experimentalphysiologie in Freiburg (1830)', *Sudhoffs Archiv*, 47 (1963), pp. 347–59, at p. 356. Likewise, in 1844, A. W. Volkmann founded a physiological institute at Halle with an annual budget of 300 thaler; yet too few documents are extant for a thorough examination of Volkmann's rhetoric and interests. See GStAM, Rep. 76va, Sekt. 8, Tit. X, Nr 39; Rep. 76va, Sekt. 8, Tit. IV, Nr 15.

[16] For the debate over whether the 'anatomisch-physiologisches Kabinett', founded in 1821 in Freiburg by K. A. S. Schultze, should be considered the first physiological institute, see E. Th. Nauck, 'Bemerkungen zur Geschichte des physiologischen Institutes Freiburg i. Br.', *Berichte der naturforschenden Gesellschaft zu Freiburg i. Br.*, 40 (1950), pp. 147–59; Vladislav Kruta, 'J. E. Purkyně as Physiologe', *Nova Acta Leopoldina*, N. F. 24, Nr 151 (1961), pp. 57–76; Rothschuh, 'Schultze'; Vladislav Kruta, 'J. E. Purkyně's account of the origin and early history of the Institute of Physiology in Breslau (1841)', *Scripta Medica*, 39 (1966), pp. 1–16, at pp. 13–14.

students to gain hands-on experience in anatomical and experimental exercises and microscopy; to allow the director and his assistants to repeat experimental discoveries made elsewhere and to conduct their own original researches; and to represent the subject (*Fach*) of physiology at the university and to publish an annual report to communicate with the larger scientific world. Such a programme would require a separate building, Purkyně argued, which should include a large lecture hall, in which anatomical and physiological preparations, instruments and models also could be stored; rooms for microscopical and chemical investigations; a library and workroom for the director; animal stalls; and apartments for assistants and a janitor.[17] He requested an initial 900 thaler for equipment (three microscopes, air pump, balance, gasometer, apparatus for electrical, hydraulic, optical and acoustic demonstrations, surgical tools, chemical apparatus and reagents), and a continuing annual budget of 240 thaler for animals and supplies and 600 thaler for salaries for assistants, a janitor and an artist. The director of this large enterprise would be the *Ordinarius* for physiology in the medical faculty, i.e. Purkyně himself. The institute, Purkyně concluded, would be a 'public and integrative part of the organism of the university'. Its clientele would include not only medical students but also other faculty, students and even scientific 'amateurs' in Breslau.[18]

In 1843, Karl Heinrich Schultz[19] (1798–1871), botanist and physiologist in the Berlin medical faculty, presented a more modest plan for an 'Observatorium for theoretical medicine'. Although he wanted to offer all medical students *Naturanschauungen* of living processes and to provide laboratory space for advanced students to prepare medical dissertations, Schultz did not request a separate building. Instead, he proposed dividing the *Observatorium* into three sections – physiological, pathological and pharmacological – using rooms, respectively, in the main university building, the Berlin Veterinary School,

[17] For a floorplan of Purkyně's institute from 1845, see Ilse Jahn, 'Diskussionsbeitrag', *Nova Acta Leopoldina*, N.F. 24, Nr 151 (1961), p. 209. For another analysis emphasising the pre-1839 background of Purkyně's institute and describing the physiologist as an educational reformer inspired primarily by Johann Heinrich Pestalozzi, see William Coleman, 'Prussian pedagogy: Purkyně at Breslau, 1823–1839' in Coleman and Holmes (eds), *The Investigative Enterprise*, pp. 15–64.

[18] See Purkyně to Altenstein, 1 June 1836 and 4 July 1839, in Jan Ev. Purkyně, *Opera Omnia*, 13 vols. (Prague, 1918–85), vol. XII, pp. 219–41. For the original documents, see GStAM, Rep. 76va, Sekt. 4, Tit. X, Nr 47, Bd I, Bl. 40r–53v, 93r–104r. The transcriptions in the *Opera* are not always exact; any required corrections will be noted.

[19] In 1848, Schultz changed his name to Schultz-Schultzenstein. To avoid confusion, I shall refer to him by the shorter name even after 1848.

and the Charité, Berlin's large city hospital. Only one section would meet each semester, so that one and a half years would be required for the full cycle. In addition to the director (who should be an *Ordinarius* in the medical faculty and skilled in experimental physiology and medical chemistry), the *Observatorium*'s staff would include several prosectors (employed at the veterinary school), an assistant (preferably a chemist), an artist, mechanic, janitor and several student assistants. To purchase twenty microscopes, Schultz requested an initial outlay of 2100 thaler. His annual budget he set at only 100 thaler plus salaries. Although he did not want to require attendance at the *Observatorium*, Schultz suggested that the subjects of experimental physiology, experimental pathology and experimental pharmacology be added to the promotion and licensing exams, and that all medical dissertations be required to demonstrate 'investigative skills'. That is, by modifying the content of medical examinations, Schultz would thrust his new institution onto the centre stage of medical education in Berlin.[20]

The third proposal came from a *Privatdozent* in Bonn, Julius Budge (1811–88). In 1846, he requested permission to establish a private physiological institute (which he also called a 'seminar') as an 'intermediate station' for medical students between the anatomical institute and the clinics. In the former, he claimed, students make only rough, quick, naked-eye observations of organs and body structure; the latter assume highly developed observational skills which are not learned in the anatomical institute. Hence, Budge's new institute would be 'practical', i.e., would emphasise the 'art of observing' and hands-on experience in microscopy, chemical analysis and physiological and physical investigations. Budge envisioned three sections – chemical, physical and physiological/anatomical – each with its own instructor who would offer a one-semester course to students who had already attended lectures in anatomy, chemistry and physics. Budge himself would lead the physiological/anatomical section; another *Privatdozent* from the philosophical faculty (Ottokar Fabian Karl von Feilitzsch) would teach the physical course; staffing for the chemical section Budge left unspecified. Even though the institute would be private and supported primarily by fees of 1.5 Friedrichs d'or per student per semester,[21] Budge none the less requested the exclusive use

[20] Schultz, 'Bericht an Ew. Excellence den Wirklichen Geheimen Staatsminister Dr. Eichhorn über ein bei der Universität zu Berlin zu errichtendes medizinisches Observatorium' [18 March 1843], GStAM, Rep. 76va, Sekt. 1, Tit. VII, Nr 9, Bd IV, Bl. 147r–155r.

[21] About 8.5 thaler, a substantial honorarium for a semester-long course.

of five rooms in the Bonn university building, an unspecified sum for apparatus, and salary for a janitor.[22]

Each of these proposals sought to establish an institution for physiology copied from an existing model. And each proposal reflected its local context and especially the marginal status of its proponent in that context. That is, each institute-builder was trying to create a niche for himself at his university as well as trying to reform physiology and physiological pedagogy.

Contexts and models

Purkyně had been called to Breslau in 1823 as *Ordinarius* for physiology and pathology, and since 1831, and possibly earlier, had struggled to build an 'institute', at least in part because of his unhappy relations with the Breslau anatomist, Adolf Wilhelm Otto (1786–1845). Purkyně's status in the Breslau medical faculty had been problematic from the beginning. That faculty and the university curator had proposed at least five better-known candidates for the position in 1822,[23] and were outraged by the appointment of the non-Prussian, little-published prosector from Prague.[24] Complaints,

[22] Budge to Eichhorn, 30 April 1846, and 'Entwurf zu Statuten eines physiologischen Seminars an der Universität Bonn', GStAM, Rep. 76va, Sekt. 3, Tit. x, Nr 58, Bd 1, Bl. 9r–13v.

[23] Including Franz von Paula Gruithuisen (1774–1852), professor of 'physical science and natural history' at a medical school in Munich, who in his *Beiträge zur Physiolognosie und Eautognosie* (Munich, 1812), pp. 344–5, had called for the creation of institutes for experimental physiology; Karl Friedrich Heusinger (1792–1883), an *Extraordinarius* in Jena who taught anatomy and physiology; and Karl Gustav Carus (1789–1865), already well-known for his books on comparative anatomy, and who in 1822 was professor of obstetrics at the medical-surgical academy in Dresden.

[24] Johann Nepomuk Rust, general surgeon at the Friedrich-Wilhelms-Institut in Berlin, had in 1822 advised his fellow Bohemian, Purkyně, how to seek the Breslau chair, and had introduced him to Karl Rudolphi, professor for anatomy and physiology at the Berlin university and powerful advisor to Altenstein in the Cultural Ministry. In October 1822, Rudolphi wrote two strongly worded letters recommending Purkyně to Altenstein for the Breslau position. The Breslau medical faculty, however, had eagerly courted von Gruithuisen, whom the Cultural Ministry apparently had even agreed to appoint pending approval from the police, something required in the aftermath of the Karlsbad Decrees. After the King approved Purkyně's appointment in January 1823, the Breslau medical faculty wrote a bitter letter complaining about this undistinguished physiologist who would not contribute to the 'honour of the faculty'. See Rust to Purkyně, 3 March 1822, in Jaroslav Jedlička (ed.), *Jana Ev. Purkyně Korespondence* (Prague, 1920), vol. 1, pp. 162–3; GStAM, Rep. 76va, Sekt. 4, Tit. iv, Nr 1, Bde viii and ix, *passim*; Erich Witte, 'Die Berufung Purkyněs nach Breslau', *Anatomischer Anzeiger*, 92 (1941–2), pp. 68–77 (this source must be used with caution, as Mikuláš Teich has kindly warned me); Vladislav Kruta, 'Purkyněs Berufung nach Breslau' in J. E. Purkyně, *Abhandlung über die physiologische Untersuchung des Sehorgans und des Hautsystems* [1823], ed. and transl. Joachim Ebert and Karel Zlábek (Halle, 1979), pp. 23–6.

sometimes contradictory, immediately arose about Purkyně's teaching. His lectures were considered too abstract and filled with *Naturphilosophie*, or too narrowly focused on the auxiliary sciences of physics and chemistry rather than on physiology in its totality. And everyone agreed his command of German was very weak. Indeed, the anatomist even urged Purkyně to add demonstrations and experiments to his lectures to boost his low student enrolments and compensate for his linguistic shortcomings.[25]

In 1824, Purkyně began what he called an 'Experimentalkolleg', demonstrating the processes of respiration, circulation, digestion, secretion, nerve and muscle actions in his physiological lectures. These lecture props were supported by small grants of 50–80 thaler per year from the Cultural Ministry, but never by a regular budget. By 1828, he had students themselves conducting microscopic investigations for medical dissertations (a trickle which became a small stream after he acquired a large Plössel microscope in 1832), his enrolments had risen, and he had begun to offer popular lectures on physiology for non-medical students.[26] At first, Purkyně used equipment and space in the anatomical institute until friction with Otto forced him to seek a room from the philosophical faculty. Evicted from this space in 1831, Purkyně first proposed an independent physiological institute with its own dedicated space.[27] But the Breslau curator refused to support this request, arguing that no other university, not even Berlin, had such an institute, and that a room for

[25] Rust, however, had especially praised Purkyně's ability to lecture in Latin and German. Witte, 'Die Berufung Purkyněs', pp. 73–4; GStAM, Rep. 76va, Sekt. 4, Tit. x, Nr 47, Bd I, Bl. 3r and 6r–11r; for lectures and attendance figures for 1824–30, see Rep. 76va, Sekt. 4, Tit. XIII, Nr 1, Bde II–IV.

[26] Between 1833 and 1840, Purkyně directed at least fifteen dissertations. For those years, the Breslau medical faculty as a whole averaged 14.6 promotions (dissertation required) per year, with an average enrolment of 60 students per semester. In other words, the other six *Ordinarien* on Breslau's medical faculty directed, on average, slightly more dissertations per year than did Purkyně. Purkyně, *Opera*, vol. II, pp. 81–4, vol. VI, pp. 6–7, vol. XIII, pp. 260–6; Bernhard Nadbyl, *Chronik und Statistik der königlichen Universität zu Breslau* (Breslau, 1861), pp. 19–22; Z. Vacek, 'The scientific work of J. E. Purkyně and its significance for the development of histology and embryology', *Physiologia Bohemoslovaca*, 36 (1987), pp. 191–202.

[27] In reviewing his career in Breslau, Purkyně wrote to Johannes Schulze on 17 December 1849; 'Zur Anregung des hiesigen physiologischen Instituts hat bei mir das Wort des verewigten Hegel das meiste beigetragen, der, als ich bei ihm über Mißverhältniß zur Anatomie Klage führte, mit fester Stimme sprach: "Sie müssen sich ein eigenes Institut errichten lassen".' GStAM, Rep. 92, Schulze Litt. P, Nr 28, Bl. 326r–327v. Yet as Vladislav Kruta, in 'G. W. F. Hegel a J. E. Purkyně', *Ceskoslovenská Akademie Věd. Sekce Filosifie a Histoire*, 13 (1965), pp. 282–4, has argued, no other extant evidence links Hegel to Purkyně's attempts to create an institute in Breslau, and it seems likely that Purkyně overemphasised the significance of Hegel's contributions to his Breslau institutional innovations.

Purkyně might be found in the new anatomical building then under construction. The anatomist, however, managed to prevent Purkyně from securing space in either the new or the old anatomy buildings, so that the physiologist was forced to use his private home for his experimental lectures and his students' independent researches.[28] Clearly, these ongoing difficulties with the Breslau anatomist helped prompt Purkyně to seek institutional independence.

The institutional forms Purkyně proposed for experimental physiology followed models already developed in other disciplines or being developed elsewhere in physiology. Lectures accompanied by experiments and demonstrations, for example, had become standard features of eighteenth-century German university curricula in natural science. According to Rudolf Stichweh, professors of *Naturlehre* by 1750 began offering lectures in experimental physics to large audiences of students from all four faculties. As much theatre as physics, these lectures helped establish the role of the 'physicist' in the early nineteenth century as a populariser and service teacher rather than as a researcher.[29] Lecture demonstrations in the medical faculty, however, remained more specialised. Since the creation of anatomical theatres at most German universities in the sixteenth century, anatomical demonstrations had become a regular part of medical education. And in 1828 when Hermann Kilian reviewed German scientific education, he found lectures in 'experimental physiology' being offered not only at Purkyně's Breslau, but also in Berlin, Bonn, Freiburg, Göttingen and Heidelberg.[30]

More novel, however, was Purkyně's vision of practical exercises in physiology. Not until well into the nineteenth century would physics students be able to acquire their own experimental skills in university-owned laboratories. Likewise, even though medical students might

[28] Even though the old anatomy building had been promised to Purkyně, Otto with the aid of Alexander von Humboldt managed to secure that space for his private residence. Von Humboldt to Altenstein, 16 January 1835, reprinted in Kurt-R. Biermann (ed.), *Alexander von Humboldt, Vier Jahrzehnte Wissenschaftsförderung: Briefe an das preußische Kultusministerium, 1818–1859* (Berlin, 1985), p. 70. For Purkyně's efforts in experimental physiology before 1836, see GStAM, Rep. 76va, Sekt. 4, Tit. x, Nr 47, Bd 1, Bl. 1r–37v; Purkyně, 'Kurzer Bericht über die Entstehung und jetzigen Stand des physiologischen Instituts in Breslau' [1841], in Purkyně, *Opera*, vol. xii, pp. 213–18, transl. in Kruta, 'Purkyně's account'; Heidenhain, 'Purkyně'; Karl Hürthle, 'Die Gründung des physiologischen Instituts in Breslau durch Joh. Ev. Purkinje', *Allgemeine medicinische Central-Zeitung*, 77 (1908), pp. 72–4.

[29] Rudolf Stichweh, *Zur Entstehung des modernen Systems wissenschaftlicher Disziplinen: Physik in Deutschland, 1740–1890* (Frankfurt, 1984), pp. 334–51.

[30] Quoted in Johannes Steudel, 'Medizinische Ausbildung in Deutschland 1600–1850' in Sigrid Schwenk *et al.* (eds), *Et Multum et Multa. Beiträge zur Literatur, Geschichte und Kultur der Jagd: Festgabe für Kurt Lindner* (Berlin, 1971), pp. 393–420, at pp. 400–2.

attend courses in the anatomical institutes entitled 'Introduction to Dissections', they would not always wield the scalpel themselves. Before Prussia in 1825 combined medicine and surgery, many university-trained students may not have touched a cadaver until their final licensing examinations. When Purkyně in his *Experimentalkolleg* began to offer his students hands-on experience, mostly with microscopes, he was thus innovating in medical education, at exactly the same time as was Liebig who also in the 1820s had begun to offer his Giessen chemistry students practical laboratory exercises.[31]

Still, Purkyně's vision of an institute for physiology copied in many ways the well-established structure of anatomical institutes – staff, fixed annual budget, collections of specimens and equipment, dedicated building or rooms. Indeed, in 1839 when seeking to justify his request for an annual budget, Purkyně explicitly compared his projected institute to an anatomical institute.[32] Purkyně's institutional innovation, then, came primarily in his *Experimentalkolleg*.

Karl Heinrich Schultz also found himself by 1843 occupying a marginal position in Berlin. After earning his medical degree at the Friedrich-Wilhelms-Institut, he had been named *Extraordinarius* in the Berlin medical faculty in 1825, exactly when Karl Rudolphi was the leading anatomist-physiologist in that faculty. In 1830, Schultz's experimental study of the flow of sap in plants won a prize at the Paris Académie des Sciences and Schultz stood perhaps at the height of his fame. He ascended to *Ordinarius*, although not for any specific subject, in 1833, the very year in which Johannes Müller was called to Berlin. Müller's arrival may have signalled the beginning of Schultz's isolation in the medical faculty even though through the 1830s he was seen as a leader for reform in the faculty and in 1840 as dean he helped call Johann Schönlein to Berlin.[33] Already in the 1820s Müller and Schultz had clashed publicly over the methods for studying the chemistry and function of blood, and over their respective experimental results. Müller advocated cautious observation and description; his opponent more freely ascribed vital forces to living

[31] Not until summer semester (SS) 1830 did Purkyně offer a course (to twenty-three students) whose title 'Die Experimental-Physiologie und das Gebrauch des Microscopes' clearly implies hands-on experience for students. His usual course, entitled only 'Experimental-Physiologie', drew the following enrolments before he opened his institute in 1839: Summer Semester 1825, 12; SS 1827, 30; SS 1828, 26; SS 1831, 10; WS 1831–2, 7; SS 1832, 18; SS 1833, 23; SS 1834, 23; SS 1836, 31; SS 1837, 32. GStAM, Rep. 76va, Sekt. 4, Tit. XIII, Nr 1, Bde. III–VII.

[32] Purkyně, *Opera*, vol. XII, p. 235.

[33] Max Lenz, *Geschichte der königlichen Friedrich-Wilhelms-Universität zu Berlin*, 4 vols. (Halle, 1910–18), vol. II, part II, p. 165; Rolf Winau, *Medizin in Berlin* (Berlin, 1987), pp. 138–9.

blood.[34] At Berlin, both men lectured on human physiology, although Müller as director of the anatomical museum and theatre had by far the stronger institutional position and attracted the lion's share of students and fees. Not until 1840 did the Cultural Ministry finally allow Schultz to examine medical candidates in the subjects of 'medical science and theoretical medicine'. In thanking the ministry for this promotion, Schultz vaguely alluded to the 'many years of belittling [*Verkleinerung*]' he had endured. By the 1850s, Schultz's salary would be the lowest of all *Ordinarien* in the medical faculty.[35] Clearly, Schultz felt slighted amidst his more prominent colleagues.

Since he taught botany and 'botanical excursions' (i.e., field observation in Berlin's various botanical gardens), Schultz did have access to state-supported institutions for his research and teaching. Convinced early of the need for specialised institutions of medical instruction, Schultz in 1825 had already urged the Cultural Ministry to establish a 'physiological institute'.[36] His 1843 proposal, however, called not for an institute but an 'observatory'. By 1843, five of the six Prussian universities possessed astronomical 'observatories'; the magnetic 'observatories' of C. F. Gauss and Wilhelm Weber had become well known, and Weber especially advocated such observatories as sites for educating university students in the art of precise measurement.[37] Yet as will be seen below, Schultz was much more interested in *Naturanschauungen* than in precise quantitative measurements. Even though he might have selected a label from an existing institution, the *Observatorium* he proposed would be quite different.

When Julius Budge arrived in Bonn as a thirty-one year old *Privatdozent* in 1842, his Jewish background (although he had converted to Protestantism, as had many Jewish intellectuals in Prussia) and youthful energy amidst the elderly Bonn medical faculty made his situation difficult. The faculty consisted of eight *Ordinarien* with an average age of fifty-seven, four of whom had been appointed to their positions at the founding of the university in 1818; a single

[34] Carl Schultz, *Der Lebensprocess im Blut* (Berlin, 1822); Johannes Müller, 'Dr C. H. Schultz, Der Lebensprocess im Blute, eine auf microscopischen Entdeckungen gegründete Untersuchung', *Isis*, 1 (1824), pp. 267–92; Brigitte Lohff, 'Johannes Müller (1801–1858) als akademischer Lehrer', unpublished Ph.D. dissertation (Hamburg, 1977), pp. 64–77.

[35] Schultz to [Altenstein], 4 February 1840, SPK, Darmst. Lb 1830 Schultz-Schultzenstein; GStAM, Rep. 76va, Sekt. 2, Tit. xv, Nr 27, Bd 1, Bl. 18v–22r. In 1854, Schultz's salary (he earned no fees!) of 1000 thaler was much lower than the average income of 2700 thaler for *Ordinarien* on the Berlin medical faculty.

[36] Schultz to Eichhorn, 10 January 1847, GStAM, Rep. 76va, Sekt. 1, Tit. vii, Nr 9, Bd v, Bl. 26r.

[37] See Weber to Sabine, 20 February 1845 in *Wilhelm Webers Werke*, 6 vols. (Berlin, 1892–4), vol. ii, pp. 274–6.

Extraordinarius; and several *Privatdozenten*. Several of the older faculty were ill and taught only irregularly; another soon would go blind. Student enrolments had dropped steadily since 1825.[38] During the 1840s, the Cultural Ministry would struggle to rejuvenate the Bonn medical faculty, widely recognised as the weakest of any Prussian university.

Budge, who in 1841 had published a massive experimental work on the function and structure of nerves, came to Bonn primarily to teach physiology. Karl Mayer, *Ordinarius* for anatomy and physiology, who at his appointment in 1819 had received annually 300 thaler to support his own research in 'experimental physiology', had already in the 1820s accompanied his physiological lectures with 'experiments and microscopic observations', and in 1837–8 had offered 'microscopical exercises in physiology'.[39] But from 1841–3, Mayer was ill and could announce only three courses, two of which were cancelled for lack of auditors. Budge quickly took the lead in teaching physiology. In addition to courses on general, human and comparative physiology, he regularly taught a course in experimental physiology which became the basis of his request for a physiological institute.[40] According to later reports, Budge offered students in the latter class practical experience in microscopy, embryology, vivisection and in some chemical analysis (of healthy and diseased urine, of the resorption of sugar injected into the bloodstream or digestive tract, and of *in vitro* conversion of starch to sugar by glandular tissue).[41]

In proposing a private physiological seminar, Budge drew on different institutional models than had Purkyně or Schultz. As Turner has shown, Prussian university chemists had for years built their own

[38] In 1825, an average of 78 medical students per semester enrolled at Bonn; by 1835, that number had declined to 61. In 1845, it would drop to 51. The nadir of 44 students was reached in 1855. Karl Schmiz, *Die medizinische Fakultät der Universität Bonn, 1818–1918* (Bonn, 1920), p. 60. Total average enrolments per semester at Bonn for the same years: 1830, 844; 1835, 682; 1840, 611; 1845, 681; 1850, 957; 1855, 778. Franz Eulenberg, *Die Frequenz der deutschen Universitäten von ihrer Gründung bis zur Gegenwart* (Leipzig, 1904), pp. 302–4.

[39] Altenstein to Mayer, draft, 29 November 1818, GStAM, Rep. 92, Altenstein AVI, Nr 14, Bl. 1; Rep. 76va, Sekt. 3, Tit. XIII, Nr 1, Bd 6; 'Tabellen der Vorlesungen', Bonn Universitätsarchiv, Rektorat U62. For a description of the 'remarkable experiments' conducted by students in Mayer's course on 'experimental physiology', see *Jahrbuch der preußischen Rhein-Universität*, 1819–21, pp. 434–6. See Johannes Dietrich Meyer, 'August Franz Josef Carl Mayer: Leben und Werk', Inauguraldissertation (Bonn, 1966).

[40] Schmiz, *Die medizinische Fakultät*, pp. 83–6; GStAM, Rep. 76va, Sekt. 3, Tit. IV, Nr 39, Bd II, Bl. 76r–82r. Between 1842 and 1850, Budge offered his course on experimental physiology nine times, with an average enrolment of thirteen students.

[41] See Budge's printed report for 1854 in GStAM, Rep. 76va, Sekt. 3, Tit. IV, Nr 39, Bd II, Bl. 149r–155v.

private laboratories into which they invited selected students for a fee, or without charge as a means of patronage. These small laboratories, rooted in private apothecary shops or profit-making pharmacy schools, had by the 1830s begun to receive some state support, but the chemistry professors tended to own most of the apparatus, and take it with them when they moved to another university. Not until the 1850s would Prussia begin to move from this personal, entrepreneurial concept of chemical laboratories to the principle of complete subsidisation and ownership by the state.[42] By calling for a private rather than a fully subsidised physiological institution in 1846, Budge moved cautiously and appeared to challenge less directly the anatomical institute, in which physiological instruction had previously been conducted.

Budge also referred to his proposed institution as a 'seminar'. At first glance, Budge's desire for a seminar is not surprising since Bonn in 1825 had opened the first seminar in natural science at any German university. Based on philological seminars already developed in the eighteenth century, these institutions were intended to train future teachers for *Gymnasien* and lower schools (*Berufsbildung*) and to support studies in natural science more generally at the university. Led by all the *Ordinarien* for natural sciences in the philosophy faculty (physics, chemistry, zoology, botany and mineralogy), the Bonn seminar students delivered to each other general lectures in the sciences, similar to those they later would give as teachers, and prepared original scientific papers, sometimes based on experiments and observations. The seminar offered limited stipends for some students, and gave all members access to a specialised library and experimental apparatus and collections of preparations for practical exercises.[43] Budge must have viewed a seminar primarily as a vehicle for practical exercises, since medical students rarely became teachers

[42] R. Steven Turner, 'Justus Liebig versus Prussian chemistry: reflections on early institute-building in Germany', *Historical Studies in the Physical Sciences*, 13 (1982), pp. 129–62, at pp. 152–5.

[43] For the original regulations of the Bonn seminar, see Johann Friedrich Wilhelm Koch (ed.), *Die preußischen Universitäten: eine Sammlung der Verordnungen*, 2 vols. (Berlin, 1839–40), vol. II, pp. 624–31. See also Stichweh, *Zur Entstehung*, pp. 364–75; Robert S. Leventhal, 'The emergence of philological discourse in the German states, 1770–1810', *Isis*, 77 (1986), pp. 243–60; Christa Jungnickel and Russell McCormmach, *Intellectual Mastery of Nature: Theoretical Physics from Ohm to Einstein*, 2 vols. (Chicago, 1986–87), vol. I, pp. 78–107; Kathryn M. Olesko, 'Commentary: On institutes, investigations, and scientific training' in Coleman and Holmes (eds.), *The Investigative Enterprise*, pp. 295–332; William Clark, 'On the dialectical origins of the research seminar', *History of Science*, 28 (1989), pp. 111–54; and especially Gert Schubring, 'The rise and decline of the Bonn natural sciences seminar', *Osiris*, 2nd series, 5 (1989), 57–93.

and in 1846 he did not envision students giving lectures in the seminar.[44] But by labelling his institution a seminar, Budge carefully sought to mould his proposal to fit as easily as possible into the institutional landscape at Bonn.

In proposing various institutional models for physiology – an institute, an *Observatorium*, and a seminar – Purkyně, Schultz and Budge each sought to tailor his innovation to the local context of his university. They all had begun teaching 'experimental physiology' in various forms, first providing demonstrations for students to observe passively, and then seeking to implement exercises in which at least some students could more actively conduct their own experiments and observations. Had Purkyně, Schultz and Budge enjoyed more co-operative relations with the directors of the anatomical institutes at their universities, their physiological exercises might well have been accommodated within those institutions. All three, for example, focused their requests for apparatus on the microscope, an instrument increasingly at home in the anatomical institutes of the 1840s. Yet ultimately physiology and anatomy would diverge into separate disciplines with separate institutional bases within medical faculties. These Prussian proposals represent early steps toward this divergence at an institutional level. The rhetoric of the proposals, even more than the local contexts and the institutional models, reveals the interests at work to reshape medical disciplines and medical education at the mid-century German universities.

Rhetoric and interests

First, a methodological proviso: reading documents in the Cultural Ministry archives requires careful attention to the rhetorical strategies of the writers and an awareness of the purposes for which the texts were written. When faculty members seek to persuade the Cultural Ministry to act (e.g. request financial support or propose candidates for teaching posts), one must assume that the prose sent to Berlin combines in complex ways the 'actual' views and interests of the faculty and what they think the cultural ministry wants to hear. That is, faculty might be expected to cloak their own interests in what they

44 In 1850, Budge would add to his institute a 'physiologischer Verein', in which at weekly meetings medical students presented experimental work they had done in Budge's physiological exercises, or reported on recent literature. Bernhard Johnen, *Bericht über Stand und Wirksamkeit des physiologischen Vereins zu Bonn* (Bonn, n.d. [1854]), in GStAM, Rep. 76va, Sekt. 3, Tit. IV, Nr 39, Bd II, Bl. 100r–101v.

consider to be the interests of the Cultural Ministry. And the ministry officials, trying to control unruly faculties, might be expected to deploy similar rhetorical strategies. Or when the ministry has decided to spend funds in a certain way, it might use different rhetorical means to persuade the Finance Ministry or the King to approve.[45] Furthermore, in many cases the parties in these negotiations also talked face-to-face, exchanges which leave no direct traces in the documentary record and for that very reason may have contained the expression of yet other interests. Determining the 'real' interests of individual faculty members, faculties as groups, or the Cultural Ministry, merely by reading documents they sent each other is hardly possible. At best, one can try to understand the rhetorical strategies adopted by each actor, and can only speculate about interests motivating those strategies.

Among the three proposals to create physiological institutes, Purkyně's rhetorical strategy of 1836, richly developed in a lengthy twenty-seven-page memorandum to minister Altenstein, is undoubtedly the most complex. As noted above, his first attempt in 1831 to establish a formal institute had been squelched by the Breslau curator.[46] But by 1836, Purkyně's prospects had brightened. Shortly before, he had discovered with Gabriel Valentin the ciliary movement in vertebrates, a widely and immediately hailed find which boosted Purkyně's already considerable reputation.[47] Not insignificantly, Purkyně and Valentin dedicated the monograph announcing their discovery to Alexander von Humboldt and Altenstein, thanking the latter privately for his support of the subject (*Fach*) of 'experimental physiology' in Breslau.[48] Equally important for Purkyně's designs, a

[45] Bruno Latour, *Science in Action* (Milton Keynes, 1987), pp. 108–11, has described such strategies as 'translating interests'.

[46] Purkyně was not the only person troubled by Friedrich Wilhelm Neumann (1763–1835), curator at Breslau since 1819. Concerning Neumann, a former Breslau librarian remembered in 1868: 'Einen engherzigeren, missgünstigeren, falscheren Regierungsmenschen habe ich nie kennen lernen.' Cited in Kruta, 'Purkyně's account', p. 3.

[47] Johannes Müller, for example, in his 1834 annual review of physiology, characterised the discovery as of 'most consequential importance'. Quoted in Mikuláš Teich, 'Purkyně and Valentin on ciliary motion: an early investigation in morphological physiology', *British Journal for the History of Science*, 5 (1970), pp. 168–77, at p. 170.

[48] Altenstein, '...durch Anschaffung eines trefflichen Mikroskopes, durch besondere Unterstützung des Fachs der Experimentalphysiologie auf hiesiger Universität', made it possible for them to make the discovery, wrote Purkyně to Altenstein, 30 November 1834, GStAM, Rep. 76vf, Litt. P, Nr 4, Bl. 34r–v. In sending the book to the Cultural Minister, Purkyně went even further: 'Möge es [the discovery of ciliary motion] dazu beitragen die Wissenschaft der Physiologie der es angehört, die erst in neuerer Zeit, noch schüchtern in den Kreis der altbegründeten mit reichen Apparaten und Sammlungen versehenen mit angemessenen Localen ausgestatteten Doctrinen der Physik, Anatomie, Zoologie, Chemie,

new curator had been appointed for Breslau who became immediately supportive of his famous physiologist.[49] Still, Purkyně's 1836 manifesto reflects a strategy of caution, as if he did not want to appear too radical in seeking to establish a new institution for physiological teaching and research.

Physiology needed such an institute, Purkyně began, because the subject (*Fach*) had undergone massive change. In some earlier unspecified time, physiologists had engaged primarily in 'idle speculations' and 'literary-philosophical' disputation. The subject had been 'discursive', a 'lecture doctrine [*Kathederdoktrin*] which dealt only with disputable concepts', an 'axiomatic teaching method'.[50] It had floated between the extremes of 'intellectual [*geistige*] commentary on anatomy' and the 'otherworldly independence of *Naturphilosophie*'. But recently, continued Purkyně, citing no specific examples, physiology had left those heights for an 'earthly and material but living and organic home'. It had become a 'demonstrative *Fach*', an 'experimental science', a 'science of experience'. Like the other experimental sciences – Purkyně listed variously anatomy, therapeutics, physics, chemistry, botany, mineralogy 'and others' (the list might be longer?) – physiology now based its practice on experiment and observation. In this new status as an 'Erfahrungswissenschaft',[51] physiology thus 'must demand [from the state], with the same right as other natural sciences, a complete set of experimental and demonstration apparatus, and a suitable locale for experiments and demonstrations and for storing instruments, models and preparations'. One might ask, of course, that the physiologist conduct experiments in his own home (as Purkyně was doing), or that he

Minerlogie [sic] einzutreten sich wegen möchte, der vorsorgenden Beachtung Ew. Excellenz näher zu bringen...'. Purkyně to Altenstein, 5 July 1835, SPK, Darmst. 3k 1825(2) Purkyně. Altenstein, although delayed by illness, read the book dedicated to him with interest, and discussed in some detail the significance of Purkyně's and Valentin's discovery. Altenstein to Purkyně, 24 April 1836, GStAM, Rep. 76vf, Litt. P, Nr 4, Bl. 44r–v.

49 In his first dealing with Purkyně, the new curator, Ferdinand Wilhelm Heinke (1784–1857), asked permission to grant 80 thaler from surplus funds to his physiologist. To persuade the ministry of this request, Heinke stressed Purkyně's successes in teaching (dissertations, twice-weekly microscopic demonstrations) and research (ciliary movement), the fact that he had received no space in the new anatomy building, and the 'extraordinary importance' of physiology for the medical sciences. Heinke also strongly supported Purkyně's 1836 proposal to the ministry. Heinke to Altenstein, 21 February 1836, 27 June 1836, GStAM, Rep. 76va, Sekt. 4, Tit. X, Nr 47, Bd I, Bl. 32r–33v, 38r–39r.

50 Rather than 'aeromatische' given in Purkyně, *Opera*, vol. XII, p. 222. See GStAM, Rep. 76va, Sekt. 4, Tit. X, Nr 47, Bd I, Bl. 42v.

51 Purkyně may have borrowed the concept of *Erfahrungswissenschaft* from Karl Burdach, *Die Physiologie als Erfahrungswissenschaft*, 6 vols. (Leipzig, 1828–40), the first four volumes of which Purkyně enthusiastically reviewed in 1833. See Purkyně, *Opera*, vol. V, pp. 117–22.

charge exorbitant student fees to cover his costs. But then this demand should be made equally of the other demonstrative subjects. Why should physiology be punished for the 'accidental' fact that it discovered its need for experimental and demonstrative apparatus later than other subjects? With such rhetoric, Purkyně asked not for radical innovation; he would have the Cultural Ministry believe that he simply wanted what had long become standard for other sciences, in both the medical and philosophical faculties.[52] He merely wanted to claim his 'rights'.[53]

Realising that physiology at nearly every university except Breslau was combined with the anatomical chair, Purkyně carefully described the independent status of physiology as the new *Erfahrungswissenschaft* and its relation to the other disciplines. A 'partly historical, partly statistical overview' of Europe's scientific institutions revealed four separate patterns for anatomy and physiology, ranging from total separation and isolation to one person simultaneously filling both roles. According to Purkyně, the former, the most common arrangement,[54] leads to one-sidedness with anatomy alone treating the material elements and physiology becoming completely abstract and literary. The latter, although it might reduce costs since apparatus can be shared, usually requires too much of one person. Much better, he implied, is the arrangement in which both physiology and anatomy have their own institutional support, and relate as 'sister sciences', united in love rather than regulations. Throughout this analysis, Purkyně referred to anatomy and physiology as clearly distinguished subjects (*Fächer*) intellectually; the problem was to provide adequately for their institutional separation. Always cautious, Purkyně

[52] Interestingly, Purkyně did not mention explicitly any other existing institutions. Of course, anatomical theatres and clinics were standard in all medical faculties by 1836; and botanical gardens, cabinets for mineralogy and physics, and some chemical laboratories also existed for use by members of the philosophical faculties. But state-supported 'institutes' (dedicated spaces, personnel beyond the professors) for physics and chemistry would begin to emerge only in the 1840s. See Stichweh, *Zur Entstehung*, pp. 376–82; Turner, 'Justus Liebig'; *Handbuch über den königlich Preussischer Hof und Staat* (Berlin, 1845), pp. 137–59.

[53] Purkyně, *Opera*, vol. XII, pp. 219, 222, 220, 224, 230 and 231. By way of comparison annual budgets for various institutions at Breslau for 1837–9 were as follows: medical clinic, 2650 thaler; botanical gardens, 2610; anatomical institute, 2398; institute for church music, 873; zoological museum, 868; mineralogical cabinet, 400; chemical laboratory, 372; physical cabinet, 348. Koch (ed.), *Die preußischen Universitäten*, vol. I, p. 307. Recall that Purkyně had requested an annual budget of 840 thaler.

[54] So strongly is Purkyně emphasising the independence of physiology that his rhetoric here hardly corresponds to reality. In 1836, only two German universities (Breslau and Königsberg) had separate chairs for anatomy and physiology. Did Purkyně think Schulze would believe that such an arrangement was 'the most common at present-day universities'? Purkyně, *Opera*, vol. XII, p. 221.

nowhere referred to specific universities or professors; nowhere did he discuss systematically how the particular subject matters of anatomy and physiology might be distinguished (even though his students were mostly writing dissertations in what might have been called microscopic anatomy). Apparently he wanted to justify the institutional separation of anatomy and physiology as modestly as possible. Interestingly, he did not exploit the already existing separation of the *Ordinarien* at Breslau by arguing that since physiology had its own chair it also needed its own institute.

Just as physiology could not be reduced to anatomy, so too could it not be reduced to the physical sciences. In some detail, Purkyně outlined the complex tasks of physiology. 'General physiology' deals with broad concepts of life; 'special physiology' includes physiological morphology, physiological physics, physiological chemistry, physiological dynamics, physiological psychology and physiological anthropology. The last of these deals with 'complete humanity as a total organism'; psychology treats the soul, consciousness and the free will;[55] dynamics considers not only physical agents such as light, heat, electricity, but also 'vital forces' and 'specific energies', drawing analogies with physical forces where possible. Embryology (morphology) requires the 'doctrine of teleology of organic forms'. Clearly, physiology has its own subject matter, expansively ranging from embryology to anthropology, and its own explanatory tools. As such, it has a 'real existence', is an 'autonomous' *Fach* (wrote Purkyně as early as 1831),[56] and thus requires its own institute.

For his final rhetorical justification for an institute, Purkyně turned to status, in both a local and larger sense. On pragmatic grounds, he wrote, it is impossible to expect the physiologist to meet his 'scientific needs' in the already established institutes of anatomy, botany, physics or chemistry. Directors of these institutes are already too busy to accommodate a physiologist, they lack space, costly instruments are difficult to share, etc. But more importantly, it is 'unworthy', even 'barbaric', to expect representatives of 'so important a branch of natural science as physiology' to work in other institutes. Any respectable, independent science deserves its own state-supported institutes at the university. Furthermore, in this 'progressive generation', in the present 'upturn of scientific life in Europe', such institutes have become the 'spirit of true science [*Wissenschaftlichkeit*]'. 'It would be doubly important', Purkyně concluded, 'if

[55] See Josef Brožek and Jiří Hoskovec, *J. E. Purkyně and Psychology* (Prague, 1987).
[56] Purkyně, *Opera*, vol. XII, p. 219.

through Your Excellency's decision the beginning of such a worthy position for physiology could occur in our Prussian state, partly on account of science and its teachers, partly on account of the good example, which like so many others, would spread from here to all sides all the more effectively.'[57]

Significantly, Purkyně in this memorandum did not try to justify a physiological institute on the grounds of its utility for medicine, the state or pedagogy. In his opening sentence, he did note that physiological demonstrations and experiments are important for the education (*Bildung*) of medical students. And he did briefly mention the clientele for the institute: not only the director, but also medical students (how they would be selected was not specified), other faculty and 'amateurs of science' would have hands-on access to the apparatus. Conspicuous by its absence, however, is any mention of the service of physiology to the medical enterprise. In his 1823 Breslau dissertation, Purkyně had introduced the concept of 'physiological praxis', stressing that healing is the 'axis' around which the 'fundamental efforts' of physiology turn.[58] All such rhetoric, however, disappeared from Purkyně's later entreaties to the Cultural Ministry. Chemistry, physics, botany – these were the sciences Purkyně emphasised as the model for the new physiology: the more physiology became like them, the less connected it seemed to medicine.[59] Furthermore, Purkyně specifically urged the state not to support physiology on grounds of utility. He suggested that the state, only recently having moved to support natural science, had acted primarily from two motives. It had first begun to underwrite those 'doctrines' which had 'obvious utility' – medicine, surgery, obstetrics, anatomy, physics, mineralogy and later chemistry. Or it had supported sciences like zoology simply because of the pleasures they offered. Physiology, however, fitted neither of these categories and thus had received minimal state aid. But a 'higher progress' occurred, Purkyně argued, when 'pure science for itself [*reinen Wissenschaft um ihrer selbst willen*]' is supported. States that had elevated themselves beyond utility would always include among their characteristic goals the

[57] Purkyně, *Opera*, vol. XII, pp. 224 and 233–4. [58] Purkyně, *Abhandlung*, pp. 108–9.

[59] In his 1839 request for staff, equipment and a regular budget, Purkyně did mention the value of physiology as the 'soul of medicine'. Every working physician creates from his own experience a 'physiological system', which may be more or less informed by 'objective physiological science', and every physician expects that all progress in medicine will come from progress in anatomy and physiology. Yet it remains the responsibility of the physician to apply the 'pure results of physiology' in medical praxis; physiologists themselves must live only for 'pure science'. Purkyně, *Opera*, vol. XII, pp. 235–6 and 241.

support of 'Wissenschaft um ihrer selbst willen.'[60] In his rhetoric, then, Purkyně called on Prussia to support the new physiology simply for its own sake.

Finally, given Purkyně's well-known interest in Pestalozzian educational reforms, recently emphasised by the late William Coleman, it seems surprising that he did not explicitly discuss pedagogy or the pragmatic Pestalozzian theme of learning through active engagement with the surrounding world.[61] According to Pestalozzi, the keystone of the epistemological process is *Anschauung*, a term used broadly by the reformer to mean both mental operations relevant to forming ideas (sense impression, observation, perception, intuition) and a more active, higher mental process which makes perceptions conscious.[62] In the 1836 document, Purkyně does occasionally refer to the new physiology as based on 'sensory *Anschauungen*', and to the importance of enhancing lectures with models or demonstrations (*Veranschaulichung*) to aid in the formation of an '*Anschauung* and concept [*Begriff*] of life'.[63] The new physiology did progress by seeing rather than by abstract philosophising, and it should be taught by seeing. But Purkyně's rhetoric here does not make this a primary *raison d'être* for an institute.

Further, such references to *Anschauung* were neither bold nor surprising in 1839. From Johann Reil at the turn of the century through some of Schelling's most enthusiastic supporters to Schönlein and the 'natural history' school of medicine, calls had abounded for a medicine or medical education based on *Anschauung*.[64] Likewise, Kenneth Caneva has identified what he aptly calls a 'concretising' tradition in early nineteenth-century physical science, based on

[60] Purkyně, *Opera*, vol. XII, pp. 225 and 231. In an 1829 public lecture, Purkyně had made the same point. Earlier, physiology like all sciences in their early states, was studied 'nur nach irdischen äußerlichen Zwecken. Erst jetzt fängt man an, sie nach reinen innern Gründen zu bearbeiten... Die Phänomenologie in der Physiologie ist rein empirisch; die Deutung ist rationell. Jedoch ist die Forderung der Wissenschaft von der des Lehrvortrags zu scheiden.' *Ibid.*, vol. II, p. 75.

[61] Coleman, 'Prussian pedagogy'. Cf. Erich Witte, 'Beitrag zur Kenntnis der Bildung von Purkinje', *Sudhoffs Archiv*, 35 (1942), pp. 348–56, and Kruta, 'J. E. Purkyně als Physiologe', p. 65, for the influence of Komensky on Purkyně's pedagogical vision.

[62] Borrowing heavily from Leibniz, Kant, Rousseau and others, Pestalozzi never systematically described his epistemological assumptions. See Kate Silber, *Pestalozzi: The Man and his Work* (London, 1960), pp. 138–9; Dieter Jedan, *Johann Heinrich Pestalozzi and the Pestalozzian Method of Language Teaching* (Berne, 1981), pp. 48–52.

[63] Purkyně, *Opera*, vol. XII, pp. 220, 222, 225 and 233. For Purkyně's later discussion of the place of *Anschauung* in microscopy, see his 'Mikroskop. Seine Andwendung und Gebrauch bei physiologischen Untersunchungen' [1844], in *Opera*, vol. III, pp. 119–54.

[64] See, for example, the quotations in Horst-Peter Wolff, 'Die medizinisch-chirurgische Lehranstalt in Magdeburg (1827 bis 1840)', *NTM*, 12 (1975), pp. 77–87, at pp. 78–9; Johanna Bleker, *Die naturhistorische Schule 1825–1845* (Stuttgart, 1981), pp. 22–4.

qualitative experimentation and demands that theories be *anschaulich*.[65] Giving all medical students hands-on experience in laboratories may have been a radical innovation in 1836, as Coleman argues. But Purkyně in his rhetoric for the Cultural Ministry went out of his way to disguise that fact.

The rhetorical strategy employed by Schultz differs sharply from Purkyně's, as did, undoubtedly, their interests. Rather than welcoming the new status of physiology among the natural sciences, Schultz deplored recent trends in his field. Explicitly concerned with pedagogy, Schultz frequently wrote of *Anschauung*. He envisioned a new type of *Bildung* based on organic principles rather than the dead, reductionist philosophy of the Greeks, a philosophy which, he later wrote, leads only to 'communism, aetheism and Judaism'.[66] Indeed, Schultz dreamed of the medical faculty replacing the philosophical faculty as the site in which all students, not just those studying medicine, could acquire the integrated, moral *Bildung* necessary for the survival of life, society and Christianity.

Even though Schultz had been calling for an independent physiological institute for nearly twenty years, his proposal in 1843 was prompted by specific circumstances. In 1842, the Berlin medical faculty had issued yet another suggestion for improving training in 'theoretical medicine' (i.e. anatomy and physiology). Prussia's *Tentamen philosophicum*, created in 1825 specifically to improve the scientific preparation of medical students before they entered the clinics, was not achieving its intended purpose. The examination did not include anatomy or physiology, and for years medical faculties had complained about students rushing to the practical courses and clinics without adequate theoretical backgrounds.[67] The Berlin faculty this time proposed a *Maßregel* (i.e., a rule intended for all Prussian medical faculties) to require students to attend sixteen specific courses before being allowed to take examinations for promotion. Only such restrictions might counter the 'material tendency' and dislike of theory among the students, reasoned the Berlin faculty.[68]

65 Kenneth L. Caneva, 'From galvanism to electrodynamics: the transformation of German physics and its social context', *Historical Studies in the Physical Sciences*, 9 (1978), pp. 63–159, especially at pp. 68–71.

66 Schultz to Cultural Minister Karl Otto von Raumer, 30 July 1852, GStAM, Rep. 76va, Sekt. 1, Tit. VII, Nr 9, Bd V, Bl. 244r–247v, at Bl. 245v.

67 See Wenig, 'Medizinische Ausbildung'.

68 Berlin medical faculty to Cultural Minister Johann Friedrich von Eichhorn, 12 October 1842, GStAM, Rep. 76va, Sekt. 1, Tit. VII, Nr 9, Bd IV, Bl. 53r–64v. By adding the proviso that all required courses must be taught by *Ordinarien* or *Extraordinarien*, the Berlin faculty proposed to eliminate the *Privatdozenten*, a radical suggestion that doomed the plan. For the

In a separate vote, Schultz strongly disagreed with his Berlin colleagues. The problem is not with the students, he argued, but with the faculty. Theoretical subjects are taught with no bridges to medical praxis. Even the natural sciences in the philosophy faculty need a 'medical tendency' to serve medical students. Further, medical theory is taught as a collection of facts, assumptions and hypotheses to be learned by rote from books. Just as 'observation and experiment' permeate clinical instruction, so too must they become the basis of instruction in theoretical medicine. This requires physiological institutes, concluded Schultz, noting their existence already in Breslau and Göttingen.[69] Berlin, however, 'is falling behind'.[70] Several months later, Schultz's seventeen-page memorandum outlining plans for an 'Observatorium for theoretical medicine' reached the Cultural Ministry.

Unlike Purkyně's, Schultz's rhetorical strategy was based squarely on his view of medical education. He attempted to justify his *Observatorium* by appealing to the needs of medicine, not those of physiology. Medicine, Schultz began, urgently requires two types of unities – of teaching and research, and of theory and empiricism. The 'true purpose of [medical] study is the application of science in life'. Since medical science is not a 'closed, finished building' but a 'continuously growing tree', so too must medical instruction change. This can only occur if the professor is also a scientific researcher. The research imperative, Schultz was claiming, belongs in the medical as well as in the philosophical faculty. The professor also must reject a purely empirical medicine and not shy away from medical theory. Every 'reasonable' physician is driven to theory simply by the need to seek reasons for his actions in natural laws. It is essential, therefore, that the medical student receive 'theoretical *Bildung*', based not on the opposition of theory and empiricism, but on their unity.[71]

To unite teaching and research and theory and praxis, Schultz continued, medical faculties must offer 'organic studies of nature',

other Prussian medical faculties' responses to the proposal from their Berlin colleagues, see *ibid.*, Bl. 68v–84r.

69 In Göttingen, Rudolf Wagner had established a physiological institute in 1842, sharing a building with the physics institute. See [Wagner], 'Ueber die Gründung physiologischer Institute und das physiologische Institut zu Göttingen', *Allgemeine Zeitung*, 1842, pp. 2587–9; [Wagner], *Ueber das Verhältniß der Physiologie zu den physikalischen Wissenschaften und zur praktischen Medizin, mit besonderer Rücksicht auf den Zweck und die Bedeutung der physiologischen Institute* (Göttingen, 1842); [Wagner], 'Ueber das physiologische Institut zu Göttingen und die damit in Verbindung stehenden Sammlungen', *Göttingische gelehrte Anzeigen*, 1842, pp. 1977–83.

70 Schultz, 'Separatvotum,' 3 January 1843, GStAM, Rep. 76va, Sekt. 1, Tit. VII, Nr 9, Bd IV, Bl. 65r–67r.

71 Schultz, 'Bericht', Bl. 147r–148v.

taught with proper pedagogical methods. The only way to teach theoretical medicine is through '*Naturanschauungen* and studies of nature', not through 'mere tradition and books'. This has been realized in anatomical, chemical and clinical instruction, but not in physiology, pathology or pharmacology (the three subjects for Schultz's *Observatorium*). Learning via experiment and experience will provide *Anschauungen* or 'living pictures' that are 'just as indelible and complete' as bookish descriptions are 'blurred and incomplete'. Learning by *Anschauungen* is easier, faster, and longer lasting than is memorising from books. *Naturanschauungen* of physiological actions are essential for all of medicine. Medical praxis is based on knowledge of the normal 'inner course of organic actions'; anatomical structures cannot be understood without a view of the development of organs (embryology); to understand deviations in illness, knowledge of the 'inner machinery of physiological processes' such as muscle and nerve action, or movement of the blood, is essential. And most importantly, unsubstantiated prejudice can most easily be combated by sensory *Anschauungen*. 'The path of research is thereby shown to students, and their desire for their own testing will be stimulated. This lays the foundation for further scientific training (*Fortbildung*), through which sensory *Anschauung* itself finally dissolves into rational theory'.[72] Here, then, is a rhetoric filled with Pestalozzian principles.

Such visualising experimentation also indicates for Schultz that reductionist physiology must be rejected. Chemical experiments treat neutral, dead matter which never exhibits the 'fire of organic activity'. Experiments on living bodies, however, always reveal a 'self-activity through the interaction of elements of form', forms which never appear in dead matter (*Stoff*). The exterior matter merely acts as a stimulus to awaken the 'energy of life'. Schultz's rhetoric here becomes animated, as he castigates those who claim life itself is merely a chemical, physical or mechanical process. Rather, these physical sciences deal only with the conditions of life and the material residue of life after death. They cannot explain the 'life principle' or the 'excitation of life [*Lebenserregung*]'. The relations between chemistry and physiology, Schultz concluded, are like those between a carrier of supplies and a field marshal in a war – an analogy guaranteed to catch the attention of a Cultural Minister who only a year later would appoint Eilhard Mitscherlich, a senior member of the Berlin philo-

[72] *Ibid.*, Bl. 151v–152v.

sophical faculty, to teach physiological chemistry in the medical faculty.[73]

In later writings on medical reform and medicine, Schultz became even more stridently anti-reductionist. Drawing upon a comprehensive philosophical dualism of life and death, Schultz developed a physiology of 'rejuvenation' (*Verjüngung*), in which polar organic forces of 'formation' and 'moulting' continually seek to perfect dead matter and make it living. Indeed, the entire cosmos consists of hierarchical levels of perfection, in which the forces of 'organic rejuvenation' constantly drive all of creation towards humanity, the final 'world goal [*Weltzweck*]'.[74] Physiological institutes such as Purkyně's in Prague or Wagner's in Göttingen are actually only chemistry and physics laboratories, and contribute little to physiology. Such institutes, for example, consider nutrition as *Stoffwechsel*, as the simple balance of chemical elements entering and leaving the animal body. For Schultz, however, nutrition is *Formwechsel*, in which 'life stimulus' and 'assimilative forces' transform dead matter into organic forms. Such laws of rejuvenation, Schultz argued, can only be learned through 'truly organic studies of nature' and by 'organic empiricism' in the medical faculty.[75]

Since the laws of rejuvenation govern not only organisms, but also society and all its organisations, medicine must replace philosophy as the path to *Bildung*. The upheavals of 1848, for example, Schultz vaguely attributed to a 'spirit of organism'. Early in 1850, only months after Prussian troops had finally crushed most revolutionary activity across the German states, he praised the 'tendency to organise

[73] *Ibid.*, Bl. 149r–150v and 152r–v; Schultz to von Eichhorn, 15 February 1844, SPK, Darmst. Lb 1830 Schultz-Schultzenstein.

[74] Schultz's rhetoric of dualism, hierarchy and organic *Bildungskraft* sounds not unlike Schelling's earlier *Naturphilosophie*. Yet Schelling's dualistic dynamics drew on forces Schultz considered 'dead', so that Schultz, who frequently criticised all 'theories of world harmony' for neglecting the fundamental split of life and death, undoubtedly considered Schelling a reductionist and a monist. See K. H. Schultz-Schultzenstein, *Der organisirende Geist der Schöpfung* (Berlin, 1851); K. E. Rothschuh, 'Ansteckende Ideen in der Wissenschaftsgeschichte, gezeigt an der Entstehung und Ausbreitung der romantischen Physiologie', *Deutsche medizinische Wochenschrift*, 86 (1961), pp. 396–402; Reinhardt Pester, 'Nachklassische bürgerliche Naturphilosophie und Wissenschaftsentwicklung in der Mitte des 19. Jahrhunderts', *Greifswalder philosophische Hefte*, 3 (1983), pp. 32–48.

[75] Schultz, *Ueber die Verjüngung des menschlichen Lebens und die Mittel und Wege zu ihrer Kultur: Nach physiologischen Untersuchungen in praktischer Anwendung*, 2nd enlarged edn (Berlin, 1850); Schultz to von Raumer, 18 April 1852, GStAM, Rep. 76va, Sekt. 2, Tit. XX, Nr 72, Bl. 27r–v. Among the most extensive experiments conducted by Schultz himself were his attempts to show that blood cells form in the lymph system. He fed rabbits diets of olive oil and water until they died, and then used the microscope to search for traces of blood formation (i.e., oil drops) in the digestive and circulatory systems. See Schultz, *Ueber die Verjüngung*, pp. 116–75.

in our time, overall in life and science, in art and handicrafts, in state and church'. New ideas of personal freedom and self-regulation of corporations, communities and families all reflect this organising principle. What is needed in these times is a 'physiology of the state, of law, of language', and finally of spirit (*Geist*) itself. Concluded Schultz in 1851: 'The formation of an organic unity in natural science through religious and scientific *Bildung* is the chief task of humanity and civilisation in our time.'[76]

For Schultz, then, a new institution for theoretical medicine would serve far greater purposes than simply meeting the needs of physiology. By making physiology *anschaulich*, the *Observatorium* would become the centre of medical education. And by teaching the 'true organising principles' for society, it would also become the centre of *Bildung* in the university. Schultz's rhetorical strategy was much more expansive and aggressive than the cautious tack taken several years earlier by Purkyně.

Budge presented the most moderate rhetoric and the shortest (only ten pages) of the three proposals. He too began by noting that for some time he had considered founding a new institute. His justification for taking the step in 1846, however, was narrowly focused and almost exclusively pedagogical – teaching medical students the 'art of observation'. The most difficult task for young students, argued Budge, is learning to observe at the sick-bed. There the cases shown to students are isolated, and physiological processes are highly disturbed by illness. Likewise, at smaller universities like Bonn, students in the anatomical institutes rarely have time to use microscopes or learn the 'most commonplace' chemical analyses. Budge's criticism of current teaching practices within Bonn's anatomical institute could not have been more direct; it might have been overly harsh.[77]

[76] *Ibid.*, pp. iii and 529–32; Schultz-Schultzenstein, *Der organisirende Geist*, p. 54; cf. K. H. Schultz-Schultzenstein, 'Schriften über Medizinalreform', *Jahrbücher für wissenschaftliche Kritik*, December 1845, cols. 873–960; K. H. Schultz-Schultzenstein, *Das organische Observatorium an der königlichen Universität zu Berlin: Erster Jahresbericht, welcher die leitende Idee des Observatoriums enthält* (Berlin, 1852).

[77] Even though the Bonn anatomist, Mayer, had in the 1830s offered 'microscopical exercises in physiology' and 'microscopical anatomy', it is unclear how well equipped his institute was for widespread instruction in the hands-on use of microscopes. In 1842, for example, Mayer received a special grant of 200 thaler from the Cultural Ministry to purchase an unspecified number of Schiek microscopes; his annual reports and budgets for 1840–5 (1500 thaler per year, with 400 going for salaries, and about 200 for cadavers, 200 for 'preparations for the museum', and 100 for 'utensils') do list regular expenditures for microscopic preparations. Funds for chemical exercises, however, were either small or nonexistent in these budgets. GStAM, Rep. 76va, Sekt. 3, Tit. x, Nr 14, Bd v, Bl. 3–110; Rep. 76va, Sekt. 3, Tit. xv, Nr 15, Bd II, Bl. 127r–163v. I would guess that 200 thaler in 1842 might have provided from five to eight Schieck microscopes.

To emphasise further the importance of skills in microscopy and chemical analysis, Budge noted how medical praxis and instruction had changed. Clinical professors, he wrote, now spend days studying pathological tissue, and employ assistants in their institutes or clinics to conduct chemical or microscopic investigations. This has greatly benefited medical science, argued Budge, citing Schönlein's clinic at the Charité (in 1842, the latter had brought the recently qualified (habilitated) chemist, Johann Franz Simon, into his clinic) and the upswing of pathological anatomy at the Austrian universities. Students must enter these practical clinics already possessing the basic skills of chemistry and microscopy, and only a physiological institute in an 'intermediate station' can offer such training at the correct point in the process of medical education.[78] Like Purkyně and in contrast to Schultz, Budge sought to support recent changes in the practice of physiology as a medical science with the creation of a new institute.

The rhetoric of the institute-builders thus reflects three broadly different justifications for their proposals: *Wissenschaft um sich selber willen*, organic *Wissenschaft* as the basis of *Bildung*, and praxis as essential in medical training. Parallel to these rationales are the three types of clientele emphasised by the proposals: future physiologists, future citizens and future physicians. How idiosyncratic, however, were Purkyně, Schultz and Budge in calling for physiological institutes? Did their faculty colleagues share their views? And what interests did officials in the Cultural Ministry hold on the matter?

In 1843, obviously intrigued by Schultz's proposal for an *Observatorium*, the new Cultural Minister, Johann Friedrich von Eichhorn and Johannes Schulze, longtime official in that ministry, requested all Prussian medical faculties to evaluate its probable success at their universities, and to suggest modifications which might enable the plan to better achieve its goals. These evaluations, from all the faculties except Berlin, provide some access to the medical faculties' perceptions of the institutional needs for physiology. And of course they also reveal rhetorical strategies deployed by the faculties as they sought to provide for the future of the medical disciplines.[79]

The faculties at Königsberg, Breslau and Greifswald supported Schultz's idea in general even as they fiddled with specific details of the institution to be created. Greifswald enthusiastically called for 'physiological experimental institutes' to be built at every university,

[78] Budge, 'Entwurf zu Statuten', Bl. 9r–11v.

[79] GStAM, Rep. 76va, Sekt. 1, Tit. VII, Nr 9, Bd IV, Bl. 176r–179r (Halle), 274r–285r (Breslau), 291r–294r (Königsberg), 301r–311v (Bonn), 312r–319v (Greifswald).

and asked to be allowed to submit their own detailed plan. Königsberg found the name *Observatorium* misleading (it sounds like a clinic) and the proposed tripartite division too extensive. They proposed instead a set of statutes for a simple 'physiological institute', to be erected in the anatomy building, in which students could conduct independent research. Breslau noted the parallels between Schultz's plan and their own institute (Purkyně's), and suggested enlarging Schultz's *Observatorium* so that all medical students could use it.

These three faculties agreed that medical education, on practical grounds, should be intuitive, experiential and *anschaulich* rather than merely descriptive and discursive. Only then could the gap between medical theory and praxis be bridged. They agreed that as an experimental science (*Erfahrungswissenschaft*), physiology deserved its own institute, just as chemistry, physics and anatomy had theirs. They agreed that it had become impossible to deliver physiological lectures without concomitant experiments and demonstrations. And they argued that since much physiological knowledge was being produced via experiment, the subject also should be taught by experiment. If, therefore, the 'spirit of observation [*Beobachtungsgeist*]' had become the foundation of medical theory and praxis, then physiology must be taught so as to stimulate that spirit among the future physicians. For these 'pro' faculties, the rhetorical rationale for institutional expansion rested primarily on pedagogy. Institutes would support physiological lectures and would offer students hands-on experience in experimentation and observation.

Interestingly, the 'pro' faculties did not comment especially on physiological methods, or on Schultz's strident anti-reductionism. Greifswald did note the need to 'translate' Schultz's views from the 'pictures and especially the similes taken from the plant kingdom, which he fancies' to the 'sober language of science'.[80] But these faculties apparently realised that squabbling with their colleague Schultz over the goal of physiology would not help persuade the Cultural Ministry to create new institutes.[81] Much more suited to that task, apparently, was rhetoric about medical education.

The medical faculties in Bonn and Halle thought Schultz's *Observatorium* would not justify the cost. Halle claimed such an institution would be redundant at their university. They reported that their anatomist (Eduard d'Alton), with three microscopes, already

[80] *Ibid.*, Greifswald, Bl. 312v–313r.

[81] The Bonn faculty did criticise Schultz's attack on physiological chemistry, noting the valuable results achieved by Mulder, Dumas and Liebig. *Ibid.*, Bonn, Bl. 301r–v.

taught experimental physiology; experimental pathology was conducted in the clinics; and pharmacology also was being taught adequately, although a pharmacological collection was needed. The elderly Bonn faculty were more categorical in their criticisms. Future physicians, they argued, need to learn how to observe, but not how to experiment, and ample opportunities for the former already exist in the clinics. Like blind empiricism, many experiments are aimless and seldom lead to satisfactory or useful knowledge. Further, they observed, the Bonn faculty since 1818 had managed to publish a good deal of experimental and observational research without the services of a special institute (a correct claim!).[82] According to the Halle faculty, students were too busy for courses in independent experimentation; they also lacked talent and interest in such work. Even in Berlin, with its large number of students and well-known Johannes Müller, very few students chose to work independently under him.[83] The Halle and Bonn faculties, then, directly denied what their colleagues in Greifswald, Königsberg and Breslau had most praised – the pedagogical necessity of physiological institutes.

These medical faculties showed some knowledge of physiological institutes already existing in 1843. Rudolf Wagner's institute in Göttingen, established only a year earlier, was mentioned by all five faculties. Purkyně's institute in Breslau was noted four times, as was the institute in Jena. Other 'institutes' in Rostock, Tübingen, Giessen and Paris (Magendie) drew comment.[84] Yet significantly, none of the medical faculties tried to prod the Cultural Ministry to action by comparing Prussian and non-Prussian attempts at institutionalisation. Intra-state competition, at least in this case, did not appear to the faculties as an important rhetorical tool to be deployed against the Cultural Ministry.

The medical section of the Cultural Ministry (a group of advisors including Schönlein and several other Berlin professors) also offered its opinion, at the request of Schulze, of the idea of establishing physiological *Observatorien* at all Prussian universities. Like the 1842

[82] For internal discussions among the Bonn faculty concerning the preparation of their report, see Bonn Universitätsarchiv, MF2005.

[83] Students rarely 'chose' to enter Müller's 'physiological laboratory'; rather, he selected those 'talents' he thought worthy of special attention.

[84] K. A. S. Schultze, who wrote the report for the Greifswald faculty, also stressed his own priority: '1821 wurde an der Universität Freiburg das erste deutsche Institut für physiologische Experimente und mikroskopische Untersuchungen von dem mit unterzeichneten Hofrath Schultze gegründet, und die dazu erforderlichen Localitäten und Fonds zum Theil von der Grossherzoglich Badischen Regierung bewilligt.' GStAM, Rep. 76va, Sekt. 1, Tit. VII, Nr 9, Bd IV, Bl. 314v–315r.

Berlin faculty suggestion for a *Maßregel*, which had prompted Schultz to make his proposal in the first place, the medical section blamed inadequate theoretical preparation on the 'material taste' of the medical students themselves. This deficiency would only be exacerbated by the 'pure empiricism' of Schultz's *Observatorium*. The problem with students was not that they could not see, but that they preferred to see rather than to think. Theory and praxis in medical education were already closely united, claimed the medical section, citing as examples the existence of botanical gardens, clinics and anatomical institutes. Physiological lectures already were everywhere accompanied by experiments. No new physiological institutes were needed, although the medical section allowed that requests from individual physiologists should at least be considered.[85] The medical section, that is, preferred a policy of 'bottom up' rather than 'top down' university reform.

And what of the rhetoric and interests within the Cultural Ministry? Can an emergent 'science policy' be identified in its responses to the three requests for physiological institutes, or in the ministry's justifications for its responses? Johannes Schulze, in verbal consultation with his ministerial advisers, made the final decisions on the requested institutes.[86] In 1837, he requested and received 3800 thaler from general state funds to renovate a building for Purkyně's institute, 700 thaler for initial equipment, and by 1844 agreed to an annual budget of 750 thaler for the same.[87] In requesting the construction funds from the Prussian king, Schulze chose to follow the same rhetorical strategy as had Purkyně in making his 1836 request. Indeed, large sections of Schulze's official justification, which went out under Altenstein's name, were taken verbatim from Purkyně's own prose.

'Physiology, longer than the other branches of natural science, has

[85] Medicinal-Abtheilung, 'Votum', 20 August 1844, GStAM, Rep. 76va, Sekt. 1, Tit. VII, Nr 9, Bd IV, Bl. 328r–333v.

[86] First drafts of all the crucial documents are in Schulze's hand; his direct control of university affairs during the 1830s and 1840s is well known. See Conrad Varrentrapp, *Johannes Schulze und das höhere preussische Unterrichtswesen in seiner Zeit* (Leipzig, 1889).

[87] A shed near the entrance to the anatomical institute was converted to Purkyně's first institute. Kruta, 'Purkyně's account'; King Friedrich Wilhelm III to Altenstein, 20 February 1838, 18 March 1840, GStAM, Rep. 76va, Sekt. 4, Tit. X, Nr 47, Bd I, Bl. 72r and 111r. The original budget approved by the king of only 300 thaler was too small to permit Purkyně to hire a regular assistant. Not until 1843 did he manage to increase the annual budget to 750 thaler. See Purkyně, 'Organischer Bericht über das physiologische Institut der Universität Breslau', 30 December 1844, in *Opera*, vol. XII, pp. 265–96, at pp. 278–80. By way of comparison, note that Schulze provided the Breslau anatomist, Otto, a total of 3500 thaler between 1837 and 1841 to publish a lavishly illustrated, multi-volume work on pathological anatomy, entitled *Museum anatomico-pathologicum vratislaviense*. GStAM, Rep. 76va, Litt. O, Nr 5, Bl. 104v–105v, 154r and 177r.

had the fate of being underestimated and ignored in its essence, even though for science itself and for practical life it is of the greatest importance.' So began Schulze's memorandum, developing as the first rationale for creating a physiological institute the recent changes in that science. He did not elaborate the contributions of physiology to the 'practical life'. Instead, Schulze described in considerable detail how physiology had advanced from submersion under anatomy, to the 'fog of *Naturphilosophie*', and now finally to the light of experience and experiments. One cannot, he assessed, conduct physiological experiments in physics or chemistry laboratories (note that by 1840, each Prussian university except Berlin had both physical cabinets or laboratories and chemical laboratories or institutes). Thus physiology needed its own space, preparations and apparatus. Going beyond Purkyně's own rhetoric, Schulze effusively praised the Breslau physiologist's research and his European reputation. He noted that already one of Purkyně's students, Valentin, had been called as physiologist to Berne. Thus, to support Purkyně's valuable researches, 'which are just as important for the advance of science as for the training [*Ausbildung*] of young physicians', a new physiological institute should be created.[88] This last phrase is the only mention throughout the memorandum of the pedagogical value of the institute. Like Purkyně, Schulze justified his support of the new venture primarily by the benefits it would bring to *Wissenschaft um sich selber willen*.

After the negative verdict from his medical section, Schulze at first refused to move on Schultz's request for an *Observatorium*, and completely abandoned any attempt to create such institutions at Prussian universities. Schultz, however, kept reiterating his request and narrowed the scope of his proposed *Observatorium* to a room in the main university building with a closet in which to store microscopes. Finally, in 1848, Schulze awarded Schultz 300 thaler to purchase several microscopes, but the political upheavals of that year delayed final approval of the funds until 1850.[89] Unlike the case of

[88] Schulze, 'Pro memoria', 9 October 1837, GStAM, Rep. 76va, Sekt. 4, Tit. x, Nr 47, Bd I, Bl. 65r–66r.

[89] See various letters between Schultz and the Cultural Ministry in GStAM, Rep. 76va, Sekt. 1, Tit. VII, Nr 9, Bd IV, Bl. 369r–370r; Bd V, Bl. 26r–70r; Rep. 76va, Sekt. 2, Tit. x, Nr 72, Bl. 1r–26r. In du Bois-Reymond's not unbiased opinion, Schulze finally gave Schultz the funds to spite Müller, who recently had refused to support Schulze's adopted son as a candidate for a faculty position in Berlin. See du Bois Reymond to Helmholtz, 18 March 1851, in Christa Kirsten (ed.), *Dokumente einer Freundschaft: Briefwechsel zwischen Hermann von Helmholtz und Emil du Bois-Reymond, 1846–1894* (Berlin, 1986), pp. 107–8; Lenz, *Universität Berlin*, vol. II, part II, pp. 161–5.

Purkyně, Schulze apparently wrote no official justification of his decision to fund what Schultz was still calling an *Observatorium*. That was perhaps just as well, for Schultz's new institution soon provoked the wrath of Johannes Müller, and by 1855 had all but disappeared after further funding from the ministry had ceased.[90]

In Bonn, unlike Breslau or Berlin, the medical faculty were given the opportunity to comment on Budge's request for the seminar. Finding the faculty deeply split, primarily because of questions over Budge's ability to direct such a venture, the Bonn university curator recommended that a leading physiologist be called as an *Ordinarius* before any state-owned institute be established. In the meantime, he suggested supporting Budge's physiological exercises as a private institute with small, extraordinary grants.[91] Schulze in Berlin agreed, and provided Budge with 50–100 thaler per year until Budge left Bonn in 1856, after Helmholtz's popularity had siphoned off most of his students. In explaining his decision, Schulze reiterated an interest which he also had exhibited when funding Purkyně's institute:

> For all good institutions what is most important is the right men; where a recognised, useful effort [i.e., person] appears, it is best not to set any insurmountable difficulties in his path. Concerning the qualifications of Budge, contested among the faculty members, only the practical attempt itself can decide. If he is worthy, the small beginning of a private institute could become a state institute; if not, the former will not long burden the university building.[92]

[90] Schultz purchased three microscopes with his 300 thaler, and operated the *Observatorium* in 1851–2, listing as 'participants', in his first annual report, all the auditors in his classes ('Medicinische Botanik und Pflanzen-Physiologie', 'Physiologie des Menschen durch Beobachtungen und Experimente erläutert', 'Encyclopädie und Methodologie der Medicin', 'Allgemeine Pathologie und Therapie nebst deren Entwicklungsgeschichte durch Beobachtungen erläutert'; note that in the winter semester, 1851–2, Schultz also announced a class on 'Arzneimittellehre durch Experimente erläutert', which, after only two students expressed interest, he did not give). When the Cultural Ministry asked the Berlin medical faculty for an evaluation of Schultz's first annual report, they exploded in disgust. Claiming (correctly) never to have been officially informed about the *Observatorium*, noting that Berlin's anatomical institute had for some time had a 'physiological laboratory', and that Müller in that laboratory had produced many of Europe's leading physiologists, the faculty, led by Müller, angrily refused to take a position on something concerning which they until then had been placed in a completely passive position. To compete with Schultz, Müller decided that henceforth he and *Privatdocent* du Bois-Reymond would offer 'physiological exercises', not merely to the most talented students they selected (as they had done for the first time in the summer semester, 1851) but to any student who would pay the fees. Schultz received no further funding for his *Observatorium*. In 1853, two of his microscopes were stolen; by 1855 he was cancelling lectures 'because the *Observatorium* is still incomplete'. GStAM, Rep. 76va, Sekt. 2, Tit. X, Nr 72, Bl. 27r–81v; Rep. 76va, Sekt. 2, Tit. VII, Nr 18, Bde I–III, *passim*; Schultz-Schultzenstein, *Das organische Observatorium*.

[91] See GStAM, Rep. 76va, Sekt. 3, Tit. X, Nr 58, Bd I, *passim*; Bonn Universitätsarchiv, MF2006.

[92] Schulze to curator Bethmann-Hollweg, 26 October 1846, GStAM, Rep. 76va, Sekt. 3, Tit. X, Nr 58, Bd I, Bl. 15r–16v.

A month later, in approving the initial 200 thaler for Budge, Schulze noted his desire to create a physiological institute in Bonn as soon as the personnel could be arranged. 'These [physiological] institutes, after their origin several years ago, have exerted a noticeable and decisively agreeable influence on the desired improvement of medical study at the given universities, and through the outstanding performances, which could not be achieved by any other ways, have placed their indispensability beyond doubt.'[93]

Hence by 1846, Johannes Schulze appeared convinced of the 'indispensability' of physiological institutes. By 1850 he had acted to realise, at least in part, each of the three proposals for erecting such institutes. Schulze's rhetoric, however, shows him more interested in supporting capable scholars than in defending a particular experimental approach to physiology or in marshalling the services of medicine to serve the state. That is, the rhetoric of personal patronage fills Schulze's memoranda. For over twenty-five years, he had been operating Prussia's universities on this principle, a policy that Altenstein had described long before in his famous reform essay of 1807. In discussing how the state should support the arts and sciences, Altenstein had written:

> It is most important to support great, powerful men for every science and art. A small number of these will alone be considerably more effective than a collection of mediocrity... Very much depends on how these men are used. If they are well chosen, they make in any case the best use of their forces, and it is merely necessary that they be given the opportunity to act [*einwirken*].[94]

During the *Vormärz*, Altenstein's Cultural Ministry frequently had been guided by such a policy.[95] In making decisions about experimental physiology in the 1840s, Johannes Schulze did not significantly alter this long-established *modus operandi*. Or at least his *modus orandi*, as revealed in the ministry documents, remained unchanged.

Conclusions

Thus ended the first wave of institute-building for physiology at the Prussian universities. One small building was renovated in Breslau, and several microscopes and miscellaneous other apparatus were purchased for Bonn and Berlin. The significance of this first wave,

[93] Schulze to Bethmann-Hollweg, 21 November 1846, GStAM, Rep. 76va, Sekt. 3, Tit. x, Nr 58, Bd I, Bl. 22r–23r.

[94] Karl Freiherr von Stein zum Altenstein, 'Denkschrift vom 11. September 1807' in Georg Winter (ed.), *Die Reorganization des preußischen Staates unter Stein und Hardenberg*, 2 vols. (Leipzig, 1931–8), vol. I, part I, pp. 364–566, at p. 457.

[95] For many revealing examples of such a policy at work, see Biermann (ed.), *Humboldt*.

however, is greater than these meagre material moves would indicate. The fate of the three proposals, made between 1836 and 1846, sheds light on several significant features of the discipline of physiology, its institutionalisation and Prussian state attitudes towards universities and experimental science. First, the complexity of the proposals – calling for functionally differentiated institutes supporting large lectures, hands-on practical exercises for all students and original research for a select few – indicates that the conception of what would become the modern university institute had emerged long before 1869 when the institutional revolution in physiology began with the dedication of Ludwig's institute. Second, the concept of physiology as an independent subject (*Fach*) was never in question, even though institutionally, physiology still was very much part of anatomy at most Prussian universities. Further, the proposals illustrate complex and integrated approaches to physiology, combining physical, chemical and anatomical/microscopical methods. The institute idea was not the exclusive preserve of advocates of a single approach to physiology. Third, these proposals for a unified physiology derived from quite diverse interests, ranging from anti-reductionist concepts of *Bildung* to *Wissenschaft um sich selber willen* to the transmission of practical skills for medical students. Fourth, judging from the medical faculties' mostly positive responses to the idea of institutes, it seems clear that the need to conduct physiological research by observation and experiment was widely recognised by 1843, and that many Prussian anatomist-physiologists already by the 1840s enhanced their lectures with experiments or visual materials. Fifth, the tentative creation of the three institutes reflected many personal and local features at each university. The only 'science policy' advocated by the Cultural Ministry was to reward 'talent' wherever it appeared among faculty members. No general plan to reform physiology emerged from the Cultural Ministry. Despite Schulze's praise in 1846 of the indispensability of physiological institutes, no more such institutes would be founded at Prussian universities for the next decade. And when du Bois-Reymond finally opened his new institute in Berlin in 1877, Prussia stood far behind other states in the institutionalisation of physiology.[96] It also took Prussia until 1872 to create independent physiological chairs for all its medical faculties. By that time, every other German-speaking university except Giessen had already separated the anatomy and physiology chairs.

[96] See Axel Genz, 'Die Emancipation der naturwissenschaftlichen Physiologie in Berlin', Diplomarbeit (Institute für Geschichte der Medizin, Magdeburg, 1976).

What about the particular timing of the first wave of institute-building? Note first that competitive market mechanisms apparently did not play any significant roles in the founding of these institutes. Unlike the pattern which would become frequent later in the century, in which a candidate would accept a call to a university only if the state would build him a new institute, none of the proposals here were linked to conditions of employment. Purkyně and Schultz had been *Ordinarien* for years before submitting their proposals. Budge's success with his physiological exercises undoubtedly helped him advance to *Extraordinarius* in 1848 and *Ordinarius* in 1855, but he never used employment as a lever to seek concessions for his institute. And none of the three institute-builders ever explicitly tied their requests to comments about institutional conditions outside Prussia.

More important for explaining the timing of the proposals, I think, was the dissatisfaction of Purkyně, Schultz and Budge with various conditions at their respective universities. All three, for complex reasons, had only limited access to the funds, space and equipment of the anatomical institutes, and personally were marginal within their medical faculties. These problems, as much as any larger plans for the development of physiology as a discipline, drove them to seek institutional space for themselves by appealing directly to Berlin. In addition, it cannot be ignored that not until 1840 had instrument manufacturers begun to produce inexpensive, high-quality microscopes.[97] Although each of the institute-builders advocated a unified approach to physiology, in practice all three stressed microscopy. These factors, plus a clear conception of physiology as an independent *Fach*, if not a discipline, helped motivate the first wave of institute-building.

Finally, what about the rhetorical strategies employed by the first wave of institute-builders? No single pattern marks the three proposals submitted by Purkyně, Schultz and Budge. Since so few specialised institutes yet existed for the medical faculties, obviously no standard ritual had emerged for requesting such support from the Cultural Ministry. Each institute-builder thus had to rely on his past experience of negotiations with Johannes Schulze and other officials in the ministry, and indeed the rhetoric of the proposals often exudes a personal tone. Likewise, no single pattern marks the responses of Schulze, who apparently could be moved by appeals to scientific

[97] Rudolf Wagner, 'Anhang zu dem vorhergehenden Artikel "Mikroskop"' in R. Wagner (ed.), *Handwörterbuch der Physiologie mit Rücksicht auf physiologische Pathologie*, 4 vols. in 5 (Brunswick, 1842–53), vol. II, pp. 441–8.

productivity, to the need for improving medical training, or to *Bildung* as the basis of the university. Schulze, who himself had been trained as a classical philologist in Friedrich August Wolf's seminar in Halle, and who, upon entering the Cultural Ministry began to attend Hegel's lectures in the early 1820s to prepare himself for dealing with the universities,[98] certainly left no traces of interest in modernising the state in his ministerial documents; neither did any of his ministerial colleagues during the *Vormärz* period under consideration. Everyone, except some of the elderly professors in Bonn, seemed to agree that experimentation in research and in pedagogy would be the future path for physiology. But no one tried to talk about experimentation as a means to train citizens for the modern state and its economic needs. In other words, the 'modernisation theory' receives little support from this case study of early Prussian physiology.

The 'competitive market' theory finds scarcely more corroboration here. The ministry was impressed by Purkyně's European reputation; declining student enrolments did worry faculty and Berlin officials alike. But funds always were scarce, and the whims of influential advisers like Rudolphi or Müller had to be satisfied. University laboratories, at least for medical science, did not emerge in this early period as important pawns in struggles between Prussia and other states for supremacy in medical education, or as bargaining chips for universities seeking to lure leading scholars to join their faculties. Instead, the early institutes were created by marginal, albeit entrepreneurial faculty able to realise neither their research nor their careerist goals in existing university institutes. By appealing directly to the Cultural Ministry in founding new institutes, these entrepreneurs were able to bypass local and collegial constraints and to achieve if not parity at least increased prestige, funding and pedagogical power for themselves and for their emerging discipline of experimental physiology. Such a strategy would remain important for the later entrepreneurs who after 1860 would play for considerably higher stakes in making the institutional revolutions within the natural sciences at German universities.

[98] Varrentrapp, *Johannes Schulze*, pp. 28–33 and 432–4.

3

The fall and rise of professional mystery

Epistemology, authority and the emergence of laboratory medicine in nineteenth-century America

JOHN HARLEY WARNER

Two parallel and not necessarily incompatible stories have dominated the historiography of the laboratory's rise to prominence in nineteenth-century American medicine. One has to do with the emergence of the laboratory as a leading source of knowledge in western medicine. The task for Americanists in elaborating this story primarily has been to relate a narrative widely known (or assumed to be known) on the broad scale of western culture to the course of change in the United States. This has involved tracing how European ideas, methods and instruments were transplanted to American soil, and how laboratory medicine took shape and acquired sometimes different meanings in the peculiar American environment. Such accounts often centre on the Americans who travelled for study to Europe, especially Germany; the intellectual excitement the experience produced in them and the allegiances to European medical ways they formed; and how they tried to put these commitments into practice after their return. The explanatory problems typically addressed include accounting for sources of resistance to the emergence of laboratory medicine in America; the introduction of an ideal of laboratory science into medical education; the sometimes different meanings ascribed to the laboratory and its methods in the American context; and, above all, why America so often seemed to lag behind Europe.[1]

The other story has to do with how, during the final decades of the nineteenth century, science – either explicitly, or as often only tacitly, that of the laboratory – gave American physicians a powerful and new source of authority. More often than not, the telling of this story

[1] The best of such studies published recently include W. Bruce Fye, *The Development of American Physiology: Scientific Medicine in the Nineteenth Century* (Baltimore, 1987); Gerald L. Geison (ed.), *Physiology in the American Context, 1850–1940* (Bethesda, Md, 1987); and Kenneth M. Ludmerer, *Learning to Heal: The Development of American Medical Education* (New York, 1985).

includes relatively little about the ideas, methods or physical artifacts of the laboratory, about how they got to America, or about how they were used once they had made the journey. The focus, instead, tends to be the ideal of science for which the laboratory came to stand. The social and economic degradation of the medical profession during much of the nineteenth century ordinarily is accepted as background, while the analysis centres on how from the final decades of the century onwards the idea of laboratory science served as a tool in professional uplift. The explanatory problem most commonly addressed here is how the rise of laboratory science in American medical culture served as a platform for elevating the power and prestige of the profession in American society.[2]

In telling these stories, historians have produced some quite sophisticated work. Much of it, though, has been distinctly marked by two problems. To begin with, the two stories have remained more separate than integrated. The rise of the laboratory as a way of knowing, a source of knowledge and a forum for intellectual endeavour in western medicine on the one hand, and the rise of the laboratory as a vehicle for fulfilling the cultural and economic aspirations of the American physicians on the other, have remained to a striking extent subjects of separate narratives. At the same time, each story has had a marked tendency to fall prey to presentism. Not only older positivist accounts that sought to trace progress but also recent work informed by the new social history have tended to have a strong teleological odour about them. Too often, accounts have been written as if the elevation of laboratory medicine in America to European standards in the one case, or the elevation of the American medical profession to its twentieth-century status in the other, are the self-evident ends to which historical narratives should lead. In looking at the place of the laboratory in American medicine, that is, some have tended to write with an eye to where American medicine in the late nineteenth century was going more than to where it had been.

This chapter seeks to show how changes in western medical science

[2] The most thoughtful studies that focus on the use of an ideal of science in professional uplift are Gerald L. Geison, 'Divided we stand: physiologists and clinicians in the American context', in Morris J. Vogel and Charles E. Rosenberg (eds), *The Therapeutic Revolution: Essays in the Social History of American Medicine* (Philadelphia, 1979), pp. 67–90, and S. E. D. Shortt, 'Physicians, science, and status: issues in the professionalization of Anglo-American medicine in the nineteenth-century', *Medical History*, 27 (1983), pp. 51–68. And see Howard S. Berliner, *A System of Scientific Medicine: Philanthropic Foundations in the Flexner Era* (New York, 1985); E. Richard Brown, *Rockefeller Medical Men: Medicine and Capitalism in America* (Berkeley, 1979); and Robert E. Kohler, *From Medical Chemistry to Biochemistry: The Making of a Biomedical Discipline* (Cambridge, 1982).

and changes in American culture interacted in shaping the options that physicians believed were open to them, and, only in the final decades of the century, made it possible for some American physicians to claim authority on the basis of an elitist epistemology that granted privileged access to knowledge. The relationship between epistemology and authority, I want to suggest, was critical in shaping the ascendancy of the laboratory in American medicine and the meanings of that process to American physicians. Equally though, this relationship was central to the culture of American physicians long before the laboratory loomed very large at all in their professional world. Rather than start my account with the period when the laboratory started to appear prominent, I will examine the shifting course of the relationship between epistemology and authority from the early decades of the nineteenth century. This is in part an attempt to avoid some of the problems of seeing the laboratory in twentieth-century medicine, and the medical profession in twentieth-century American society, as the endpoints for a narrative written looking backwards. At the same time, it is an effort to move away from the tendency to see the emergence of laboratory medicine as the emergence of scientific medicine, for in the appraisal of physicians throughout the first two-thirds of the nineteenth century, after all, their medicine already was scientific. I will argue that while medical epistemology in America broadly followed European trends, the timing and meaning of change in the United States had as much to do with the role assigned to special knowledge in conferring authority in American culture as it did with changes in available medical knowledge and method, including the laboratory and the distinctive ways of knowing it represented.

Starting in the 1820s and continuing until the outbreak of the Civil War, the medical profession in America came under aggressive popular attack. The challenge grew in part out of the earlier republican critique of professional aristocracy that had its roots in the American Enlightenment, expressed in the programme of Thomas Jefferson and Benjamin Rush for the simplification and dissemination of medical knowledge. But criticism of the professions, including medicine, came to be infused with a new political urgency and power. The rising democratic impulse in American politics was evident in the ascendancy of the Jacksonians, and in their levelling campaign against monopoly, special privilege and chartered corporations. Characterised by a romantic longing for the values of an earlier, simpler American way of life, the Jacksonians targeted privileged groups, aristocracy, paper money and monopolies as signs of the growing corruption of society. The scepticism of claims to special knowledge and authority conferred by formal education that Alexis de Tocqueville described so clearly when he visited the United States in 1831 informed a growing popular indictment of what one sectarian healer typically denounced as 'King-craft, Priest-craft, Lawyer-craft, and Doctor-craft'.[3]

The assault upon the medical profession was expressed most forcefully in the campaign against professional monopoly, in which adherents of the botanical medical sect Thomsonianism formed a vocal and influential lobby. 'The medical monopoly deserves to be abolished', demanded one botanic practitioner in 1841. 'The law which deprives one class of men of their rights and gives special privileges to another, is not just. It violates the first principles of democracy.'[4] Echoing the theme of liberation that pervaded the rhetoric of Democratic politicians, sectarian medical reformers called for emancipation of the American people from their oppression by established medicine. 'There is not a greater aristocratic monopoly in existence, than this of regular medicine – neither is there a greater humbug', one reformer charged. 'False and dangerous must be that science which exists – not from any truth or utility in itself, but from legislative enactments, cunning, and deception, which strictly speaking *enslave the people* to it and its votaries.'[5]

[3] The phrase comes from Wooster Beach, founder of the botanical medical sect Eclecticism, and appears in his journal *The Telescope*, which was devoted to radical religious and political causes; quoted in Joseph F. Kett, *The Formation of the American Medical Profession: The Role of Institutions, 1780–1860* (New Haven, 1968), p. 105. On attitudes towards knowledge and authority in antebellum America, see Lee Benson, *The Concept of Jacksonian Democracy: New York as a Test Case* (Princeton, 1961); Daniel H. Calhoun, *Professional Lives in America: Structure and Aspiration, 1750–1850* (Cambridge, Mass., 1965); Karen Halttunen, *Confidence Men and Painted Women: A Study of Middle-Class Culture in America, 1830–1870* (New Haven, 1982); Lawrence Frederick Kohl, *The Politics of Individualism: Parties and the American Character* (New York, 1989); Edward Pessen, *Jacksonian America: Society, Personality, and Politics* (Homewood, Ill., 1969); Edwin C. Rozwenc, *The Meaning of Jacksonian Democracy* (Lexington, Mass., 1963); Arthur M. Schlesinger, Jr., *The Age of Jackson* (Boston, 1945); and George R. Taylor, *The Transportation Revolution, 1851–1860* (New York, 1951).

[4] 'Medical monopoly', *Botanico-Medical Recorder*, 9 (1841), p. 309. And see 'Memorial of the American Eclectic Medical Convention', *Eclectic Medical Journal*, 2 (1849), pp. 50–61; 'The monster threatened', *Boston Thomsonian Manual and Lady's Companion*, 5 (1838–9), p. 153; 'Address', *Western Medical Reformer*, 4 (1844), pp. 1–2; and 'The two systems', *Water Cure Journal, and Herald of Reforms*, 17 (1854), pp. 98–9.

[5] John King, 'The progress of medical reform', *Western Medical Reformer*, 6 (1846), pp. 79–82 at pp. 80–1.

What has been too little emphasised in the historical reading of the rhetoric of the Thomsonians[6] and of like-minded radical critics who followed such medical sects as hydropathy,[7] is the extent to which it was based upon a caricature of the regular medical profession. Far from enjoying a monopoly, *de facto* or *de jure*, regular physicians functioned within a medical market-place that was remarkably open. In representing the profession as a bastion of monopoly in American society, critics were constructing a straw villain they could easily attack using prevalent polemical conventions rather than depicting social reality. Their assault on medical monopoly is best regarded as a symbolic crusade. It was an outlet for anti-authoritarian sentiment, certainly; but the authority being assailed was not so much that derived from a legal monopoly as from claims to the exclusive possession of special knowledge. Underlying the crusade against monopoly was a deeper animus against all claims to distinction based on the possession of special learning or privileged access to knowledge.

[6] There is still no book devoted to Thomsonianism and later botanic sects in America, but the useful literature on the movement and its assault upon medical orthodoxy includes Alex Berman, 'The impact of the nineteenth century botanico-medical movement on American pharmacy and medicine', unpublished Ph.D. dissertation (University of Wisconsin–Madison, 1954); Alex Berman, 'The Thomsonian movement and its relation to American pharmacy and medicine', *Bulletin of the History of Medicine*, 25 (1951), pp. 405–28 and 519–38; Alex Berman, 'Wooster Beach and the early Eclectics', *University of Michigan Medical Bulletin*, 24 (1958), pp. 277–86; Barbara Griggs, *Green Pharmacy: A History of Herbal Medicine* (London, 1981); Kett, *Formation of the American Medical Profession*, pp. 97–131; Ronald L. Numbers, 'The Making of an Eclectic physician: Joseph M. McElhinney and the Eclectic Medical College of Cincinnati', *Bulletin of the History of Medicine*, 47 (1973), 155–66; and William G. Rothstein, *American Physicians in the Nineteenth Century: From Sects to Science* (Baltimore, 1972), pp. 125–51.

[7] See Elizabeth Barnaby Keeney, Susan Eyrich Lederer and Edmond P. Minihan, 'Sectarians and scientists: alternatives to orthodox medicine' in Ronald L. Numbers and Judith Walzer Leavitt (eds), *Wisconsin Medicine: Historical Perspectives* (Madison, Wis., 1981), pp. 47–74; Susan E. Cayleff, *Wash and Be Healed: The Water-Cure and Women's Health* (Philadelphia, 1987); Jane B. Donegan, *'Hydropathic Highway to Health': Women and Water-Cure in Antebellum America* (New York, 1986); and Harry B. Weiss and Howard R. Kemble, *The Great American Water-Cure Craze: A History of Hydropathy in the United States* (Trenton, N.J., 1967). On the broader health reform movement and its criticism of orthodox medicine, see Stephen Nissenbaum, *Sex, Diet, and Debility in Jacksonian America: Sylvester Graham and Health Reform* (Westport, Conn., 1980); Ronald L. Numbers, *Prophetess of Health: A Study of Ellen G. White* (New York, 1976); and Martha H. Verbrugge, 'The social meaning of personal health: the Ladies' Physiological Institute of Boston and Vicinity in the 1850s' in Susan Reverby and David Rosner (eds), *Health Care in America: Essays in Social History* (Philadelphia, 1979), pp. 45–66. Homeopathy shared in the assault upon orthodox monopoly, theory and practice, but was not marked by an animus against professionalism; see Harris L. Coulter, *Divided Legacy: A History of the Schism in Medical Thought*, 3 vols. (Washington, D.C., 1973), vol. III: *Science and Ethics in American Medicine, 1800–1914*; Harris L. Coulter, *Homoeopathic Influences in Nineteenth-Century Allopathic Therapeutics: A Historical and Philosophical Study* (St Louis, 1973); Martin Kaufman, *Homeopathy in America: The Rise and Fall of a Medical Heresy* (Baltimore, 1971); and Kett, *Formation of the American Medical Profession*, pp. 132–64.

The force that propelled this assault was most dramatically expressed in the campaign against medical licensing. Starting in the 1830s, the Thomsonians and their Jacksonian allies led a drive in the state legislatures for the repeal of all medical licensing laws. Liberally deploying the anti-monopoly rhetoric of free trade and egalitarianism that had such powerful resonances in American society, they persuaded the legislatures to virtually abolish legal regulation of medical practice. By mid century, only a few traces of a licensing system remained, and, as Matthew Ramsey has concluded on the basis of an extensive trans-national study, 'The American medical field was the freest in the Western world.'[8]

By and large, what the licensing laws that existed before repeal had provided was an honorific distinction between licensed and unlicensed practitioners. The penalties for unlicensed practice, even when enforced, often were trivial – as in the loss of the right to sue in court for uncollected fees. The highly successful battle against licensing could not do away with medical monopoly in America, for there was none to be abolished; instead, it did away with the honorific distinction claimed by regular physicians. And that was precisely its aim. The chief target was the *honorific* distinction that had been granted regular doctors on the basis of the claim to special knowledge and special access to knowledge that came from education in the regular medical tradition.[9]

Recognising this is important, for it underscores the fact that the assault upon the medical profession was above all an effort to undermine the idea that specialised professional knowledge should constitute a valid source of distinction and authority in American society. It was an attack on professional mystery, the possession of profound secret knowledge concealed from or unknowable to ordinary citizens, and on claims to authority by merit of its possession. Samuel Thomson, the founder of Thomsonianism, typically asserted in the preface to his *New Guide to Health* that while other realms of knowledge such as religion and politics 'are brought where "common people" can understand them; the knowledge and use of medicine, is in a great measure concealed in a dead language, and a sick man is

[8] Matthew Ramsey, 'The politics of professional monopoly in nineteenth-century medicine: the French model and its rivals' in Gerald L. Geison (ed.), *Professions and the French State, 1700–1900* (Philadelphia, 1984), pp. 225–305, at p. 251.

[9] On licensing and its decline, see Samuel Lee Baker, 'Medical licensing in America: an early liberal reform', unpublished Ph.D. dissertation (Harvard University, 1977); Kett, *Formation of the American Medical Profession*, pp. 1–96; Rothstein, *American Physicians*, pp. 63–100; and Richard Harrison Shryock, *Medical Licensing in America, 1650–1965* (Baltimore, 1967).

often obliged to risk his life, where he would not risk a dollar'.[10] Insisting that 'the spirit of the medical profession must be revolutionised, to be in harmony with the spirit of the times', reformers endlessly called upon doctors to abandon 'their Latin Diplomas and antique technicalities'.[11] Physicians' use of Latin was assailed as but one visible sign of their attempt to keep knowledge of medicine inaccessible to the public, something expressed more profoundly in their needlessly intricate theorising about the body in health and disease. The mystification of medicine by the profession, like the claim that it had privileged access to knowledge, was illegitimate, and any prestige physicians held by merit of it should be taken back by the people.

Accompanying the assault on professional mystery came the proclamation of an alternative – and assertively more democratic – medical epistemology. Common experience, commanded by the ordinary man and woman, was a sufficient guide to health and healing and, moreover, the only source of truly authentic medical knowledge. 'In the science of medicine, I assure you, there is no mystery', one botanic practitioner writing to the public urged in 1834. 'There is nothing incomprehensible about it'.[12] As another botanic put it, the 'unfathomable arcana of medicine' should be replaced by simple truths.[13] What was beyond the ken of ordinary people could not constitute sound knowledge. Direct experience of nature, an epistemology of both common sense and common experience, would inform medicine characterised by truth and simplicity. 'We wish to see the healing art brought home to our own firesides, and rendered so plain and simple, that it can be understood by all', one Thomsonian editor advised. 'It is as easy to cure disease, as it is to make a pudding', he claimed, insisting that in medicine there should be 'no mysticism – no bombast – no monopoly'.[14] Contrasting hydropathy with or-

[10] Samuel Thomson, *New Guide to Health; or Botanic Family Physician* (Boston, 1835), p. 5.

[11] B., 'Medical despotism', *Western Medical Reformer*, 6 (1847), pp. 265–70, at p. 266.

[12] Daniel H. Whitney, *The Family Physician, or Every Man His Own Doctor* (New York, 1834), p. iv. It is telling that calls for the demystification of American medicine re-emerged most forcefully with the anti-establishment sentiment of the 1960s and 1970s. Consider, for example, calls from the women's movement for women to regain control of their own bodies. 'We must work on, and along with, doctors and nurses to demystify and deprofessionalize medicine', one feminist health manual demanded (The Boston Women's Health Book Collective, *Our Bodies, Ourselves: A Book By and For Women* (New York, 1976; 1st edn 1971), p. 249).

[13] Samuel North, *The Family Physician and Guide to Health* (Waterloo, N.Y., 1830), p. iii.

[14] *Boston Thomsonian Manual and Lady's Companion*, 5 (1838–9), p. 137.

thodox medicine, another reformer echoed, 'Our science is not buried in technicalities, nor our practice veiled in mystery.'[15]

Critics underscored the evils of the putative mystification of medical knowledge by the regular profession by pointing to its dire effects on the people's health. It kept a knowledge of healing and the laws of healthful living from the public. As one health reformer charged, orthodox doctors

> do not aim to enlighten mankind in regard to their physical well being, but rather seek to envelop their processes of cure in deep and impenetrable mystery. This mystery possesses a magic charm for the uninitiated and ignorant. You have only to look about you to become aware of the credulity and superstition with which the Medical Profession is regarded.

It was the health reformer's task, she continued, 'to sow far and wide the seeds of truth that will eventually germinate and b[e] the means of redeeming the world from ignorance that so effectually blinds the mass of its inhabitants'.[16] A hydropathic practitioner similarly noted that 'the medical profession has arrogated to itself all knowledge having important relation to health – virtually saying, we, and we alone, are the conservators of the bodies of men'. Orthodox doctors held this knowledge as 'too sacred, or too occult for the common understanding'.[17]

More than simply making medical knowledge appear beyond the grasp of common Americans, though, the highly wrought, speculative systems of regular physicians, critics asserted, led to dangerous practice. 'False theory and hypothesis', Thomson claimed, 'constitute nearly the whole art of physic.'[18] The target critics most violently denounced was orthodox heroic therapy. Regular doctors, in their view, exemplified the corruption of established medicine by quite literally poisoning the American people. What led to this deluded practice in the first place was their purportedly blind reliance on rationalistic theories instead of on experience. Speculative systems of pathology and therapeutics not only represented the core of the regular physician's special knowledge, but also the source of his

[15] 'Address of the American Hydropathic Convention to the people of the United States', *Water Cure Journal, and Herald of Reforms*, 10 (1850), pp. 79–81, at p. 81.

[16] Ellen M. Snow, 'Duties of physicians', *Water Cure Journal, and Herald of Reforms*, 21 (1856), pp. 55–6, as quoted in Regina Markell Morantz, 'Nineteenth century health reform and women: a program of self-help' in Guenter B. Risse, Ronald L. Numbers and Judith Walzer Leavitt (eds), *Medicine without Doctors: Home Health Care in American History* (New York, 1977), pp. 73–93, on p. 76.

[17] G. H. Taylor, 'Medical credulity', *Water Cure Journal, and Herald of Reforms*, 16 (1853), p. 75. And see 'Physic and prevention', *Water Cure Journal, and Herald of Reforms*, 11 (1851), pp. 90–1.

[18] Thomson, *New Guide*, p. 35.

misguided, murderous bleeding and purging. And, accordingly, sectarian critics routinely illustrated their medical writings and lectures by examples of cases 'treated by the murderous systems'.[19] By placing their faith in complicated, rationalistic systems, regular physicians not only kept knowledge of healing from the public, but also misguided their own practice by obscuring from themselves nature's simple truths.

The persistent message of assaults upon the regular profession was that medical knowledge should be simplified, stripped of all needless embellishments, and that access to it should be opened up. Once this happened, critics maintained, the authority regular physicians claimed by merit of their singular command of medical truth and access to it would, properly, disintegrate. No longer would regular physicians be able to use artificially intricate medical knowledge to exploit and defraud the public. A better, simpler epistemology of common experience would improve health care, banish the evils of heroic drugging, and foster a healthier, more democratic and more fittingly American social order. As in the rhetoric of other Jacksonians, the theme of return was central in the polemics of popular medical reformers – return that is to truth, simplicity, nature and a more authentically American way of life.[20] Allegiance to an ideal of medicine grounded in direct experience of nature would lead to redemptive reforms in medicine and society alike.

Historians have pointed out that the popular assault upon the medical profession in America was a significant source of change in regular medicine. In doing so, they have tended to identify the forces of the market-place as the engines of medical reform. As the attack on orthodox ways led to a popular outcry against heroic drugging, this argument generally goes, regular physicians tailored their goods to the demands of the market, making their therapies increasingly milder to render them less vulnerable to sectarian ridicule and more palatable to paying patients.[21] Unmistakably there is truth in this account. Yet,

[19] George Washington Bowen, 'Notes taken on lectures given by Chas. D. Williams on the Institutes and Practice of Homoeopathy, Cleveland Institute of Homoeopathy, 1851–2', (Western Reserve Historical Society, Cleveland, Ohio).

[20] This point is developed in David J. Keblish, 'Thomsonianism: a romantic movement of restoration and the "Thomsonian Paradox"', unpublished B.A. thesis (Yale College, Yale University 1988). Marvin Meyers suggested that a theme of return is one element evident in the rhetoric of all Jacksonians in *The Jacksonian Persuasion: Politics and Belief* (Stanford, 1957).

[21] See, for example, Rothstein, *American Physicians*. On therapeutic change, see Charles E. Rosenberg, 'The therapeutic revolution: medicine, meaning, and social change in nineteenth-century America' in Vogel and Rosenberg (eds), *The Therapeutic Revolution*,

sectarian attacks exerted at the same time a conservative influence on regular medicine that was itself an important force in the creation of medical orthodoxy. The socio-economic and intellectual siege upon orthodox medicine urged regular practitioners to turn inward in order to find in established tradition a stable core of professional definition and distinctiveness. In the realm of practice, this conservative influence led regulars to proclaim their allegiance to the traditional therapies that had come under attack more stridently than ever before, transforming bloodletting and mineral drugs into symbols of orthodox identity.[22]

A similar impulse among regular physicians in the face of popular attack was to loudly reaffirm the necessary complexity of their medical knowledge. Georgia physician Paul Eve could typically tell medical students gathered for their commencement ceremony in 1849 that the source of 'the unfavorable opinion entertained by the public for the medical profession is, that as a science it is the most difficult, obscure and complicated of all human learning. No other occupation in life involves such varied and minute knowledge.'[23] The importance of initiation into the special knowledge that distinguished the regular profession was formalised in the new institutions set up to define and preserve orthodoxy. Emblemising the conservative response to the attack on orthodox knowledge, in 1847 the newly created American Medical Association wrote into its Code of Ethics that 'no one can be considered as a regular practitioner' unless he had been educated in regular medicine, mastering 'the aids furnished by anatomy, physiology, pathology, and organic chemistry'.[24] Assaults on the regular profession and the repeal of licensing urged regular physicians to underscore what defined the orthodox faith and distinguished them as singularly qualified healers.

Yet the popular critique of professional mystery may have had a

pp. 3–25, and John Harley Warner, *The Therapeutic Perspective: Medical Practice, Knowledge, and Identity in America, 1820–1885* (Cambridge, Mass., 1986).

[22] John Harley Warner, 'Medical sectarianism, therapeutic conflict, and the shaping of orthodox professional identity in antebellum American medicine' in W. F. Bynum and Roy Porter (eds), *Medical Fringe and Medical Orthodoxy, 1750–1850* (London, 1987), pp. 234–60, and John Harley Warner, 'Power, conflict, and identity in mid-nineteenth-century American medicine: therapeutic change at the Commercial Hospital of Cincinnati', *Journal of American History*, 73 (1987), pp. 934–56.

[23] Paul F. Eve, *An Introductory Lecture, Delivered in the Medical College of Georgia, November 6th, 1849* (Augusta, 1849), p. 22.

[24] 'Code of medical ethics', *Transactions of the New York State Medical Association*, 1 (1884), pp. 570–84, at p. 577, is taken from the American Medical Association's Code, which was drafted after it was founded in 1847 and adopted by many local and state medical societies.

still far more profound influence in shaping regular American physicians' attitudes towards established medical knowledge and expectations about how new knowledge should be gained. More than its direct influence on regular thought and behaviour, it created a socio-economic and intellectual environment that shaped the ways physicians responded to and assimilated other sources of change. In particular, I want to suggest that the popular assault on the medical profession and its knowledge was one important force in shaping epistemological change in regular medicine: it gave the turn from rationalism toward empiricism that so marked western medicine during the first half of the nineteenth century a special meaning in the American context. The peculiar situation of the medical profession in antebellum American society intensified the symbolic meanings regular physicians came to attach to an ideal of empiricism they derived largely from the Paris Clinical School, and helps explain why they so ardently embraced that ideal in the first place.

During precisely the decades when the assault upon the regular profession arose and came to thrive, from the 1820s to the outbreak of the Civil War, American physicians in increasing numbers travelled to Paris to supplement the medical training available in their own country. At least 700 of them studied in Paris between 1820 and 1860, and the influence of these migrants was far out of proportion to their number, for on their return they were the ones who tended to become professors in American medical schools, editors of journals and contributors to the professional literature. Historians have well catalogued the elements of French medicine they brought back, such as a stress on the stethoscope and physical examination, tissue pathology, systematic clinical instruction and autopsy, clinical scepticism, the anatomo-clinical viewpoint and clinical statistics. But historians have given much less attention to how very selective the Americans were in what they sought to transplant into their native soil, and little at all to the different meanings such elements of French medicine could take on in the American context.[25]

[25] An extensive literature on Americans and French medicine includes Henry Blumenthal, *American and French Culture, 1800–1900: Interchanges in Art, Science, Literature, and Society* (Baton Rouge, La., 1975), pp. 402–67; Russell M. Jones, 'American doctors and the Parisian medical world, 1830–1840', *Bulletin of the History of Medicine*, 47 (1973), pp. 40–65 and 177–204; Russell M. Jones, 'American doctors in Paris, 1820–1861: a statistical profile', *Journal of the History of Medicine and Allied Sciences*, 25 (1970), pp. 142–57; Russell M. Jones, 'Introduction' in *The Parisian Education of an American Surgeon:*

What is singularly striking about the relationship between American physicians and the Paris Clinical School is the extent to which the Americans embraced and celebrated the empiricism they found expressed there. Indeed, they portrayed it as the most notable feature of French medicine. What Americans were pointing to was the sensual empiricism of the French medical idéologues, a radical reaction against the Enlightenment rationalism of the old medical regime.[26] But ordinarily they expressed it in simple terms: the empiricism of French medicine stood for an allegiance to fact, to truth, to knowledge attained and verified by direct observation and analysis of nature. American disciples of the Paris Clinical School tended to make a stark dichotomy between rationalism on the one hand, linked with hypothesis, reasoning and grand unified systems of pathology and therapeutics, and empiricism on the other, associated with observation, a sceptical attitude towards established knowledge and hostility to theory. Orthodox physicians who proclaimed the empiricist faith were troubled by the common use of the term 'empiric' as a derisive epithet for the quack, and at times urged their brethren to call unqualified healers and mountebanks something else. The empiricism which elite regular practitioners brought from France, exemplified by direct observation of symptoms in the living body and pathological lesions in the deceased, was an epistemological stance they believed promised to transform medicine only through the committed labour of educated physicians consecrated above all to medical truth.

But even though empiricism was one important element of the French programme for medicine, this does not explain why Americans so vigorously took it up and so prominently featured it in their plan for transforming medicine. That medical Americans in Paris should take note of the Parisian commitment to empiricism was perhaps inevitable; that they should see it as the most important feature of French medicine and energetically make it their own was not. The English who studied medicine in Paris during the same period, for example, also took note of Parisian empiricism, but dwelled on it far less. As I have suggested elsewhere, in telling about what the Parisian

Letters of Jonathan Mason Warren (1832–1835) (Philadelphia, 1978), pp. 1–69; and Richard H. Shryock, 'The advent of modern medicine in Philadelphia, 1800–1850', in Richard H. Shryock, *Medicine in America: Historical Essays* (Baltimore, 1966), pp. 203–32.

26 Of the large literature on the French medical empiricism that was a resource for Americans, see Erwin H. Ackerknecht, *Medicine at the Paris Hospital, 1794–1848* (Baltimore, 1967), and George Rosen, 'The philosophy of ideology and the emergence of modern medicine in France', *Bulletin of the History of Medicine*, 20 (1946), pp. 328–39.

medical world was like and what was most significant about it, the English tended to place relatively more emphasis on the institutional arrangements, professional organisation and value system that made up French medical polity, while Americans tended to stress above all its epistemology.[27]

During the second quarter of the nineteenth century, American physicians elevated empiricism to a symbol of professional uplift. At a time when regular physicians widely believed their profession had come to occupy a degraded position, many saw in an ideal of empiricism the promise of not just conceptual change but professional salvation. To those who travelled to Paris, the strident empiricism they perceived as an outgrowth of the French revolution in medicine promised a fresh start in reconstructing medical knowledge. Just as Americans saw their nation forging a new social and political order, so radical empiricism offered a basis for creating a new medical tradition, and its very newness may have enhanced its symbolic value in the American context. Many regular practitioners shared the perception one Boston physician expressed when he asserted in 1836 that 'disease has never, until quite recently, been investigated'. Direct observation was just beginning to expose 'the incomprehensible mysticism and absurd speculations of the closet dogmatists upon the nature of disease'.[28] The leaders among regular physicians loudly reconsecrated their profession to science, but they made it clear that science meant empiricism. Confidently and publicly proclaimed, an allegiance to empiricism was to be the hallmark of a new order for medical knowledge and for the medical profession.[29]

Empiricism adopted as a symbol and plan for professional uplift was neatly suited to the prevailing socio-political tenor of American culture. In taking up empiricism as the chart by which the medical profession would steer its course, regular reformers set themselves on a tack in some respects remarkably parallel to that of their critics.

[27] John Harley Warner, 'The medical migrant's baggage unpacked: Anglo-American constructions of the Paris Clinical School' in Ronald L. Numbers and John V. Pickstone (compilers) *British Society for the History of Science and the History of Science Society. Programs, Papers, and Abstracts for the Joint Conference, Manchester, England, 11–15 July 1988* (Madison, Wis., 1988), pp. 213–20.

[28] L. M. Whiting, 'Investigation of disease', *Boston Medical and Surgical Journal*, 14 (1836), pp. 181–90, at p. 181; emphasis removed.

[29] John Harley Warner, 'The selective transport of medical knowledge: antebellum American physicians and Parisian medical therapeutics', *Bulletin of the History of Medicine*, 59 (1985), pp. 213–31, and Warner, *The Therapeutic Perspective*, esp. pp. 37–57. And see Richard H. Shryock, 'Empiricism versus rationalism in American medicine, 1650–1950', *Proceedings of the American Antiquarian Society*, n.s. 79 (1969), pp. 99–150.

French empiricism, after all, could represent direct observation of fact open for all to see rather than shrouded as a professional mystery, and therefore offered regular reformers a rallying point and symbol of professional advancement that promised to be exceptionally resilient to the prevailing animus against claims to privileged access to knowledge. It provided what could be framed as an epistemology of common experience, an epistemology singularly well calculated to withstand attacks from monopoly-bashing exponents of Jacksonian Democracy like the Thomsonians. To be sure, the direct observation of nature of the Thomsonians was far from identical to the direct observation of nature of Paris-returned elite American physicians. The clinic and autopsy table offered a context for observing nature quite different from that envisioned by those who spoke only of the domestic bedside. Nevertheless, both versions of medical empiricism turned upon a vigorous insistence on the primacy of direct experience. Regular physicians took up the empiricist faith of their assailants and used it to mount a counterattack against them. 'We go for *science*, in medical practice and in medical reform', one physician wrote in 1839, at once denouncing the Thomsonians and proclaiming his orthodox faith. 'And by science in medicine, we mean large experience, not theory.'[30]

The rhetorical forms physicians used in putting forward the empiricist programme for reform point to commonalities between regular practitioners and their critics that went deeper than simply a shared emphasis on experience. Like the Thomsonians, regular doctors made the theme of return central in their reformist rhetoric. For orthodox reformers, as much as for their critics, empiricism was envisaged as a vehicle by which medicine would be returned to nature, purity, simplicity and truth. Regular physicians had in mind not so much a restoration of the values of a simpler, ancestral American society as a return to the medicine of the Hippocratics, which American empiricists, like their French counterparts in the tradition of Condillac and Cabanis, tended to idolise. In depicting an allegiance to empiricism as a vehicle for return to a better way, regular physicians found a parallel and a rejoinder to the most powerful polemical device critics used against their profession.[31]

[30] W. A. A., 'Thomsonism', *Boston Medical and Surgical Journal*, 19 (1839), pp. 379–83, at p. 382. I am indebted to Jon Harkness for helping me to see the coexistence of different versions of medical empiricism. Helpful too is Harold J. Cook, *The Decline of the Old Medical Regime in Stuart London* (Ithaca, 1986).

[31] The cult of Hippocrates that emerged among antebellum American physicians and the way it shaped the reception of experimental science deserve close study.

More than a commitment to empiricism alone, the epistemological stance that Americans took from France included equally a strident opposition to rationalism. And regular reformers in the United States used it in an energetic campaign of their own to demystify established medical knowledge. An assault upon rationalism pervaded regular physicians' programmes for reconstructing medical knowledge, but it can best be seen in their drive to demolish rationalistic systems of practice, a process of tearing down that many saw as the necessary prerequisite to any plan for rebuilding. The rationalistic systems of pathology and therapeutics inherited from the Enlightenment came to represent the causes of the profession's degradation. From the 1820s through the remainder of the antebellum period, a crusade against rationalistic systems fought in the name of empiricism gave regular medical reformers a rallying point and a project for reform. The task of those who had taken up the ideal of empiricism, as the Paris clinician Pierre Louis aptly characterised it in a letter to one of his Boston students, was to construct 'a barrier against the spirit of system'.[32] Elite orthodox reformers, no less than their critics who preached medical democracy, engaged in a self-conscious campaign to rid medicine of rationalistic structures, to banish all vestiges of speculation.

In empiricism, then, regular reformers saw a key to uplifting the knowledge, practice and authority of the medical profession. The debasement of the profession – epitomised by the strength of sectarians – could in large measure be explained by a misguided allegiance to rationalism. Rationalistic systems of practice encouraged therapeutic extremism, the heroic bleeding and purging that was a main target of sectarian attacks. Reformers also blamed the notorious disunity of the regular profession on rationalism, since conflict among those who advocated competing systems was a leading source of discord within regular ranks. Empiricism would rid the profession of the therapeutic overkill associated with rationalistic systems and thereby scotch sectarian criticism of regular practice. It would also reduce professional division and encourage a unified professional front. Above all, careful empirical observation would improve regular practice, enabling regular physicians to better compete against sectarians and shoring up the profession's standing in the eyes of the public. Using empiricism as a vehicle for improving practice, reformers believed, could bring uplift in a society prepared to honour

[32] P. C. A. Louis to H. I. Bowditch, Paris, 5 February 1840 (Francis A. Countway Library of Medicine, Boston).

natural merit but antagonistic to artificial distinctions in rank. Empiricism would transform practice and in the process elevate the standing and authority of the medical profession in American society.[33]

It would certainly be wrong to suggest that the socio-political context of medical practice in the United States caused physicians to take up an ideal of empiricism: during the first half of the nineteenth century a shift from rationalism toward empiricism was evident in varying degrees throughout western medicine. But there is ample reason to say that the peculiar socio-economic, political and intellectual milieu of antebellum America redoubled the meaning this particular epistemological stance held for regular medical reformers. It made a commitment to empiricism matter more to them and let them see in it greater promise.

Regular doctors obviously did not share the antiprofessional animus of their critics, nor were they willing to concede that all people were equally able to interpret the secrets of nature. They did agree with their assailants, however, that relying on direct experience of nature was the best guarantee of good practice. They also agreed that the theoretical edifices of rationalistic medicine were dangerous and must be torn down. Most of all, though – and to an extent that may have been singular to American medicine – they agreed that practice, not the possession of or access to special knowledge, was in the final analysis the source of the medical practitioner's authority and identity. In a largely unregulated medical field, proclaiming an allegiance to the distinctive symbols of orthodoxy, such as the value of bloodletting and mineral drugs in principle, and interacting with patients and other practitioners in ways that displayed a commitment to medical tradition, were the outward signs that identified the regular physician and claimed for him whatever authority the public accorded his profession.

Historians have long stressed the tension between the democratic allegiances of antebellum society and the aspirations of the professions for distinction and special privilege, and to the extent that the professional identity of regular physicians was enhanced by membership in an exclusive society, possession of particular educational credentials, or licensing, this is fitting. Yet American physicians embraced a concept of their identity and authority as professionals that was in considerable measure in harmony with egalitarian ideals.

[33] Warner, 'Selective transport', esp. pp. 224–8, and Warner, *The Therapeutic Perspective*, esp. pp. 37–57 and 185–206.

Similarly, historians have seen it as paradoxical that professional leaders did not put up a more determined fight against the repeal of medical licensing laws. But licensing was not critical to what it meant to be a professional physician, as they understood it. The repeal of licensing did not undermine the American physician's professional identity and authority, which were rooted not in legal or institutional structures but in practice. It was in this context that empiricism seemed to offer such a promising basis for uplifting the authority of the profession.[34]

In the empiricist programme, the laboratory was seen to hold little promise for advancing medical practice or authority. In French medicine during the first half of the nineteenth century, as Erwin Ackerknecht and others have stressed, the leading figures of the Paris Clinical School tended to dismiss the basic sciences as irrelevant to their plan for medical reconstruction. More recent revisionist interpretations have pointed out that the dominant Parisian medical ethos actually had a constructive influence in shaping the experimental laboratory work pursued in spite of it.[35] Yet this does not alter the overriding fact that until mid century, the leading clinicians remained sceptical and often antagonistic towards medical claims for the basic sciences, and kept laboratory work on the margins of the Parisian medical world. So too, American physicians influenced by French ways, who tended to make an allegiance to empiricism even more persistently central to their plan for reform, saw the laboratory only on the dim fringes of their vision of medicine's future. The singular strength of their commitment to empiricism was matched by the firmness of their dismissal of the basic sciences from plans to better practice.

The regular physician and reformer Elisha Bartlett, for example, wrote his treatise on *The Philosophy of Medical Science* (1844) as a self-conscious American manifesto of medical empiricism. He vigorously rejected the proposition that physiological investigations could

[34] This is expanded upon in John Harley Warner, 'Anglo-American professional reform and the French medical model', paper given at the Annual Meeting of the Organization of American Historians, Reno, Nev., 27 March 1988.

[35] Ackerknecht, *Medicine at the Paris Hospital*, esp. pp. 3–12, 121–7. John E. Lesch gives the fullest expression of the revisionist view in *Science and Medicine in France: The Emergence of Experimental Physiology, 1790–1855* (Cambridge, Mass., 1984); Ann Laberge makes the point for the case of medical microscopy in 'Dr Alfred Donné and the microscopic analysis of human milk', paper presented at the Annual Meeting of the Southern Historical Association, Norfolk, Va., 10 November 1988.

lead to an understanding of disease. 'By what conceivable process of reasoning – by what imaginable steps of logical deduction – could a knowledge of the former have led us to a knowledge of the latter?' he demanded.[36] So too, '*all* our knowledge of the relations between diseases and their remedies, or modifiers, is solely and exclusively the result of direct observation'.[37] Reasoning from pathology was delusive. 'Therapeutics is not founded upon pathology. The former cannot be deduced from the latter. It rests wholly upon experience. It is, absolutely and exclusively, an empirical art.'[38] The reliance of earlier ages on reasoning had led to what Bartlett called 'the abominable atrocities of wholesale and indiscriminate *drugging*', with dire consequences for 'the innocent victims to *rational* physic'.[39] Medical hypotheses and theories

> have only rendered more obscure and difficult what was sufficiently so before their intervention; and they have ever impeded the progress of the science which they professed to promote. Not only so, but they have almost always acted injuriously upon the practical application of the science of medicine... They have, in many instances, converted the science from an instrument of good, to an engine of positive ill – a means of inflicting upon men the very evils, which its true objects and aim are to remove.[40]

With clear implications for the medical relevance of reasoning from the basic sciences, Bartlett concluded that

> so far as medical science has any just title to the appellation; and so far as medical art possesses any rules, sufficiently positive to be worth anything, it is owing, exclusively, to the diligent, unprejudiced, and conscientious study of the phenomena and relationships of disease. The sole tendency of every departure from this study, – the sole tendency of every attempt to refer these phenomena to certain unknown and assumed conditions, for the purpose of rendering them *rational*, has been to hinder the progress and improvement of the science and the art. So has it ever been, so will it ever be.[41]

By undermining the 'hypothetical explanations' of rationalistic systems, one reviewer wrote in praise, Bartlett's book 'tears off the veil which has been thrown over false science, and exposes it in all its deformities'.[42] In the final analysis, empiricists such as Bartlett tended

[36] Elisha Bartlett, *An Essay on the Philosophy of Medical Science* (Philadelphia, 1844), p. 94. And see Erwin H. Ackerknecht, 'Elisha Bartlett and the philosophy of the Paris Clinical School', *Bulletin of the History of Medicine*, 24 (1950), pp. 43–60.

[37] Bartlett, *Philosophy of Medical Science*, p. 108.

[38] *Ibid.*, pp. 113–14; emphasis removed. [39] *Ibid.*, p. 290. [40] *Ibid.*, p. 182.

[41] *Ibid.*, p. 218.

[42] J. C. N[ott], Review of 'The philosophy of medical science, by Elisha Bartlett', *New Orleans Medical and Surgical Journal*, 1 (1844–5), pp. 490–2, at pp. 491 and 492. Bartlett's programme of radical empiricism was not of course uniformly admired; see, for example,

to see laboratory study of basic science placed in aid of medical understanding as part of the useless embellishment of medical knowledge the critics of their profession were assailing, and which they themselves sought to place beyond the medical pale.

This is not to say that American physicians committed to empiricism were necessarily opposed to the pursuit of laboratory science. Laboratory work in physiology or chemistry, like work in geology, paleontology or taxonomic botany, might well be regarded by medical colleagues and by some among the public as an admirable expression of the individual physician's cultural participation. The cultivation of science and perhaps leadership in a scientific society, no less than participation in civic lending libraries, museums and other learned societies, could win for the individual physician community respect and esteem, not so much as a healer but as a citizen. Oliver Wendell Holmes typically recommended to young physicians in 1853 that microscopical research offered a constructive way to occupy the abundant leisure time on their hands while waiting for their first patients.[43] By and large, however, basic science was not seen as very pertinent to reforming medical practice, and therefore it was regarded as a doubtfully promising source of authority for the profession. Special learning might be admirable, but in antebellum America expert knowledge was not in itself a culturally compelling source of authority. As a speaker reminded the graduating class of medical students at Harvard in 1870, their success in American society 'depended fully as much upon what they were as upon what they knew'.[44]

Throughout the nineteenth century, some American physicians entered the profession in the first place principally for their love of science. Medicine was widely acknowledged to be the best occupational choice for a man who wanted to pursue science in a society that afforded few opportunities to take it up as a profession, and physicians as a group were prominent among the cultivators of science.[45] Scientific investigation was acceptable and perhaps ad-

review of 'Elisha Bartlett, an essay on the philosophy of medical science', *Western Lancet*, 3 (1844–5), pp. 386–8.

[43] Oliver Wendell Holmes, 'Microscopic preparations', *Boston Medical and Surgical Journal*, 48 (1853), pp. 337–42.

[44] 'Letter from Boston', *Cincinnati Lancet and Observer*, 13 (1870), pp. 234–8, at p. 235.

[45] Among the most useful treatments of the place of science in antebellum American culture are George H. Daniels, *American Science in the Age of Jackson* (New York, 1968) and Alexandra Oleson and Sanborn C. Brown (eds), *The Pursuit of Knowledge in the Early American Republic: American Scientific and Learned Societies from Colonial Times to the Civil War* (Baltimore, 1976). And see Edward C. Atwater, '"Squeezing Mother Nature":

mirable, as long as it did not interfere with the physician's obligations as a practitioner. However, science – of whatever sort – was to remain clearly subordinate to practice. When in 1833 the young Bostonian James Jackson, Jr. wanted to emulate the research model presented by his mentor in Paris, Pierre Louis, and proposed to devote several years to investigation in the clinic before starting practice, for example, his physician-father saw no choice but to reject his plan. 'In this country', the father later explained,

> his course would have been so singular, as in a measure to separate him from other men. We are a business doing people. We are new. We have, as it were, but just landed on these uncultivated shores; there is a vast deal to be done; and he who will not be doing, must be set down as a drone. If he is a drone in appearance only and not in fact, it will require a long time to prove it so, when his character has once been fixed in the public mind.[46]

Science – including work in fields like chemistry and experimental physiology – was a legitimate and usually estimable pursuit for Americans who professed to be physicians, but not as their primary endeavour.[47]

Thus at mid century, when laboratory science had risen to prominence in the culture of German medicine both as an element in the education of physicians and in their claim to professional authority and esteem, the laboratory remained very much on the margins of American medicine. Part of the explanation for this may have been material, as many historians have pointed out, for in medicine as in other spheres, the United States lacked the financial and institutional resources at the disposal of scientific investigation in the Old World.[48]

experimental physiology in the United States before 1870', *Bulletin of the History of Medicine*, 52 (1978), 313–35.

[46] James Jackson, *A Memoir of James Jackson, Jr., M.D. with Extracts from His Letters to His Father: and Medical Cases, Collected by Him* (Boston, 1835), pp. 55–6.

[47] In the medical context, at least, it is a presentistic conception of science that has informed the widely accepted thesis that Americans were indifferent to basic science; see Richard Harrison Shryock, 'American indifference to basic science during the nineteenth century' in *Medicine in America: Historical Essays* (Baltimore, 1966), pp. 71–89, and the use of the indifference thesis to explain American neglect of laboratory science in Phyllis Allen Richmond, 'American attitudes toward the germ theory of disease (1860–1880)', *Journal of the History of Medicine and Allied Sciences*, 9 (1954), 428–54, and Phyllis Allen Richmond, 'The nineteenth-century American physician as a research scientist' in Felix Marti-Ibanez (ed.), *History of American Medicine: A Symposium* (New York, 1959), pp. 142–55.

[48] See Ronald L. Numbers and John Harley Warner, 'The maturation of American medical science' in Nathan Reingold and Marc Rothenberg (eds), *Scientific Colonialism, 1800–1930: A Cross-Cultural Comparison* (Washington, D.C., 1987), pp. 191–214. On the German physiology that provides the contrast, see, for example, Joseph Ben-David, *The Scientist's Role in Society: A Comparative Study* (Chicago, 1984; 1st edn, 1971); William Coleman and

Yet this is at best only a partial explanation, and the marginal place assigned to the laboratory had deeper roots in the nation's culture.

The laboratory appeared to be a rather impotent source of knowledge for the American medical profession. So long as both the identity and the authority of physicians were rooted in practice, the possession of extensive scientific knowledge in itself was not a powerful source of professional authority. And so long as the regular profession's leading reformers pursued an ardent empiricist crusade, basic science was not regarded as likely to have much potential in uplifting practice when measured up against clinical experience. Above all, so long as rationalism was seen as dangerous to the profession's practice and politics alike, reformers were unlikely to see reasoning from basic laboratory science as a blueprint for medical reconstruction. American empiricists sought to eschew the iatrochemical and iatrophysical indulgences of medicine's rationalistic past. Most agreed that physiology, for example, might have a legitimate place in medicine as a mnemonic device and source of explanation; but it was not a reliable guide to changing practice. And in America, to some measure in contrast with Germany, the real test of the power of science to confer authority in medicine rested in its ability to direct intervention.

During the decades after the Civil War, as more and more American physicians in search of supplementary medical training chose to spend time in Germany instead of France, an increasing number returned to proselytise the ways of laboratory medicine to the American profession. The story of their studies in Germany, the allegiances they formed there to Germanic ideals not just of medicine but of higher education in general, and the ways they sought to transmit these ideals to their own country has been well told and well documented. In most accounts, their efforts have been regarded as the high-road to progress, the pathway by which American medicine became scientific. In other accounts, most of them recent, their work has been cast as the beginning of a process leading to the triumph of reductionism and dehumanisation of American medicine. In any event, usually the

Frederic L. Holmes (eds), *The Investigative Enterprise: Experimental Physiology in Nineteenth-Century Medicine* (Berkeley, 1988); Karl E. Rothschuh, *History of Physiology*, trans. and ed. Guenter B. Risse (Huntington, N.Y., 1973); and Arleen Tuchman, 'Experimental physiology, medical reform, and the politics of education at the University of Heidelberg: a case study', *Bulletin of the History of Medicine*, 61 (1987), 203–15.

scepticism that met those who sought to bring laboratory medicine to a place of prominence in America has been framed as resistance to science, whether that science has been regarded as a forward-looking source of betterment or an oppressive tool of capitalist values.[49]

What deserves far more attention than it has received, however, is that those who urged the laboratory and its ways encountered much more than just scepticism from practising physicians. They were met not merely by apathy, indifference or suspicion born of a short-sighted American pragmatism, but by active, energetic, urgent and committed opposition and attack. It is the vehemence of the opposition to claims made on behalf of the laboratory in medicine that must be explained in order to understand what was seen by practising doctors to be at stake in the bid to make the laboratory a central feature of American medicine.

It was here that the ardent American commitment to empiricism became crucial. Certainly the most common objection brought by practitioners who opposed the rise of the laboratory was simply that it offered no practical yield. But the most energetic opposition was powered by much more than this alone. Many saw in the proposition that medicine should be regrounded in the laboratory a subversion of empiricism and dangerous revival of rationalism. The laboratory, and particularly reasoning from the bench to the bedside, threatened to remove medical knowledge from the realm of common experience, not only that of the public but also that of most regular practitioners. Critics brought up under the banner of empiricism saw in the laboratory the potential for the remystification of medical knowledge. One historian, in an important study of the rise of experimental physiology in American medicine, has stated a widely held view in asserting, 'Those who wanted to reform American medicine hoped to endow it with the authority of science.' They 'sought to make American medicine scientific'. What this ignores is that most physicians believed American medicine already was scientific; but for them, science meant empiricism. They also held a different conception of the proper relationship between epistemology and authority, one in which overzealous claims on behalf of the laboratory threatened to

[49] Of a large body of literature on the American physicians who studied in Germany, the best studies include Thomas Neville Bonner, *American Doctors and German Universities: A Chapter in International Intellectual Relations, 1870–1914* (Lincoln, Nebr., 1963); Donald Fleming, *William H. Welch and the Rise of Modern Medicine* (Boston, 1954); and Robert G. Frank, Jr., 'American physiologists in German laboratories, 1865–1914' in Geison, (ed.), *Physiology in the American Context*, pp. 11–46. And see the sources cited in n. 2.

undermine the authority of the medical profession, not to 'endow it with the authority of science'.[50]

It was not the laboratory itself, but the claims made for its authority over medical practice that were seen as especially threatening and assailed accordingly. Bartlett, in his manifesto of medical empiricism, had implicitly dismissed the laboratory as a source of knowledge about practice but had not explicitly denounced it. There was no reason to: when he wrote in the 1840s, the laboratory was making no pressing claims to dominance in American medicine. Vehement assaults appeared only when some clinicians, such as Roberts Bartholow and Horatio C. Wood, started in the 1870s and 1880s to claim that knowledge produced in the laboratory was the proper platform for uplifting medical practice. 'Physiological investigation', one admirer of Wood could assert in 1875, 'has certainly achieved more exact progress than clinical experience.'[51] Once claims for the promise of the laboratory had been boldly stated, however, there was reason for those who saw danger in such a plan to raise their voices in protest.[52]

The language employed by those who denounced claims made on the laboratory's behalf is telling. Typically, one medical editor in 1876 assailed the author of a new book on materia medica for his reliance on the dictates of experimental physiology rather than on empiricism and the test of experience. 'The practitioner, at the bedside of his patient', he charged, 'does not care to indulge in medical metaphysics... No! He leaves that all to the speculative medical experimentalist.' He continued,

> In his attempts to solve mysteries, known only to the Infinite, the modern speculator makes bold assertions, not guaranteed by a single fact, and [,] with an audacity unparalleled, will no doubt shortly give the medicinal effects of religion on the human soul, describing the essence of the vital spark, its chemical constituents, and number of newly discovered elements contained therein. His task is as hopeless as that of the infant trying to grasp the crescent moon to see what makes it shine.[53]

In stigmatising the physician who relied on the experimental laboratory as 'the modern speculator', this critic clearly identified the

[50] Fye, *Development of American Physiology*, pp. 1 and 3. On the shifting meaning of science in American medicine, see John Harley Warner, 'Science in medicine' in Sally Gregory Kohlstedt and Margaret W. Rossiter (eds), *Historical Writing on American Science: Perspectives and Prospects* (Baltimore, 1985), pp. 37–58.

[51] 'Wood's therapeutics', *Boston Medical and Surgical Journal*, 93 (1875), 645–6, at p. 646.

[52] Warner, *The Therapeutic Perspective*, pp. 235–83.

[53] T. C. M[inor], Review of 'Materia medica and therapeutics. By Roberts Bartholow', *Cincinnati Lancet and Observer*, 37 (1876), pp. 838–54, at p. 842.

new rationalists with the eighteenth- and early nineteenth-century builders of those rationalistic systems that half a century of empiricist crusading had endeavoured to banish from American medicine. 'The speculative medical experimentalist', like the speculative system builder, sought to ground medical knowledge upon an unsound foundation. The perceived danger was that faith in the laboratory could undermine the gains of the empiricist revolution in medical epistemology, and that, as a consequence, the quality of medical practice would suffer and the profession would lose the claim to authority it had found in an allegiance to empiricism.

There can be no doubt, of course, that the division between strident empiricists and strident proselytisers of laboratory medicine tended to follow generational lines. In the polemical exchanges that flourished from the 1870s to the 1890s, often older French-trained American physicians argued with their younger German-trained counterparts. Those who urged laboratory medicine often aspired to careers in a new kind of American academic medicine they sought to pattern after the German style. In order to occupy posts in medical schools as laboratory researchers and instructors, they first had to lobby for their creation.[54] Those who opposed the claims made for the laboratory, on the other hand, often were those who had consecrated their careers to fighting at the empiricist barricade against 'the spirit of system', and who saw in laboratory medicine an insidious source of subversion within orthodox ranks. As these older physicians retired from their teaching posts, climbed down from positions of leadership in medical societies and turned the editorship of journals over to younger hands, the energetic opposition to the laboratory they had voiced faded.

However, this cannot simply be reduced to a clash between young progressives who for the first time were exposed to laboratory medicine and old reactionaries still confined within the mental world of the clinic. The experimental laboratory in such areas as chemistry and physiology was far from new to western medicine in the final third of the nineteenth century. Changes within science and medicine alone are insufficient to account for the new allegiance some American physicians pledged to the laboratory or for the significance for the medical profession they attached to it. What needs to be explained is what permitted Americans to engage in a new kind of discourse about the laboratory that had been scarcely possible in the antebellum period.

[54] See Fye, *Development of American Physiology*; Kohler, *From Medical Chemistry to Biochemistry*; and Ludmerer, *Learning to Heal*.

Sociologist Paul Starr has suggested that the new and compelling claims to authority the American medical profession made in the name of laboratory science can be understood as 'the renewal of legitimate complexity'. As 'the American faith in democratic simplicity and common sense yielded to a celebration of science and efficiency', doctors were able to claim a new measure of cultural authority over a public impressed by the achievements of laboratory medicine and ready to accept that it was complex beyond their mastery.[55] 'The renewal of legitimate complexity' is a phrase that very aptly describes in part what happened in the long run. But it does not aid our historical understanding of why American doctors began *when they did* to claim a new measure of authority on the basis of laboratory medicine. To begin with, Starr's account requires certain positivist assumptions that are unnecessary to historical explanation. It was not, as he argues, the development of science itself that 'broke the confidence' of the American public in their earlier conviction that 'the seeming complexity of medicine was artificial' and that 'medicine could be brought within reach of "common sense"'.[56] For their part, doctors did not need the laboratory to persuade themselves that they had an effective, scientific medicine. This they had throughout the nineteenth century, and it was only the notion of what constituted scientific medicine that changed. More than this, the timing of Starr's account is off. He situates the restoration of legitimate complexity in the changes of the Progressive Era, the period from the 1890s to the early twentieth century when, in the wake of what he regards as the evident triumphs of germ theory, laboratory medicine came to be prominently institutionalised and the profession's legal position and social status were greatly elevated. In fact, though, to understand what enabled these turn-of-the-century changes we must start by understanding why some doctors could first begin to see in the laboratory a new and powerful source of authority; we must, that is, look to earlier shifts in assumptions about the relationship between knowledge and authority.

What permitted a new kind of discourse about the laboratory to emerge when it did was in part a shift in attitudes towards the place of knowledge in American society that started to become evident as early as the 1870s and 1880s. Popular insistence that all knowledge

[55] Paul Starr, *The Social Transformation of American Medicine* (New York, 1982), p. 140.
[56] *Ibid.*, p. 59.

worth knowing should be within the command of the common man and woman waned during the postbellum decades, as did the assault upon those who claimed special knowledge and ways of knowing. The socio-political forces that had helped give empiricism its special meaning in antebellum America diminished, and, accordingly, so too did the symbolic power of empiricism itself. 'Americans after 1870', Burton Bledstein has noted, 'committed themselves to a culture of professionalism.'[57] The command of specialised knowledge unfathomable to the public at large was one attribute of the new professional ideal that began to take shape. 'In contrast to the empiricists, the professional person grasped the concept behind a functional activity, allowing him both to perceive and to predict those inconspicuous or unseen variables which determined the entire system of developments', Bledstein explains. 'The professional penetrated beyond the rich confusion of ordinary experiences, as he isolated and controlled the factors, hidden to the untrained eye, which made an elaborate system workable or impracticable, successful or unattainable.'[58] Bureaucratic organisation and specialised compartmentalisation of work became increasingly prominent in postbellum society, as in the efforts to attain efficiency through expertise in civil service reform and scientific charity work. In fields ranging from engineering to forestry, professional associations proliferated, giving members a distinctive badge of their special knowledge. The multiplication of institutions for higher education during these decades was but one sign of the elevated value assigned by some to specialised knowledge and advanced learning. Americans – especially in the growing new middle class – came more and more to acknowledge the intellectual and social propriety of specialisation. So too, there was an increasing willingness on the part of some to recognise the worth of specialised professional knowledge beyond their ken. The inner workings of this knowledge, its production and its assessment might remain mysterious to most Americans, but it won for those who showed evidence of mastery over it some measure of both esteem and authority.[59]

[57] Burton J. Bledstein, *The Culture of Professionalism: The Middle Class and the Development of Higher Education in America* (New York, 1976), p. 80. [58] *Ibid.*, pp. 88–9.

[59] On changing American attitudes towards special knowledge in the Gilded Age and Progressive Era, see George M. Fredrickson, *The Inner Civil War: Northern Intellectuals and the Crisis of Union* (New York, 1965), esp. pp. 183ff.; Richard Hofstadter, *The Age of Reform: From Bryan to F.D.R.* (New York, 1955); Richard Hofstadter, *Anti-Intellectualism in American Life* (New York, 1962); Morton Keller, *Affairs of State: Public Life in Late Nineteenth Century America* (Cambridge, Mass., 1977); Alexandra Oleson and John Voss (eds), *The Organization of Knowledge in Modern America, 1860–1920* (Baltimore, 1979); Charles E. Rosenberg, *No Other Gods: On Science and American Social Thought*

This gradual change in American culture by no means caused the medical profession to embrace laboratory medicine, but it did permit some American physicians to engage in a new kind of discourse about the relationship between epistemology and authority. A growing valuation of special knowledge that might not be accessible to all Americans gave the laboratory heightened cultural legitimacy in the final quarter of the nineteenth century, just as a different climate had given empiricism such forceful and special cultural meaning in the antebellum period. It was within this context that some physicians began to celebrate the promise of the laboratory for bringing about a thoroughgoing cognitive and social transformation of their profession.

In order for the medical profession to come to regard the laboratory as the wellspring of a new claim to authority, not just one supplementary source of scientific information, doctors needed to persuade themselves that the particular kind of knowledge produced in the laboratory – a special knowledge removed from the experience of most practitioners and their workaday routines at the bedside – could serve as a solid basis for authority that did not jeopardise medical integrity. This step demanded fundamental transformations in professional thinking. What broader cultural changes gave physicians was not just a society newly receptive to claims to authority based on special knowledge, but also a framework within which to sort out and define a new kind of professional meaning for the laboratory.

Some did come to accept the idea that laboratory knowledge could serve as a source of authority and status for their profession, a step enabled and encouraged by the broader shifts in American attitudes towards knowledge. Gerald Geison has suggested that from the late nineteenth century onwards, 'the experimental sciences, like Latin in an earlier era, have given medicine a new and now culturally compelling basis for consolidating its status as an autonomous "learned profession", with all the corporate and material advantages that such status implies'.[60] As esteem increased for the special learning science represented, claims to scientific expertise offered a promising source of status. S. E. D. Shortt, too, has drawn attention to the extent to which physicians uplifted their profession's status by using

(Baltimore, 1976), esp. pp. 135–72; Laurence R. Veysey, *The Emergence of the American University* (Chicago, 1965); and Robert H. Wiebe, *The Search for Order, 1877–1920* (New York, 1967).

[60] Geison, 'Divided we stand', p. 85.

'not the content but the rhetoric of science'.[61] He has urged that 'by forcing the rhetoric of science into the social vocabulary of the period, physicians secured a vehicle for their professional recognition'.[62] This is an important and apt description of what happened, yet at best a partial explanation of why. Broader changes in attitudes towards knowledge did not simply give the medical profession an excuse for coming up with arcane learning that would sustain new claims to elite, expert status. Locating the shifting intellectual allegiances of physicians solely in the market-place – urging that cultural change created an opportunity some shrewd doctors grabbed – fails to take seriously the intense debates about medical epistemology that practising physicians engaged in during the final decades of the nineteenth century.

Those who sought to ground professional authority in the laboratory had first to come to terms with the underlying shift in professional identity it implied, from a primary rooting in practice to one in special knowledge. And this involved fundamental alterations in their understanding of the relationship between science and professional identity, and between science and professional morality. The fine texture of their deliberations must be explored elsewhere.[63] What is important to recognise here is that those practising physicians who embraced an ideal of laboratory science found the justification for their programme not in science itself, but in the promise of science to direct clinical action. To the extent to which the avowed foundation of professional identity shifted, it was premised on a new conceptualisation of the relationship between science and practice. Those who looked to the laboratory pinned their hopes on an image of the physician as an expert in natural science in a measure new in nineteenth-century America, and claimed an accountability to science

[61] Shortt, 'Physicians, science, and status', p. 43. But also see Christopher Lawrence, 'Incommunicable knowledge: science, technology and the clinical art in Britain 1850–1914', *Journal of Contemporary History*, 20 (1985), 503–20, which provides an alternative perspective, yet to be explored for the American context.

[62] Shortt, 'Physicians, science, and status', p. 62.

[63] See Barbara Gutmann Rosenkrantz, 'The search for professional order in 19th-century American medicine' in Ronald L. Numbers and Judith Walzer Leavitt (eds), *Sickness and Health in America: Readings in the History of Medicine and Public Health* (Madison, Wis., 1985), pp. 219–32, and an earlier version of this article (bearing the same title but sufficiently different to demand attention as well), in *Proceedings of the XIVth International Congress of the History of Science* (Tokyo, 1975), vol. IV, pp. 113–24; John Harley Warner, 'Ideals of science and their discontents in late nineteenth-century American medicine', *Isis*, 82 (1991), pp. 454–78, and Warner, *The Therapeutic Perspective*, pp. 258–83. And on the structure of these relationships at mid century, see Martin S. Pernick, *A Calculus of Suffering: Pain, Professionalism, and Anesthesia in Nineteeth-Century America* (New York, 1985).

as the chief sanction for their actions. Like their critics committed to clinical empiricism they maintained that the physician was more than just a natural scientist, but they accorded to science a different place in the fulfilment of that further role. They partly shed the notion that the regular physician's identity and integrity were best guaranteed by interactions with patients and other practitioners in accordance with shared traditional values. Instead, they claimed an allegiance to science and its power to guide effective intervention as the ethical sanction for their programme and the foundation for their definition as physicians.

This assumption that faith in science would be the best guarantee of medical practice and progress alike underlay the shift in claims to professional authority from a grounding in experience towards one in expertise. It increasingly enabled physicians to claim special knowledge as the core of their professional identity, with the assurance that from good science, good practice would follow. Privileged access to knowledge in the laboratory became an especially powerful basis for claiming this authority. For Americans trained in medicine during the postbellum decades, it was increasingly possible to take up reasoning – from the laboratory to the bedside – as an ideal, while the commitment to empiricism of earlier decades lost both its cultural force and professional significance.

What physicians actually gained from their new allegiance to laboratory medicine before the 1890s was principally a growing power to explain the processes of disease and therapy. For the first generation who gave over their hearts and minds to the ways of the laboratory, it was a source of deep frustration that no potent symbol of the therapeutic fruitfulness of basic laboratory science appeared quickly, such as later would come with diphtheria antitoxin, salvarsan or the antibiotics.[64]

But there were reasons for medical practitioners to embrace experimental science as a channel for medical progress other than the cultural authority and status it promised. Certainly the medical relevance of the laboratory was proselytised most vigorously by aspiring academics who sought to create teaching and research posts that would enable them to pursue scientific work as a career. Intellectual fascination with science and career goals combined in fuelling their rhetoric. But practising physicians too had some reason to believe the laboratory might be able to deliver the goods promised

[64] Warner, *The Therapeutic Perspective*, pp. 258–82.

them as well. Newly used therapies arguably generated by experimental research were few, true; but perhaps as important, during the 1870s and 1880s, some of them, notably chloral hydrate and the salicylates, became extraordinarily prominent in actual practice. Physicians were also aware of the growing power of experimental science to explain the processes of the body in health and disease. Clinicians recognised the rapid advancement of the basic sciences; and some pointed to the fact that in experimentation, physiological processes, for example, were manipulated, not just passively observed, as support for their conviction that experimental medicine would bring therapeutic control of pathophysiological processes. Further, starting as early as the 1850s, but intensifying during the 1860s and 1870s, there was growing pessimism among American doctors about the future promise of the empiricist programme: it had successfully demolished the past errors of rationalistic systems, but had offered frustratingly little new to replace them. Even some who had been activists in the empiricist cause began to voice concern that its fruitfulness was exhausted. By the 1880s, laboratory science offered virtually the only plan on the market for which rapid clinical progress was promised, the only course that a young practitioner could enter into with exuberant optimism. The promise that laboratory science would transform medical practice rested, for a time, largely on optimistic faith, but that faith was not entirely blind.[65]

Increased authority based on a commitment to laboratory science did not wait on its demonstrated yield, however. From the final quarter of the nineteenth century and even more so during the Progressive Era – a period of faith in the authority of educated, expert elites – the command of laboratory science did serve as an effective platform for uplifting the American medical profession. Laboratory training became a hallmark of progressive – and increasingly exclusive – medical education, and institutional changes gave the laboratory a place of prominence in American medical schools. Further, by re-enacting medical licensing laws, the states gave legal recognition to the special authority physicians claimed by merit of their expert knowledge.[66] The public placed its faith in scientific

[65] John Harley Warner, 'From specificity to universalism in medical therapeutics: transformation in the nineteenth-century United States', in Yosio Kawakita *et al.* (eds), *History of Therapy* (Tokyo, 1990).

[66] On the transformation of the profession, see Ronald L. Numbers, 'The fall and rise of the American medical profession' in Numbers and Leavitt, (eds), *Sickness and Health*, pp. 185–96; George Rosen, *The Structure of American Medical Practice, 1875–1941*, ed. Charles E. Rosenberg (Philadelphia, 1983); Charles E. Rosenberg, *The Care of Strangers: The Rise*

knowledge as authoritative in itself, and largely relinquished earlier claims to comprehend that knowledge or the processes by which it was produced and validated by professionals.[67]

Advocates of the laboratory in the late nineteenth century saw it, of course, as a force in medicine for replacing speculation with fact, impressions with an exact method, superstition with positive knowledge. They regarded it as an instrument for dispelling mystery. Experiments were a more rigorous form of experience; nature's secrets were disclosed in the laboratory as they had been at the bedside, with perhaps even greater precision. The intriguing suggestion has even been made recently that in selectively importing German laboratory ways into American medicine, American exponents of the laboratory sought to 'democratise' it by, for example, the mass production of physiological apparatus for use in instructing medical students. 'In their cheaper, durable, quantity-produced forms', according to this argument, 'scientific instruments became symbolic of American anti-elitism. The laboratory itself became "democratized;" since students now had their own instruments, they could experience for themselves the relations between techniques and concepts in scientific research.'[68] The laboratory was a force to lay medicine open.

But viewed not in contrast to Europe but in comparison with earlier decades in America, it is unmistakable that the laboratory functioned as a force for elitism. The shift of laboratory medicine from Germany to America may well have involved democratisation, but the move within American medicine from the antebellum preoccupation with empirical observation to laboratory medicine later in the century most certainly went in the opposite direction. The laboratory provided the material and cognitive basis for an elitist epistemology and a regrounding of medicine on a decidedly privileged body of knowledge

of America's Hospital System (New York, 1987); and Starr, *Social Transformation*, pp. 79–144.

[67] See John C. Burnham, *How Superstition Won and Science Lost: Popularizing Science and Health in the United States* (New Brunswick, N.J., 1987).

[68] Merriley Borell, Deborah J. Coon, H. Hughes Evans, and Gail A. Hornstein, 'Selective importation of the "exact method": experimental physiology and psychology in the United States, 1860–1910', in Numbers and Pickstone (compilers), *Programs, Papers, and Abstracts*, pp. 189–96, at p. 193; and see Merriley Borell, 'Instruments and independent physiology: the Harvard Physiology Laboratory, 1871–1906', in Geison (ed.), *Physiology in the American Context*, pp. 293–321. The important insight of Borell *et al.* into the ways the experimental laboratory was recast in its transit from Europe to America merits close exploration.

accessible to only a small proportion of Americans. It entailed privileged knowledge rooted in a privileged epistemology that to most patients made medical knowledge increasingly a mystery. While Americans at large might revere its products and those who commanded them, most were more and more removed from the processes by which medical knowledge was produced.

Certainly American medicine in the nineteenth century broadly followed European trends – the general shifts that characterised western medicine as a whole. Yet it is clear from the finer structure of American patterns that change often took place according to a different timetable and sometimes had substantially different meanings in the American context. Just as French medical influence interacted with a democratic ethos in antebellum America to elevate empiricism to its eminent position, so later in the century the European example and changing attitudes toward knowledge in American culture operated together in the emergence of laboratory medicine. The socio-political climate of antebellum America gave an ideal of empiricism an especially powerful meaning to the regular medical profession. It also redoubled the animus against all trappings of mystification in medicine. This inclined regular physicians to oppose anything bearing the scent of rationalism, and may have made them especially and more persistently resistant to claims made for the medical relevance of laboratory knowledge. During the postbellum decades, however, with changing American attitudes towards knowledge in general and specialised epistemologies in particular, some regular physicians were able to embrace the laboratory as a font of precisely the kinds of special knowledge and special ways of knowing that would set professional knowledge apart from that of the lay community and bring to the medical profession rich rewards in terms of authority, status, economic security and clinical power. The mystification of medical knowledge, if not held up as an ideal, was accepted as a necessary attendant of intellectually and socially desirable change. The acceptance of this new ethos involved fundamental alterations not only in public expectations of the medical profession, but also in doctors' perceptions of their science and art. It was out of these shifting nineteenth-century popular and professional conceptions of the relationship between epistemology and authority that laboratory medicine came to be elevated to its position of hegemony in the Progressive Era – came, that is, to be a central feature in the blueprint for an elitist reconstruction of American medicine drawn by such reformers as Abraham Flexner.

4

Anaesthetics, ethics and aesthetics

Vivisection in the late nineteenth-century British laboratory

STEWART RICHARDS

Introduction

As a part of its centennial celebrations in 1976, the Physiological Society organised at its July meeting in Cambridge a number of historical exhibitions and demonstrations in the Wren Library of Trinity College and in the Physiological Laboratory itself. It was an impressive occasion which successfully rekindled something of the aura of the late nineteenth and early twentieth-century laboratory, providing for the historically minded practitioner a unique opportunity to empathise with British physiology during the period of its metamorphosis from a secondary branch of anatomy to an experimental school of pre-eminent reputation. The atmosphere was peculiar to that of the physiological laboratory. Thus, in celebrating the classical experiments it was necessary to display, and to maintain for several hours, some elaborate whole-animal preparations and complex mechanical instrumentation (see Fig. 1) in such a way as to raise a number of prima facie questions about the morality of its means. To most late twentieth-century observers the initial doubts were quickly allayed by the utilitarian ends such methods had, in the event, served; and also, of course, by the realisation that the application of modern anaesthetic techniques ensured that no pain was experienced by the animals employed. Any uneasiness that persisted was then attributable only to sensory impressions – not the

Acknowledgements: I am grateful to Maurice Crosland for helpful suggestions on an earlier version of this paper, to discussants at the Cambridge conference and, in particular, to the Editors, Andrew Cunningham and Perry Williams. Thanks are also due to the archivists at the Wellcome Institute for the History of Medicine in London, and at the University and the National Library of Scotland in Edinburgh, for permission to consult unpublished material in their care and to make quotations where appropriate. The work was supported by a grant from the Royal Society for research in the history of science.

least of which, on a stifling day during a long hot summer, were olfactory – that amounted to a feeling of revulsion, perhaps akin to that of many individuals (not opposed on moral grounds to therapeutic surgery or to the killing of animals for food) in relation to the operating theatre or the abattoir.

Subsequent reflection upon this experience suggested its relevance to the historical analysis of experimental physiology by the singular insights it provided into the minds both of the physiologists and of their antivivisectionist opponents. Indeed, it is because the practices of physiologists were perceived in the late nineteenth century as highly controversial that we are obliged, in attempting to understand them in the context of history, to consider both ethical and aesthetic factors as indispensable for the construction of any but a partial account. In this sense the science of physiology is emphatically more complex than such reductionist models as 'organic physics' or 'animal chemistry' might imply. A somewhat different, somewhat 'committed', historiography is therefore necessary if we are to gain an appreciation more representative of its essential nature than the naive and positivistic accounts of most historians and scientists would suggest. Empathetic exposure to the peculiar atmosphere of the physiological laboratory, while not in itself sufficient, is nevertheless a necessary condition for the reconstruction of historical authenticity.[1]

This chapter attempts to bridge the divide between the pro-physiologist and anti-vivisectionist positions by examining the very site of their struggle, namely the laboratory itself, and the ethical and aesthetic character of the activities there pursued. Its essential conclusion is that whilst many of the attacks by antivivisectionists were emotive misrepresentations, the simple displacement and utilitarian arguments offered by the physiologists failed to deflect the

[1] In my paper, 'Drawing the life-blood of physiology: vivisection and the physiologists' dilemma, 1870–1900', *Annals of Science*, 43 (1986), pp. 27–56, I have explored these questions more fully and offered a more detailed defence of my historiographical perspective. An example of the conventional approach, taken from the *Proceedings of the Physiological Society* for its centennial meeting, is to be found in two articles on nineteenth-century physiology by an eminent modern physiologist. We are told that George Hoggan's famous letter (written to the *Morning Post* of 2 February 1875) gave 'the most lurid and horrifying descriptions of his period as an assistant in Bernard's laboratory', yet when Bernard's own experimental notebooks are discussed there is no mention of the cruelty of his methods or of the moral dilemmas they raised. These aspects are conveniently segregated, and we are informed simply that 'Bernard exorcised the chimera of vital force and the capriciousness of nature from physiology and replaced them by determinism – the theory that vital processes are determined by physicochemical conditions'. See J. T. Fitzsimons, 'Physiology during the nineteenth century' and 'The experimental notebooks of Claude Bernard', *Journal of Physiology*, 263 (1976), 16P–25P, at 25P, and 37P–41P, at 40P.

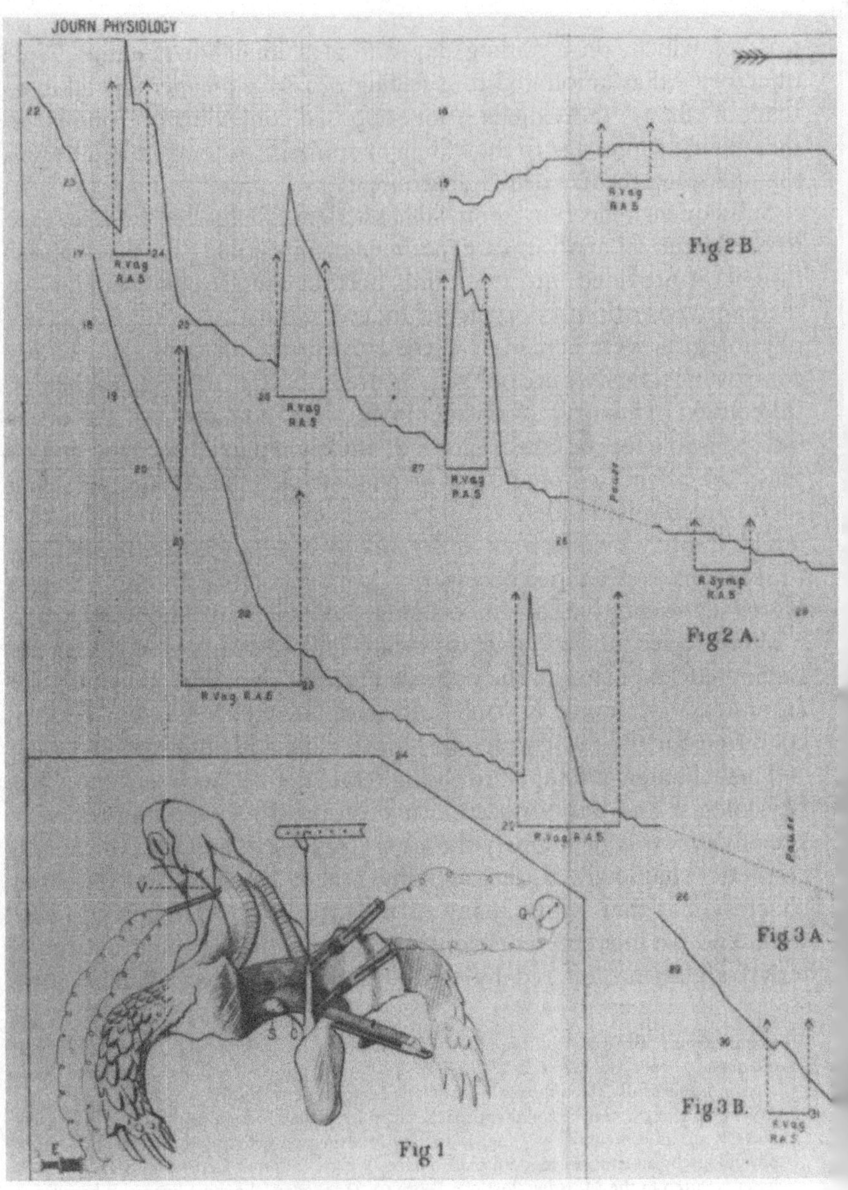

Fig. 1. An experimental demonstration first conducted in 1887 by W. H. Gaskell, and reconstructed as part of the Centenary Celebrations of the Physiological Society in 1976. The box shows the experimental set-up, in which a tortoise has electrical stimulation applied to its vagus nerve. The main diagram shows the results of the demonstration: a kymograph trace, taken from the galvanometer attached to the quiescent muscle of the heart. (See *Journal of Physiology*, 263 (1976), pp. 60P–63P.)

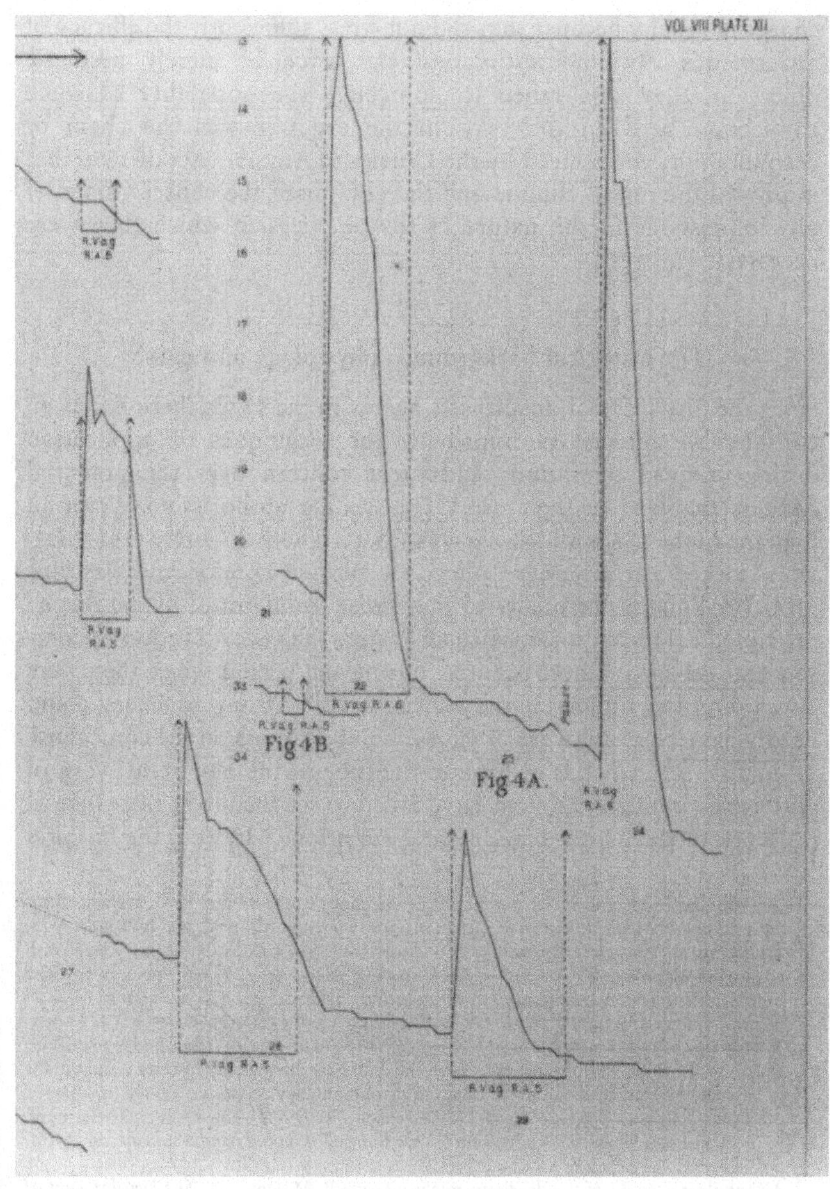
VOL VIII PLATE XIII
Fig 4B.
Fig 4A.

charge of cruelty because they did not stress sufficiently the efficacy of anaesthetics. By underestimating the force of merely aesthetic objection, they also failed to appreciate the possibility of some connection between the two. In the event it was the chain of accountability introduced by the Cruelty to Animals Act of 1876 that improved the moral climate and thereby raised the consciousness of physiologists as to the nature of the practices in which they were necessarily engaged.

The historical background: physiology and pain[2]

Since the discovery of anaesthetic agents in the 1840s there had been considerable interest in improving the techniques of application during surgical operations and great concern over the potential dangers involved in their use.[3] The leading authority in Victorian England in the 1860s and 1870s was Joseph Thomas Clover (1825–82), who worked at University College Hospital in London and was thus probably known personally to the 'great triumvirate' of the British physiological renaissance, Michael Foster, John Scott Burdon-Sanderson and Edward Albert Schäfer, during the period when they were developing the subject at the college itself.[4] At any rate they could hardly have been unaware of Clover's publications on the clinical use of volatile anaesthetics at around the time of the first great wave of antivivisectionist fervour, or have failed to see the direct relevance of his work to their own experimental ambitions.[5] Indeed, the hospital

[2] The standard references on the British vivisection question are R. D. French, *Antivivisection and Medical Science in Victorian Society* (Princeton, 1976), and N. Rupke (ed.), *Vivisection in Historical Perspective* (London, 1987). See also M. N. Ozer, 'The British vivisection controversy', *Bulletin of the History of Medicine*, 40 (1966), pp. 158–67. The movement's influence on the growth of physiology is discussed in G. L. Geison, *Michael Foster and the Cambridge School of Physiology* (Princeton, 1978), esp. chapter 2; J. Turner, *Reckoning with the Beast: Pain and Humanity in the Victorian Mind* (Baltimore, 1980), esp. chapter 6; L. G. Stevenson, 'Science down the drain: on the hostility of certain sanitarians to animal experimentation, bacteriology and immunology', *Bulletin of the History of Medicine*, 29 (1955), pp. 1–26; and L. G. Stevenson, 'Religious elements in the background to the British antivivisection movement', *Yale Journal of Biology and Medicine*, 29 (1956), pp. 125–57.

[3] An excellent account of the developments is given in B. M. Duncum, *The Development of Inhalation Anaesthesia, with Special Reference to the Years 1846–1900* (London, 1947).

[4] Geison, *Michael Foster*, p. 6. On Clover, see Duncum, *Inhalation Anaesthesia*, esp. p. 459, and R. K. Calverley, 'J. T. Clover: a giant of Victorian anaesthesia' in J. Ruprecht, M. J. van Lieburg, J. A. Lee and W. Erdmann (eds), *Anaesthesia: Essays in its History* (Berlin, 1985), pp. 18–23.

[5] See, for example, *Lancet* (1868, 1), p. 231; *British Medical Journal* (1876, 2), pp. 74–5; *British Medical Journal* (1877, 1), pp. 69–70.

had for many years been a centre for interest in anaesthetics, ether having been first used there in December 1846 (when the young Clover was present), while John Snow (1813–58) – who had carried out many pioneering experiments on animals, and enjoyed the distinction of having twice administered chloroform to Queen Victoria in the 1850s – served there as the first Specialist Anaesthetist. Dudley Wilmot Buxton (1855–1931) also specialised in anaesthesia there from 1885, publishing his important and successful textbook *Anaesthetics: Their Uses and Administration* three years later.[6]

There can be no doubt that the introduction of anaesthetics was to be as important for physiology as it was for surgery, a factor which renders all the more surprising the delay of a quarter of a century before their availability encouraged the growth of the new experimental school.[7] By minimising extraneous variables associated with the reactions to pain, anaesthetics made practicable a host of experiments that hitherto had been no more than theoretical ideals, and by overcoming a major part of the ethical problem they made such experiments acceptable. As Cranefield puts it, 'there can be no doubt that people who [would] otherwise have shunned experimental physiology... were led to take it up because it no longer required the use of surgical procedures in the absence of anaesthetics'.[8]

Not that many did so. Before 1870 experimental physiology was a very minor activity indeed and, to make matters worse, the tiny community of enthusiasts soon found themselves at the centre of a vociferous campaign of vilification that sought to expose the supposedly unsatisfactory condition of their private morals and public accountability. Were anaesthetics really used, the antivivisectionists wanted to know, and, if so, were they used effectively? The intensity of the debate reached two notable peaks, the first during the events leading to the Royal Commission on animal experiments and the resulting Cruelty to Animals Act of 1876, and the second just after the meeting of the Seventh International Medical Congress (IMC) in London in 1881.[9] In the first instance the antivivisectionists were clearly in the ascendant, the physiologists unsure and anxiously defensive. When, by the imminent passage of the Act, their freedom to experiment was to be restricted to that gaining the approval of the

[6] Duncum, *Inhalation Anaesthesia*, pp. frontispiece, 17–21, 132–4, 161–5 and 464–73.

[7] The reasons for this delay have been discussed by Geison, *Michael Foster*, pp. 13–47.

[8] P. F. Cranefield, *The Way In and the Way Out: François Magendie, Charles Bell and the Roots of the Spinal Nerves* (New York, 1974), p. 54.

[9] See N. Rupke, 'Pro-vivisection in England in the early 1880s: arguments and motives' in Rupke (ed.), *Vivisection*, pp. 188–208.

Home Secretary, so that they would 'sigh in...bondage' and be 'liable at any moment...to be arrested by legal prohibition',[10] their response was to establish the Physiological Society of Great Britain in an attempt to represent the interests of a *new* physiology that necessarily demanded experiments, some of which might cause pain, but all of which were justified by their potential consequences for clinical practice.

But it was to be another five years before an efficient campaign of self-defence was organised by the scientists, a campaign that was launched with the unanimous support of the IMC and the British Medical Association (BMA) and quickly became a standard-bearer in the wider movement concerned to propagate the prestige and authority, not merely of scientific medicine, but of science itself. Yet even with such formidable allies – or perhaps because their support rendered any more sophisticated arguments unnecessary – the physiologists clung only to a crude utilitarianism which emphasised how much more was the suffering inflicted for such trivial purposes as fashion, diet or sport than that caused in the laboratory in the pursuit of new knowledge or medical advance. 'If the former are justifiable, the latter must be so',[11] they seemed satisfied to conclude, no attempt being made to probe the conditional proposition more deeply or, what would have been more profitable, to defend their own activities by reference not to others yet more dubious, but rather in terms of the anaesthetic precautions which could largely defuse the moral debate.

The use of anaesthetics prior to 1876

By far the most comprehensive 'official' source of evidence on the employment of anaesthetics in experimental physiology at this time was the Royal Commission, first announced by the Home Secretary, Richard Cross, in May 1875. It is not necessary here for us to examine this evidence in detail, although that given by John Colam, Secretary of the Royal Society for the Prevention of Cruelty to Animals (RSPCA), and a fierce opponent of painful experiments, must be mentioned as the most important. His society had adopted the moderate position – very helpful to the Commissioners in their

10 M. Foster, Inaugural Address to the Physiology Section of the International Medical Congress, in *Transactions of the International Medical Congress, Seventh Session*, 4 vols. (London, 1881), vol. I, p. 218.

11 G. Gore, *The Utility and Morality of Vivisection* (London, 1884), p. 20.

struggle to find a judicious balance between medical utility and humanitarian zeal – that experiments performed under anaesthesia were permissible on the ground that without pain there could be no cruelty and without cruelty there was no moral issue at stake. Colam was someone who could hardly be accused of bias towards physiology and had considerable experience of visiting laboratories, of witnessing experiments and, when not satisfied, even of employing the 'surveillance of detectives'. He affirmed that anaesthetics were generally used, that laboratory practices in England were 'very different indeed from [those] of foreign physiologists', and that he did not know 'of a single case of wanton cruelty'.[12] His evidence supported Foster's claim that British physiologists were substantially more 'tender' in their treatment of animals than their continental mentors, and the Commissioners' overall conclusion was that the situation in this country was broadly satisfactory.[13] After all, the physiologists, even before the emergence of significant antivivisectionist opposition, had themselves set out voluntary guidelines for responsible research. Anaesthetics, they had agreed, should always be used when possible and never omitted for purposes of teaching; new physiological truths should be sought only by experienced investigators in properly equipped laboratories; and living animals should never be used for veterinary teaching or for the mere pursuit of manual dexterity.[14]

But despite these persuasive reassurances, the Commissioners were sufficiently astute to realise that physiology 'from its very nature is liable to great abuse'. It could not be doubted, they said, that 'inhumanity may be found in persons of very high position as physiologists' (quoting the case of Magendie) and this was the reason why a society that could not possibly ban it altogether was obliged to subject it to legal monitoring and control.[15] This was a wise and important decision which transcended the recorded evidence in order to acknowledge not what things seemed to be but what they might conceivably become. Its cautionary note is borne out, moreover, in the shape of further evidence which, though contemporary, was not made available to the Commissioners. This was evidence suggestive of a certain credibility gap between the published reports of experiments and the experiments themselves, or between the 'demonstrations' arranged to reassure visitors (such as Colam) and other investigations

[12] *Report of the Royal Commission on the Practice of Subjecting Live Animals to Experiments for Scientific Purposes* (C 1397), *Parliamentary Papers* (hereafter *P.P.*) 1876, XLI, p. 277, Qs. 2410–14. [13] *Ibid.*, Qs. 2410–14.

[14] *Report of the British Association for the Advancement of Science* (*Edinburgh*) (London, 1872), p. 144. [15] *Royal Commission on ... Experiments*, p. xvii.

pursued behind closed doors. Thus, for example, the laboratory notebooks of William Rutherford (and William Vignal, his French collaborator) for 1875 show that he performed some forty-four experiments, mostly on dogs, without mention of anaesthesia but with frequent reference to curare, which was injected to paralyse the muscles (and hence provide reproducible control conditions for flow measurements from the cannulated bile duct); however, this was done in the full knowledge that it did not produce insensibility.[16] Before the Royal Commission, Rutherford stated that a similar number of animals had been used during the previous year, but claimed that about half of his research experiments were performed on animals rendered insensible. However, when asked if he kept a record of all his experiments, he could answer only, 'Most of them, not all', so that one member of the Commission felt that in his work 'there was evidence of very great abuse and of serious cruelty'.[17] With the introduction of the 1876 Act, this at least would have had to change.

Rutherford was one of that new generation of British physiologists keen to exploit the new career opportunities by building a reputation on the basis of technical training received on the Continent. His Edinburgh mentor John Hughes Bennett had established in 1862–3 a 'school of Practical Physiology' for medical students, but it was Rutherford himself who introduced the first genuine experimental course.[18] Bennett, like William Sharpey, the University College mentor of Foster and Burdon-Sanderson, recognised the need for systematic experimentation upon living animals but was unwilling to do it himself, referring to the 'loathsome manipulations' (for biliary fistula) necessarily performed in the course of the investigations of his so-called Edinburgh Mercury Committee of the 1860s.[19] Again it was Rutherford who had carried out most of these operations and it was he who took the brunt of the criticism – especially in view of the fact that the experiments had been performed on dogs (the species guaranteed to elicit antivivisectionist abuse) and many were acknowledged to have been without anaesthetics, owing to their unacceptable influence on the rate of biliary secretion. So relentlessly

[16] W. Rutherford and W. Vignal, 'Researches on biliary secretion', vol. I, 1875. Edinburgh University Library, GEN 2007/11.

[17] *Royal Commission on... Experiments*, Qs. 2993, 2841 and 2885.

[18] *British Medical Journal* (1862, 2), pp. 162–71, esp. p. 163; *British Medical Journal* (1876, 2), p. 259; *Edinburgh University Calendar*, 1866–7, p. 74.

[19] J. H. Bennett, 'Report of the Edinburgh Committee on the action of mercury on the biliary secretions', *Report of the British Association for the Advancement of Science* (*Norwich*) (London, 1868), pp. 187–232.

was he attacked through a period of almost twenty years that the experience undoubtedly had a powerful adverse influence on his career.[20] Yet Rutherford was determined that his work was justified by its contribution to the 'scientific treatment of disease of the liver, and [that] while steadily pursuing this great object we have been most careful to avoid the infliction of all pain that was not absolutely necessary'.[21] Thus he admitted the charge of pain but not that of cruelty. Besides, he was convinced that none of his experiments entailed as much pain as that (unnecessarily) inflicted by the operation for castration 'constantly performed on horses and oxen' without anaesthetics, and which engendered no such outcry because, he suggested with wounded irony, it was *not* carried out in the name of science.[22]

Of Rutherford's contemporaries we know enough of Burdon-Sanderson to suggest an ethical position that was strikingly similar. Burdon-Sanderson was editor of the notorious *Handbook for the Physiological Laboratory* which, appearing in 1873, had encouraged the new generation of physiologists to employ vivisectional methods hitherto associated only with continental laboratories, and which had failed lamentably to spell out a coherent policy on anaesthesia.[23] One of the formative experiences of his life had been spent in what Claude Bernard himself described as his 'ghastly kitchen' and it remains for us to speculate with Shakespeare's physician Cornelius whether such practices as trying:

> the forces
> Of these thy compounds on such creatures as
> We count not worth the hanging (but none human),

had not 'ma[d]e hard [his] heart'.[24] At any rate, like Rutherford's, Burdon-Sanderson's notebooks indicate that prior to 1876 he experimented routinely on dogs (to investigate the circulatory effects of asphyxia), sometimes using curare, sometimes morphine, although this was evidently administered only after an animal had 'struggled

[20] See S. Richards, 'Conan Doyle's "Challenger" unchampioned: William Rutherford, FRS (1839–99), and the origins of practical physiology in Britain', *Notes and Records of the Royal Society*, 40 (1986), pp. 193–217, esp. 204–5.

[21] W. Rutherford, 'On the physiological action of drugs on the secretion of bile', *Transactions of the Royal Society of Edinburgh*, 29 (1880), pp. 133–264, at p. 261.

[22] *Scotsman*, 4 May 1885, p. 6.

[23] On the *Handbook* and its influence, see Richards, 'Drawing the life-blood', and S. Richards, 'Vicarious suffering, necessary pain: physiological method in late nineteenth-century Britain' in Rupke (ed.), *Vivisection*, pp. 125–48.

[24] C. Bernard, *An Introduction to the Study of Experimental Medicine*, trans. H. C. Green (New York, 1927; original French edition, 1865), p. 15; *Cymbeline*, I, vi.

much while it was being secured' on the table. In one instance he noted that the animal 'never... became insensible', and in another that 'before the usual operation [involving "two large incisions in each flank"] had been completed the effect passed off – and the animal was excited'.[25] These experiments would almost certainly not have been permitted under the Cruelty to Animals Act, and once it was on the statute book there is no evidence that Burdon-Sanderson attempted to perform any like them again.

The influence of the Cruelty to Animals Act 1876

There is thus some suggestion that for two leading physiologists of the day the effect of the Act, while it was hardly, as Foster claimed, 'to cripple physiological research in this country', must have been to alter somewhat the direction of its advance by at least requiring of its licensees a more considered and a more open appraisal of the criteria upon which the justification of experiments rested. The Act's basic condition was that anyone intending to perform experiments on living vertebrates was first required to submit to the Home Secretary an application for a licence, endorsed by a president of one of the leading scientific or medical bodies of the country and by a professor of medicine or a medical science. If granted, the licence would permit experiments *under anaesthesia* in registered places only, and subject to scrutiny by the Inspector appointed by the Home Secretary. It required renewal on an annual basis. Justification of experiments was to be in terms of the 'advancement by new discovery of physiological knowledge or of knowledge which will be useful for saving or prolonging life or alleviating suffering'. Experiments without anaesthesia, those which permitted recovery from the effects of anaesthesia, or which were performed as demonstrations to students or for the testing of previous discoveries, required in addition a certificate countersigned by an appropriate authority. Similar restrictions applied to *any* experiment on cats, dogs, horses, asses or mules.

In Rutherford's case it is difficult to know whether his own sensibilities were heightened by the Act's focusing on the problem of pain, but there appears to be little doubt that its effect was to change his laboratory practice in such a way as to reduce suffering. The official records show that his work continued to be controversial, for

[25] Sanderson's experimental notebooks of 1866–7 are in the National Library of Scotland at MS 20505/4/13/18.

he was refused certificates A and E (for experiments without anaesthesia, on dogs) in January 1877, gaining them only at the end of 1880 (though his work was not greatly impeded, for much of it was simply transferred to France).[26] Almost twenty years later he still retained an interest in the subject of bile secretion, although by then his technique had improved. Whereas the original method of temporary biliary fistula had, he admitted, 'implied production of pain', he could now implant a permanent fistula under anaesthesia and make his observations later (under certificates B and E) in conditions that would be painless.[27]

Of course, suggestive evidence relating to just two well-known physiologists is hardly sufficient to answer the important question as to whether introduction of the Cruelty to Animals Act changed, as well as reflected, attitudes to experiments. In our own day it has been shown that there is a significant difference in sensitivity between those biomedical scientists who expect to perform experiments on animals unhindered or subject only to informal 'codes of practice' (for example in the United States), and those who are accustomed to legal constraint (in the United Kingdom).[28] A century ago, evidence on this question was already publicly available in the shape of the annual returns to the Home Office of all individuals licenced to experiment under the Act. Gerald Yeo, Rutherford's successor as professor of physiology at King's College, London, used these figures for the years 1878–80 to estimate that appreciable pain had been caused to only sixteen animals (twelve by Rutherford himself) during this time. Putting it another way, he claimed that for each hundred experiments, seventy-five were absolutely painless by virtue of being performed under terminal anaesthesia; about twenty caused as much pain or discomfort as a vaccination (he said nothing of possible consequences of the material injected); four caused the pain associated with antiseptic healing of a wound (itself inflicted under anaesthesia); and, finally, about one in a hundred, where the use of anaesthetics was inadmissible, might cause 'pain equal to that accompanying an ordinary surgical operation on the human body...'.[29]

[26] French, *Antivivisection*, p. 187; and *British Medical Journal* (1877, 1), p. 79.

[27] Rutherford's application for the certificates, dated 7 April 1896, is in Edinburgh University Library at GEN. 2007/5.

[28] J. Hampson, 'Legislation: a practical solution to the vivisection dilemma?' in Rupke (ed.), *Vivisection*, pp. 314–39, esp. pp. 331–5.

[29] G. Yeo, 'The practice of vivisection in England', *Fortnightly Review*, 31 (1882), pp. 352–68, at p. 359. By this time, few 'ordinary' surgical operations were performed without anaesthesia.

Table 1. *Experiments performed in the years after the Cruelty to Animals Act 1876*

	Total number of expts[a]	No. potentially painful (certs. A & B)	No. causing pain[b]	Percentage of painful expts
1878	481[c]	117	40	8.3
1879	270	59	25	9.3
1880	311	114	47	15.1
1881	270	122	37	13.7
1882	406	259	30	7.4
1883	535	177	15	2.8
1884	441	221	16	3.6
1885	800	510	96	12.0
1886	1095	671	41	3.7
1887	1220	744	71	5.8
1888	1069	684	8	0.7
1889	1417	814	—	—
Totals	8315	4492	426	Mean 5.1

Notes:
[a] All of these were 'calculated to give pain' according to the terms of the Act, but those not accounted for under certificates A and B (second column) were required to be performed under anaesthesia, without recovery.
[b] In the majority of cases the pain caused was probably of a minor kind. Many of the animals were frogs.
[c] At least 200 of these were estimated by the Inspector 'scarcely to come within the scope of the Act at all'.
Source: Home Office Returns (annual).

Analysis of the published figures for the period from the first relevant Home Office return to the end of the 1880s gives the results summarised in Table 1. Overall, there was a steady rise in the number of experiments performed, although a large, but declining, proportion of these were taken to be painless because the animals were required, under the conditions of the licence alone, to be under anaesthesia throughout and killed before recovery. There was no reason, said the Inspector, to suppose that this condition was 'not in all cases carefully attended to'.[30] The remaining experiments, however, were potentially painful because they were performed under additional certificates which permitted work without anaesthesia (A) or recovery of consciousness after an operation requiring it (B). Whether they

[30] *Home Office Returns*, 1879, *P.P.* 1880, LVI, p. 627.

actually caused pain was not always easy to determine, nor do the Home Office data provide any relevant insights. All that we have are the assurances of the first Inspector, George Busk, FRS, FRCS (1876–86), a University College colleague of Burdon-Sanderson and Schäfer. He was an eminent individual in the medical and scientific circles of the time and, it seems, he was appointed by the Home Secretary essentially to represent their interests.[31] Busk would allow no doubts as to the painless nature of the licence-alone experiments, on the grounds of statements received from the operators themselves, and of their personal characters, of his own occasional observations, and of his consideration of the experiments' nature and probable effects. He accepted, that is, that anaesthetics were not only applied but applied effectively. His successor, John Eric Erichsen, FRS, FRCS (1886–96), a distinguished surgeon, professor of that discipline at University College and a 'moderate' member of the Royal Commission, confirmed Busk's view, saying that the licensees 'spare no trouble by the use of anaesthetics, and the employment of strict antiseptic precautions, to secure freedom from suffering in the animals experimented upon'.[32] This, implied Erichsen not unreasonably, must be obvious to anyone with an adequate understanding of physiological and related research and an unbiased willingness to evaluate its true nature.

> If anaesthetics are imperfectly or inadequately administered, so as to stop short of producing complete unconsciousness, the animal would become so excited and restless, as to render impossible the performance of any experiment requiring careful and delicate manipulation, for which purpose complete anaesthesia is an indispensable requisite. The experiments performed under the licence are always done in the laboratories or lecture theatres of large public institutions... often in the presence of many persons, and always in places readily accessible to anyone connected with the institution, who might wish to satisfy himself as to the completeness of the anaesthesia. We have accordingly the guarantees afforded by motives of humanity, considerations of convenience, and conditions of publicity for the complete anaesthisation of the animals as required by the Act.[33]

Busk had been adamant that in cases where anaesthetics were not used or where recovery was permitted afterwards, suffering was 'trifling', 'wholly insignificant' or 'of the most trivial nature'.[34] The

[31] French, *Antivivisection*, p. 179. For further information on Busk see the *Dictionary of National Biography*.

[32] French, *Antivivisection*, p. 96; *Home Office Returns*, 1888, *P.P.* 1889, LX, p. 666. On Erichsen, see the *Dictionary of National Biography*.

[33] *Home Office Returns*, 1889, *P.P.* 1890, LVIII, p. 505.

[34] *Home Office Returns*, 1882, *P.P.* 1883, LIV, p. 565; for 1881, *P.P.* 1882, LII, p. 706; and for 1883, *P.P.* 1884, LXII, p. 274.

great majority of such experiments involved nothing more than simple inoculation, with consequences either negligible or rapidly fatal; otherwise, such pain as was caused was typically that of inflammation associated with wound-healing, which was in any case always scrupulously minimised by the use of antiseptic precautions.

Busk does seem to have been conscientious in administering the Act, for when Schäfer suggested to him that simple inoculation experiments, being painless, should require neither licence nor certificate, he affirmed that the contrary had been determined by the law officers 'on the ground that the mere operation is only the beginning of what may prove to be a long and painful malady'.[35] Aware of the potentially distressing consequences of so simple an act, Erichsen, immediately upon coming to office, attached a special condition to the licence of all who performed these experiments to the effect that, after the main result had been attained, an animal that was in pain was to be killed at once under anaesthesia.[36] Although this well-advertised and welcome condition, together with Busk's blanket statements, may have had the effect of stifling details of those few experiments that did cause acute pain or prolonged suffering, it seems that on the whole the Inspectors' position was more accurate than that of the antivivisectionists who attacked them.[37] We do, moreover, have some more specific evidence of how they implemented their responsibilities in relation to the work of their colleague, Schäfer, at University College.

Schäfer's licence, the third to be issued, was signed by Richard Cross on 24 October 1876. On 2 January 1877 Busk wrote to him pointing out that he (Busk) was required under the Act to visit all registered places; he requested a list of dates and times of when Schäfer planned to be experimenting.[38] Unfortunately we do not know whether he then made a specific appointment or was in the habit of visiting unannounced, as would have been more in the spirit of the Act. However, the conditions attached to the licence certainly do not give the impression of lackadaisical administration. Schäfer's experimental work was confined to certain named rooms in University College and he was warned that if granted a certificate exempting him from the use of anaesthetics there would be other 'such conditions as

[35] Busk to Schäfer, 16 November 1885. Contemporary Medical Archives Centre, Wellcome Institute for the History of Medicine, London, ESS/B27/13.

[36] *Home Office Returns*, 1886, *P.P.* 1887, LXVI, p. 402.

[37] See, for example, *Zoophilist*, 6 (1886), pp. 4–5, and F. P. Cobbe and B. Bryan, *The Vivisection Returns, 1884: An Inquiry into their Value* (London, 1884), p. 5.

[38] Busk to Schäfer, 2 January 1877. Wellcome Institute, London, ESS/B27/10.

the Secretary of State may hereafter think fit to press'. Thus when the licence was extended in December 1877, and thereafter, Schäfer was restricted to twenty experiments a year under certificate B. After October 1881 he was further required to report to the Inspector after only six such experiments, or earlier if the inquiry had been completed; but this was relaxed in 1884 to a report after each ten, with a maximum of fifty a year. In March 1887 Erichsen added the 'pain condition' mentioned above, although the exact wording states that the animal was to be killed only if 'severe pain has been induced'.[39]

This vigilant regulation of Schäfer's activities was perhaps just as well for he was engaged in controversial ablation and lesion experiments (involving several different organs) much loathed by the antivivisectionists and employing the use of dogs and cats which, he said, 'bear such operations better than rodents'. In the mid-1880s he undertook, in collaboration with Victor Horsley, a long series of such experiments on no less than seventy-six monkeys. These required removal of part of the skull, acute observations on the effects of stimulating various brain loci with induction shocks and subsequent removal of large parts of the brain. This was followed by stitching and repair of the dura mater, bone and integument, and antiseptic dressing. Of course, the whole procedure was performed under anaesthesia (ether), and many of the animals recovered well, suffering from various forms of paralysis and ataxia but evidently not from pain. Survival times varied from a few hours to weeks or months, a few monkeys having to be killed owing to sickness.[40]

The after-effects of many of Schäfer's operations must have caused substantial distress, even if not actual pain, yet they were perfectly permissible under the licence and certificate B, and obviously regarded as of great clinical interest. In 1898 he received a warning letter from the Home Office noting that he had exceeded by three the ten experiments allowed under his certificate. The Secretary of State, it said, was willing to allow that this had occurred through 'inadvertence in failing to remember the limitation, but he must press upon you the obligation of making yourself fully acquainted with the Conditions of your licence'.[41] Thus, in practice, such conditions seemed concerned more with recording the (often generous) numbers of experiments allowed than with evaluating the nature and consequences of their

[39] Schäfer's licence and related correspondence is in the University of Edinburgh Library at GEN. 2007/5. All of the above quotations come from this source.

[40] See Schäfer's experimental notebook for the period January 1884 to November 1886. Wellcome Institute, London, ESS/B17/11.

[41] University of Edinburgh Library, GEN. 2007/5.

methods, and it was just this anomaly that gave to the critics the impression that the Act simply provided *carte blanche* for the licensees to do largely as they wished, while at the same time *protecting* them from the danger of prosecution under laws which preceded the 1876 Act. Thus, said one of them:

> with a licence and certificate in his pocket, Dr Legg may again mutilate, in order to induce disease in cats..., some of them lingering three *weeks*... before they died; or Dr Rutherford... may again open living dogs, dissect out their bile ducts, and keep them in this state under curare for 18 *hours*; or Dr Ferrier may again saw open his... monkey's skull; or Dr Gamgee and Mr Priestley may again torture animals with irritant poisons... In the face of such doings what becomes of the *anaesthetic* plea?[42]

Other sources of published data which might throw light upon this elusive problem include laboratory guides to practical physiology and the journals concerned with research. It has been shown elsewhere that Burdon-Sanderson's *Handbook*, a volume that met with outrage from the antivivisectionist camp and a great deal of soul-searching among witnesses before the Royal Commission, advocated some 137 experiments that would have been classified as 'calculated to give pain' under the 1876 Act, and would therefore have required a licence with or without appropriate certificates. A maximum of ninety-one of these were estimated actually to cause some pain, about 15 per cent of all the experiments described.[43]

A similar analysis of the first ten volumes of the *Journal of Physiology* (which commenced publication by the Physiological Society in 1878) and which cover the same years as the Home Office statistics (Table 1), is given for comparison in Table 2. Of 270 papers, some 90 describe experiments that, in Britain, would have been covered by the Act, and about 36, or 13 per cent might well have caused some pain. Once again, these are maximum figures, estimated on the basis of the methods employed (particularly with respect to anaesthesia) and their likely consequences. When anaesthetics were applied, it was assumed that they were applied effectively; on the other hand, when they were not specified it was assumed that they were not used. The similarity between results from the *Journal* and the *Handbook* is striking and supports in a general way the invariable contention of the licensees and their supporters. This, as expressed by the Association for the Advancement of Medicine by Research (AAMR), was that the great majority of experiments at the time were

[42] A. F. Astley to Editor, *Zoophilist* 2 (1 May 1882).
[43] Richards, 'Vicarious suffering', pp. 139–40.

Table 2. *An analysis of the* Handbook for the Physiological Laboratory *(1873)*[a] *and the* Journal of Physiology *(Vols. 1–10, 1878–1889) in terms of painful experiments*

	No. of expts[b]	No. 'calculated to give pain'[c]	No. with anaesthetics or 'pithing'	No. causing pain[d]	
				Under curare	No precautions specified
			Handbook		
	622	137	46	32 (8)	59 (37)
%	100	22	7	15	
			Journal		
	270	90	54	6 (4)	30 (11)
%	100	33	20	13	

Notes:

[a] From Richards, 'Vicarious suffering, necessary pain: physiological method in late nineteenth-century Britain' in N. Rupke (ed.), *Vivisection in Historical Perspective* (London, 1987), p. 140.

[b] For the *Journal*, this figure represents the number of published papers (each of which often described a series of individual experiments).

[c] Note that the 1876 Act did not apply to invertebrates.

[d] In these columns, the first figures refer to total numbers of experiments; those in parentheses to experiments on mammals (mostly cats, dogs and rabbits).

painless (being performed on man as well as animals; on isolated animal tissues and organs; or on animals under full surgical anaesthesia and killed before recovery), whilst even when pain was occasioned it was scarcely of significance because all practitioners worked on the principle of gaining the 'greatest possible result... at the least possible cost of suffering'.[44] Incidentally, it is also of passing interest that of thirty-six potentially painful experiments described in the *Journal*, twenty were performed in North American laboratories, eleven in Britain and five on the Continent. Thus, even despite the fact that foreign (especially Continental) physiologists naturally favoured their own national journals, some 69 per cent of all experiments reported during these years, and likely to cause pain, were performed in overseas laboratories.

That the proportion of painful experiments described in these two sources is almost three times that suggested by the Home Office statistics is not an indication that the latter were intentionally misleading, but merely a reflection of the far greater range of experiments covered (*all* of those 'calculated to give pain'). The distinction is clarified in the published figures for 1887 onwards by means of three categories: the physiological experiments performed for purely scientific purposes but usually of relevance to medicine; the pathological for the study of the processes of disease; and, finally, the therapeutical for the investigation of the action of drugs. Thus of 1220 experiments in that year, only 237 were said to be physiological, while of those admitted to have caused pain (71 in all), only 2 were in this category.[45]

Moral progress in the laboratory

> ... [E]ven in England until comparatively recent times, the torture of harmless animals was thought an innocent pleasure. Men of science have not always risen above the average humanity and moral enlightenment of their age and country. But speaking of this country, and of modern times, it may safely be said that no charge of wanton, needless, or excessive sacrifice of animals can be, or indeed ever has been, seriously alleged...[46]

Such was the conclusion of the AAMR in 1883, during the triumphant period after the International Medical Congress; but such also had been that of the exhaustive Royal Commission of 1875. The reason, it was said, was to be found in the discovery (by science itself) of

[44] 'Facts and considerations relating to the practices of scientific experiments on living animals, commonly called vivisection', *Nature*, 27 (1883), pp. 542–6, at p. 546.

[45] *Home Office Returns*, 1887, *P.P.* 1888, LXXX, p. 471.

[46] 'Facts and considerations', p. 543.

anaesthetics which, in humane and skilful hands ensured that pain was 'altogether prevented, [or] in the remaining cases greatly mitigated'.[47] The suffering unavoidably inflicted by Harvey, Boyle, Hales, Hunter and Bell was, accordingly, something unnecessary and unknown in the modern British laboratory.

The problem was that the antivivisectionists remained unconvinced, powerfully influenced as they were by the famous letter sent by George Hoggan, MD, to the *Morning Post* in 1875, in which (on the basis of continental experiences) he described anaesthetics as 'the greatest curse of vivisectable animals... far more efficacious in lulling public feeling towards the vivisectors than pain in the vivisected'.[48] His was a view that would be echoed in countless later, and less responsible diatribes; for anaesthetics, it was claimed, were 'the Will-o'-the-wisps of Science destined to mislead sincere but imperfectly informed Antivivisectionists, and to lure them into the bogs and quagmires of physiological deception off the straight, hard road of Abolition'.[49] Yet such assertions could be sustained only because the scientists, even after the unanimous backing of the IMC, were so ineffective in exploiting the anaesthetic argument, which should have been the hard core of their defence against charges of cruelty and immorality. As Rudolf Virchow had plainly seen in his address to the Congress, 'the criterion is pain [and] everything by which, in the way of experiments, pain is inflicted on an animal is torture of animals, and so far immoral, and contrary to religion'.[50] But as we have seen, generally reliable data on the use of anaesthetics – which were already available to the scientists of the day – strongly suggest that the problem of pain was a great deal less omnipresent by the late nineteenth century, and in particular after the impact of the Cruelty to Animals Act of 1876.

Had the scientists only capitalised on this new situation – no matter how much they resented the implication that the Act was necessary to regulate and educate them in the pursuit of their legitimate activities – they might have suffered harassment a good deal less severe and less prolonged than was in fact the case, and thus been obliged to expend less of their time and energy rebutting accusations of immorality that could hardly any longer be sustained by the evidence. As time progressed, even some of the most influential 'animal rights' campaigners were ready to be convinced on this question. Thus in

[47] *Royal Commission on... Experiments*, p. xvii.
[48] *Morning Post*, 2 February 1875; *Zoophilist*, 4 (1 May 1884).
[49] *Zoophilist*, 4 (1 May 1884). [50] *Nature*, 24 (1881), pp. 346–52, at p. 351.

evidence to the second Royal Commission (which was established early in the new century to review the working of the 1876 Act), John W. Graham, the Principal of Dalton Hall, Victoria University, Manchester, representing three antivivisection societies, stated quite unequivocally that his objection was only to cruelty. 'If cruelty can be avoided – certainly avoided, and surely avoided – I am satisfied; then I should rejoice in the experiments.'[51] Similarly, Stephen Coleridge, for the National Anti-Vivisection Society (then said to be the largest in the world) stated that:

> My objection to vivisection begins and is centred on the question of pain. If an animal can be placed under complete anaesthesia, and destroyed before it recovers consciousness, personally I have no objection to that vivisection at all; and anything that might be discovered thereby could be to the benefit of humanity and welcomed by myself.[52]

Finally, Sir Guillum Scott and Sir Frederick Banbury, for the RSPCA, again emphasised that the opposition of their Society was to painful experiments alone; where no pain was caused, the question of cruelty did not arise.[53]

In order to make good their new advantage, the task of the physiologists was to confirm that, in the use of anaesthetics, expertise had grown apace with experience. We have seen that several of them had worked in a medical environment where the anaesthetic question must have been frequently discussed, and it is hardly possible that they would have failed to exploit appropriate technical improvements for their own experimental work. Burdon-Sanderson, in fact, as early as 1869 had himself performed some research on the physiology of the use of nitrous oxide as an anaesthetic, while Schäfer, in the late 1870s, experimented in the use of atropine as a preventive of the cardio-inhibitory effects of chloroform and, much later, worked with nicotine and extracts of the 'suprarenal capsules' as intravenous stimulants for use in emergencies under anaesthesia. Other prominent physiologists actively interested in the action of anaesthetics included William Gaskell, Leonard Hill and Augustus Waller.[54] Thus it cannot be argued that the experimentalists worked in isolation from the wider

[51] *Royal Commission on Vivisection, 2nd Report, Evidence* (Cd 3462), *P.P.* 1907, XLI, p. 817, Qs. 5944–5.

[52] *Ibid., 3rd Report, Evidence* (Cd 3757), *P.P.* 1908, LVII, p. 283, Qs. 10709–10.

[53] *Ibid., 4th Report, Evidence* (Cd 3955), *P.P.* 1908, LVII, p. 559, Q. 19488.

[54] See *Transactions of the Odontological Society of Great Britain*, NS 1 (1869), pp. 53–4; *Journal of Physiology*, 18 (1895), pp. 230–79, and *Transactions of the Society of Anaesthetists*, 1 (1898), pp. 54–5; and *British Medical Journal* (1891, 2), pp. 1088–95; (1893, 1), p. 105; (1897, 2), pp. 1474–5; and (1898, 1), pp. 1057–61.

medical interest in anaesthetics, and their position might have been made relatively secure during the 1880s by which time ether and chloroform had long been routine in hospital practice.

Yet they hardly achieved this before the beginning of the new century. In evidence to the second Royal Commission, Sir James Russell, the Home Office Inspector for Scotland and the Northern Counties of England since 1890 was certain that marked improvements had taken place in the administration of anaesthetics during the thirty-year period. Like others, he made the important point that animal experimenters tended to use *deeper* levels of anaesthesia than was usual with human patients because it was of vital importance that there should be no movements which might disturb measuring apparatus or break delicate glass cannulae inserted into blood vessels or the trachea, and also of course because the death of an animal from overdose was a very much less serious matter than that of a patient.[55] Francis Gotch, Waynflete Professor of Physiology at Oxford since 1895, and a long-established colleague of Burdon-Sanderson, could vouch for the efficacy of general anaesthetics from personal experience, having been obliged to undergo a severe operation himself lasting two and a half hours. He also had no doubts as to the value and effectiveness of two disputed 'narcotics', chloral and urethane, whilst the anaesthetic status of another, namely morphine – when given in a lethal dose – was stoutly defended by Lauder Brunton and Ernest Starling. According to the latter, morphine was however normally used only as an adjunct to chloroform and/or ether which, in a mixture with alcohol (then known as ACE), had proved to be an exceptionally reliable anaesthetic for use in long-term operations.[56]

Even thirty years after having been disallowed as an anaesthetic by the 1876 Act, curare remained controversial, although it was still used in conjunction with anaesthetics as a muscle relaxant. Such use, said the Commissioners, needed 'great watchfulness lest return to sensibility should take place while the influence of the curare would prevent the exhibition of some of the signs of such return', and for this highly sensitive reason they recommended that if its use were to be

[55] *Royal Commission on Vivisection, 1st Report, Evidence* (Cd 3326), *P.P.* 1907, XLI, pp. 649, 729 and 736.

[56] *Ibid., 4th Report, Evidence* (Cd 3955), *P.P.* 1908, LVII, p. 559, Qs. 13588 and 13591; *3rd Report, Evidence* (Cd 3757), *P.P.* 1908, LVII, p. 283, Q. 6801; and *1st Report, Evidence* (Cd 3326), *P.P.* 1907, XLI, p. 649, Qs. 3607 and 3610. 'ACE', a mixture of 1 part alcohol, 2 parts chloroform and 3 parts ether, was first suggested in about 1860 by George Harley (1829–96), a former lecturer in physiology at University College, and then the professor of medical jurisprudence. See Duncum, *Inhalation Anaesthesia*, pp. 256–7.

permitted at all, an Inspector should be present throughout the experiment.[57] But this problem aside, the Commissioners undoubtedly felt that the case for the painlessness of the great majority of experiments, and for the humanity of the licensees, had been decisively made. They were sure, moreover, that a great deal of the antivivisectionist propaganda was exaggerated and sensationally distorted.

We desire... to state that the harrowing descriptions and illustrations of operations inflicted on animals, which are freely circulated by post, advertisement or otherwise, are in many cases calculated to deceive the public, so far as they suggest that the animals in question were not under an anaesthetic. To represent that animals subjected to experiment in this country are wantonly tortured would, in our opinion, be absolutely false.[58]

If then, it is true that the great majority of animal experiments were painless, what remained of the antivivisectionists' moral case? The same trend of moral progress that had led to the abandonment of torture in the seventeenth century as a means of obtaining judicial evidence had also, in the nineteenth, prompted opposition to painful vivisection as a basis for the acquisition of physiological knowledge. Both practices had been criticised not because their ends were the accumulation of unreliable evidence (which must often have been the case) but because their means could no longer find justification. With the introduction of anaesthetics into animal experiments the force of this criticism was minimised and, since animals were widely sacrificed in other connections in the name of human interests (and with inevitable deprivation and suffering), the knowledge that was gathered from 'vivisection' was increasingly seen as sufficiently important to continue the research. Its importance, of course, was in connection with clinical medicine, a link which, once made, soon had the effect of also justifying the few experiments that caused acute pain, as well as the many that required no anaesthesia but which might cause prolonged distress in the shape of disease. Suffering of these kinds was said to be necessary and hence justified as the price of human progress. Thus the success of science in finding its own answers to the accusations of painfulness – anaesthetics – and of self-indulgent curiosity – medical application – gave to the experimentalists a credibility that was simply too great and too far-reaching for the antivivisectionists to counter. With the erosion of the ground of their moral argument (and until, in more recent times, the advocacy of more controversial non-medical justifications) only the out-and-out abo-

[57] *Royal Commission on Vivisection, Final Report* (Cd 6114), *P.P.* 1912–13, XLVIII, p. 401, para. 83.

[58] *Ibid.*

litionists remained to advocate a cause that, for consistency, demanded not only strict vegetarianism (which few espoused) but also outright opposition to the exploitation of animals for any human interest whatsoever.

The aesthetic objection

Fierce hostility to experimental physiology continued long after it was fallacious to characterise it as cruel and immoral. This raises the question of whether the motivation for much of the antivivisection fervour was in reality derived from covert foundations that were a good deal less rational than the ethical principles which always occupied the foreground of the debate. If this were the case, it might explain why the science of physiology (which before the era of anaesthetics had clearly been vulnerable to ethical objections) was still charged in these terms throughout the remainder of the century despite clear evidence that the 1876 Act had accelerated a trend of moral progress which, in Britain, had in any case always been apparent.

Accordingly, the suspicion must be that, for many, opposition to physiological research was based primarily (if unconsciously) on a revulsion generated by the supposed aura of the laboratory as a hybrid product, as it were, of the operating room and the slaughterhouse. It was a deeply affective environment, a place peculiarly devoted, it seemed, to premeditated destruction and death, whose reputation was always intensified by the very word 'vivisection', which in the popular mind had become indelibly associated with ideas of ruthless interrogation, offensive air and, above all, with blood. In such circumstances it is no simple matter to identify a distinction between ethical and aesthetic judgements, but the difference is perhaps to be found in the potential to universalise. To say, 'I wouldn't do that' (because it is wrong) is different from saying, 'I couldn't do that' (because it is repulsive), in the sense that the first has to do with the nature of evil and with recommendations concerning human conduct, whereas the latter speaks only of an individual's personal sensibilities and temperament. Thus one's *inability* to work in a physiological laboratory cannot be a moral argument against experimenting upon animals, although one's *unwillingness* to do so may be. Either motive may ensure that one does no such work, but it was of the simple distinction between them that the antivivisectionists seemed never to be aware.

But this is not to suggest that in this they were unusual. Under the heading, 'The Moral Question', the second Royal Commission acknowledged that even painless experiments might well be *distasteful* to some individuals, 'especially when performed on certain classes of animals'. The different claims of various species would be made by 'civilised humanity' on the basis of 'the degree of association with or affinity or utility to man'. Recognition, it said, should be duly accorded to the 'reality and worthiness of such underlying *sentiment* which would secure a special reservation for animals coming within the aforesaid limits'. Thus, it was concluded, the anthropoid apes, together with dogs and cats, should be given equivalent protection to that provided under the 1876 Act to horses, asses and mules.[59]

Yet the sentiment of distaste gave grounds only for an aesthetic judgement, not for one that could be consistent in universal (moral) terms. Even a system of relative ethics which granted 'rights' to animals only in proportion to the evolutionary development of their species, and which therefore distinguished between painful experiments upon amphibia and reptiles on the one hand and on mammals and birds on the other (arguing on Sherrington's principle that 'where life ranks highest, there it can suffer most'), could hardly distinguish the suffering of rats or rabbits from that of dogs, cats, or even primates, except on grounds of irrational 'sentiment'.[60] However, it is possible that some confusion on this issue served the interests of the antivivisectionists, for as the grounds for moral objection shifted and weakened they were the more anxious to elicit support of a merely emotional kind. In this connection it was unfortunate that the physiologists were often their own worst enemies, giving the impression that, whatever the improved moral status of their work, its aesthetic environment would continue to be profoundly disturbing to many. Michael Foster, for example, in his most public utterance to the IMC chose to defend and define his science with a quotation from the preface to Willis's *Cerebri Anatome Nervorum Descripto et Usus*: 'For either in this way, namely through death and wounds, through dissection and, as it were, by a Caesarean operation, will truth be brought to light or otherwise will it lie for ever hid.'[61]

Whatever is to be made of this seemingly coarse and unsavoury aspect of the physiologist's work, and of its influence upon public evaluation of his profession, we are left uneasily to wonder what, if

[59] *Ibid.*, paras. 96–7 and 118 (italics added).
[60] C. S. Sherrington, *Man on his Nature* (London, 1955), p. 286.
[61] Foster, Inaugural Address, p. 218.

any, connection might conceivably exist between aesthetic and ethical sensibilities. We have seen that such 'founding fathers' of British physiology as Sharpey and Bennett supported experiments upon animals, yet could not perform them. Essentially the same was true of Darwin and Huxley.[62] There is thus a sense in which these individuals were professionally flawed, for their theoretical conviction that the new physiology was essential for the benefit of mankind would have been rendered impotent in practice by their inability to carry it out. It is important to emphasise that these were cases in which the end was recognised to be a sufficient ethical justification for the means, yet where the means could not be implemented because they engendered a paralysing sense of aesthetic revulsion. But in the present context what might be of even greater interest would be evidence as to the possibility that the converse proposition might also be true. That is, might those *not* innately incapacitated by temperament to perform experiments have been enabled, by the eroding indifference born of repeated exposure, to perform not only those they knew to be painless, but also those they considered expedient (perhaps for the advancement of reputation and career) despite the necessity for pain?

George Hoggan certainly thought so of those embroiled in the ghoulish atmosphere of Bernard's laboratory, where 'the great aim [was] to keep up with, or get ahead of, one's contemporaries in science'. No student could protest for fear of being 'hooted, mobbed, and expelled from among his fellows for doing so, and any rising medical man would only achieve professional ruin by following a similar course'. 'Were the feelings of experimental physiologists not blunted,' he said, 'they could not long continue the practice of vivisection.'[63] W. A. B. Scott, a young London physician, claimed something similar for Burdon-Sanderson's University College laboratory of 1871 where, he said, anaesthetics were 'certainly' not administered for the duration of all experiments and where work of dubious moral status was performed for 'notoriety', 'zealous students [doing] it in pursuit of medals and scholarships and to get mentioned favourably in periodicals'.[64] It was all too uncomfortably suggestive of that nightmare conjured up by Lewis Carroll, in which 'successive generations of students, trained from their earliest years to the repression of all human sympathies, shall have developed a new and

[62] For the position of Darwin and Huxley on this issue, see Richards, 'Drawing the life-blood', pp. 52–4.
[63] *Spectator*, 48 (1875), pp. 177–8.
[64] *Royal Commission on...Experiments*, Qs. 5194 *et seq.*

more hideous Frankenstein – a soulless being to whom science shall be all in all'. And it gave credence to the suspicion that the University College laboratory really was the model for that of Dr Moreau ('as bad as Gower Street – with its cats').[65]

Foster's choice of quotation (above), together with the many instances of blood-encrusted operations so openly and clumsily described in Burdon-Sanderson's *Handbook*, may be further tentative evidence along these lines, suggesting, perhaps, that if familiarity encouraged indifference, indifference might remove moderation. In private correspondence, too, the jocular insensitivity of the one and the undefended ingenuousness of the other come across clearly. Thus Foster hoped that Ludwig in Leipzig would let Henry Newell Martin 'poke about' and teach Schäfer 'all his dodges etc.'. 'Remember I shall be delighted to hear from you', he added, 'whenever a rabbit dies and you have unexpectedly time on your hands'. And Burdon-Sanderson, having spent a day in Goltz's laboratory in Strasburg, wrote with restrained enthusiasm of his dogs 'deprived of their motor convolutions. Several of them exhibited the characters of dog idiocy in great perfection...also an admirable example of a dog without cerebellum'.[66]

Conclusion

It is the purpose of these examples to represent the ethical and aesthetic character, indeed the inescapable essence, of laboratory physiology in the late nineteenth century; a science in which the use of increasingly complex apparatus and techniques tended to objectify the experiments and direct attention away from the animal itself. To ignore or to deny this is to distort the nature of a science which demanded of its practitioners a special kind of psychological commitment sufficiently powerful to bracket off not merely aesthetic, but in some circumstances, ethical misgivings also. That the evidence for insensitivity on the part of the physiologists comes largely from the period prior to 1876 strongly suggests that the Act of that year *was* necessary to guide and regulate their activities and that (despite the disillusionment of the antivivisectionists as to its relative 'weakness') its effect in improving their moral awareness was considerable. A science with undoubted potential for 'great abuse' was now obliged

[65] L. Carroll, 'Some popular fallacies about vivisection', *Fortnightly Review*, 17 (1875), pp. 847–54, at p. 854; and H. G. Wells, *The Island of Dr Moreau* (London, 1946; 1st edn, 1896), p.52.

[66] Foster to Schäfer, 21 July (1873?), Wellcome Institute, London, ESS/B5/4; and Burdon-Sanderson to Schäfer (n.d.), ESS/B11/8.

to operate at a new level of accountability. Though to many it would always remain aesthetically repellent, its lingering reputation for ethical irregularities became – with the refinement of its anaesthetic techniques and its accumulating relevance to clinical medicine – ever harder to sustain.

5

Scientific elites and laboratory organisation in fin de siècle *Paris and Berlin*

The Pasteur Institute and Robert Koch's Institute for Infectious Diseases compared

PAUL WEINDLING

During the 1880s and '90s there emerged a new form of medical research laboratory. Research institutes with a national ethos were established outside the context of universities and oriented towards public health and hospital therapy. Entrepreneurial initiatives by researchers found a positive response among state officials and the public. The foundation of such institutes was spurred on by the hope that bacteriology could provide solutions to the apparently intractable health problems of burgeoning cities. Moreover, the rise of imperialism and international competition meant that a great deal of international prestige was at stake with regard to major medical discoveries. Since the 1870s, scientists in Berlin (as capital of a recently unified Germany) had been seeking to challenge the role of Paris as the centre of science and culture. There was a scramble for a stake in the hitherto uncharted and invisible world of bacteria, or (to use the French term popularised by Pasteur after 1878) of microbes. There were also undercurrents of professional imperialism as a new species of professional specialist – the bacteriologist or microbiologist – found an institutional niche.

By the mid-1890s each European metropolis could boast of a central laboratory for bacteriological research (Table 3). In this chapter I will compare the organisation of two of the most prestigious of these institutes: the Pasteur Institute and Koch's Institute for Infectious Diseases (Institut für Infektionskrankheiten). These institutes represented a new organisational form of a research institute without responsibilities for teaching medical students, but linked to facilities

Table 3. *Medical research institutions in European metropolises*

Location	Year	Institution	Director
Paris	1888	Pasteur Institute	Pasteur
Berlin	1891	Institute for Infectious Diseases	Koch
St Petersburg	1892	Institute for Experimental Medicine	Nencki
London	1893	British Institute of Preventive Medicine	Ruffer
Vienna	1894	Serotherapeutic Institute	Paltauf

for therapy and preventive medicine. There resulted rifts with universities and with established professional institutions. These broader contexts and concerns shaped the everyday pattern of social and intellectual life in the laboratories.

Historical analysis of the siting, equipping and organisation of laboratories raises a number of controversial issues. Laboratories have been called by Bruno Latour 'theatres of proof'. He analyses how Pasteur created a style of discourse to which there could be no opposition. Latour ascribes a sweeping victory to Pasteur and his disciples.[1] This, however, is open to challenge. At the level of medical theory, microbiology (and bacteriology and germ theory) remained subject to continued criticism from environmentalist and hereditarian perspectives. It can also be argued that Latour's philosophical approach neglects crucial features of the micro-level of the internal organisation of research institutes and of scientific practices, as well as the macro-level of the politically complex process of the expansion of public health and hygiene institutes. Latour argues that the Pasteurian laboratory was a source of power detached from the social environment with 'nothing to do with doctor–patient relations or the scrutinization of cities'. This view has been criticised by social historians who suggest that reform of public health administration was already underway in France. It should also be noted that during the 1890s bacteriologists were challenged by theories of social medicine (or social hygiene) in France and Germany.[2] Although the

[1] B. Latour, *The Pasteurization of France*, trans. Alan Sheridan and John Law (Cambridge, Mass., 1988; original French edition, 1984).

[2] L. Murard and P. Zylberman, 'De l'hygiène comme introduction à la politique expérimentale (1875–1925)', *Revue de Synthèse*, ser. 3, no. 115 (1984), pp. 313–41.

secondary literature on Robert Koch lacks the epistemological sophistication of Latour, there have been similar assumptions of an overwhelming victory of Koch's bacteriology. However, the well-entrenched chemical and environmental concerns of the Pettenkofer school in Germany circumscribe any claims for a 'triumph of bacteriology'. It is necessary to locate the major national institutes within political, administrative and professional contexts, as represented by public health laboratories for routine investigation of the urban and natural environments. The extent to which there was a 'pasteurisation' or 'hygienisation' of everyday behaviour – in terms of food consumption, housing design and sexual behaviour – raises complex issues beyond the scope of this chapter.

Origins of the Pasteur Institute

After Pasteur's much publicised success in treating rabies from July 1885, the Pasteur Institute was proposed in March 1886, and opened in March 1888. It was funded by public subscription, and the organising committee included such bankers as Christophle of the Crédit Foncier, and Baron Alfons de Rothschild.[3] The institute was a private foundation, but was accorded official support and facilities by the state and municipality.[4] A grand total of 1,940,000 francs were collected. That the institute integrated diverse social interests was suggested by the publicising of how donors came from all social classes, varying from humble artisans to royalty and the commercially successful such as Madame Boucicaut, the owner of the Bon Marché department store.[5] Because of the inadequacies of the system of state funding of science through prizes, there was a need to tap additional sources of support.[6] A new factor of importance was public involvement, and there was a financial incentive in the sensationalising of medical discoveries.

While philanthropic donations were the most important source of funding, there were substantial professional and state contributions. Pasteur donated the income from rabies vaccine, and profits from the treatment of anthrax and chicken cholera, amounting to 25,000

[3] 'Inauguration de l'Institut Pasteur', *Annales de l'Institut Pasteur*, 2 (1888), pp. 1–29.

[4] A. Delaunay, *L'Institut Pasteur* (Paris, 1962).

[5] J. Mery, *Histoire des Legs à l'Institut Pasteur* (Paris, 1987). Different figures are given in R. Vallery-Radot, *La vie de Pasteur* (Paris, n.d.; 1st edn, 1900), p. 548, where it is stated that 2,586,680 francs were collected.

[6] H. Paul, *From Knowledge to Power: The Rise of the Science Empire in France 1860–1939* (Cambridge, 1985), pp. 288–93.

francs. The Ministries of Education and Agriculture provided a subsidy of 40,000 francs for the running costs of the institute. The proclamation of major discoveries was also useful in drumming up prize money from the coffers of academies and other more traditional funding agencies. International contributions were made by francophile states: 100,000 francs were donated by the Tsar of Russia and other contributors were the Emperor of Brazil and the Sultan of Turkey. German researchers and official representatives were conspicuously absent from the grand opening ceremony attended by 600 people. Only the dissident bacteriologist Ferdinand Hueppe (who was alienated from Koch and high-ranking officials) sent congratulations.[7]

The rapidity of the foundation of the Pasteur Institute is striking, particularly when compared to the much more protracted process of finding donors for the Lister Institute in London. Geison has pointed out that the success of the rabies cure could well have been exaggerated as it was difficult to establish whether a dog really was rabid. Rabies was a comparatively rare disease.[8] Latour observes that given the low numbers treated for rabies, it was astonishing how quickly 'credibility was converted into capital'. Yet the investment in the institute might be seen as a shrewd speculative venture.[9] The institute was a piece of entrepreneurship by Pasteur which was designed to satisfy the appetite for personal glory, nationalism and international humanitarianism – a medical equivalent to other 'national' but private ventures such as the Eiffel Tower of 1889 (Eiffel drew profits for twenty years from this), and de Lesseps' Panama Canal (that crashed in 1889). The major donors, who were immortalised by their busts decorating the entrance hall, had shrewdly invested in what was to be an expanding and highly durable enterprise.

The foundation of the Pasteur Institute came towards the end of Pasteur's life, representing a final bid to establish a research school of microbiology.[10] Pasteur was determined that his institutional brainchild should establish its independence from the state, municipalities and medical faculties. This was facilitated by the law of 1875 establishing the liberty of higher education.[11] The institute's location

[7] *L'Inauguration de l'Institut Pasteur le 14 Novembre 1888 en présence de M. Le Président de la République: Comte rendu* (Sceaux, 1888).

[8] G. L. Geison, 'Louis Pasteur' in *Dictionary of Scientific Biography* vol. x (New York, 1974), pp. 350–441.

[9] Latour, *Pasteurization*, p. 101.

[10] C. Salomon-Bayet (ed.), *Pasteur et la Révolution Pastorienne* (Paris, 1986), pp. 48–9.

[11] R. Fox and G. Weisz, 'The institutional basis of French science in the nineteenth century' in Fox and Weisz (eds), *The Organization of Science and Technology in France 1808–1914* (Cambridge, 1980), p. 20.

on the periphery rather than in the centre of Paris expressed the intention of maintaining distance from the state bureaucracy and the university. That the siting gave the institute autonomy and that most funding came from private sources were thus symptomatic of the prevailing liberalism of the first decades of the Third Republic. Pasteur's associates in the venture, Charles Chamberland, Emile Duclaux and Emile Roux had liberal inclinations, as shown by their subsequent support for Dreyfus.[12] Roux was also sympathetic to a type of free-thinking positivism that depended on the expertise of the scientist, closeted in the laboratory but at the same time dictating codes of public health and hygiene. As Latour observes, the *Annales* of the Pasteur Institute, begun a year before the opening of the institute itself, expressed the broad-ranging and expansive nature of the Pasteurian programme with their diversity of topics amenable to laboratory analysis.[13]

Medical science was a symbol of the Third Republic. The Pasteur Institute combined a multiplicity of personal interests with a national ethos, making it as much of a compromise between diverse interests as the highly polarised but enduring Third Republic. The buildings were constructed in the style of Louis XIII, giving a sense of harmony with the nation's cultural traditions, and yet were modern in their purpose. The institute's status as a 'national' – but independent – centre was conveyed by the opening ceremony on 4 November 1888 when it was visited by Sadi Carnot, the politically moderate President of the Republic, who had survived the nationalist surge of support for General Boulanger.[14] Political support for the institute expressed how hygiene was regarded as a means of securing social progress: medical science was to integrate the extremes of the political left and right. The appeals stressed the number of small donations by workers and petty officials. At the same time the institute was symptomatic of how laboratory scientists were seeking autonomy and status rather than being held as dependent clients of the state. As Pasteur emphasised, while his efforts only converted an elite to medical and scientific work, this elite could change the nation's destiny in their effects on the nation's economy and population.[15] While always financially precarious, a multiplicity of sources of income meant that the scientists remained masters of their destinies.

[12] On Chamberland and Duclaux, see *Dictionary of Scientific Biography*.

[13] Latour, *Pasteurization*, pp. 100–2, fig. 2–3.

[14] *L'Inauguration*, op. cit.

[15] Vallery-Radot, *Pasteur*, pp. 598–60.

Origins of Koch's Institute for Infectious Diseases

Pasteur's opening address at his institute stressed its public utility as 'a dispensary for the treatment of rabies'.[16] The Pasteur Institute spawned numerous dispensaries for the treatment of rabies, notably in Russia but also in virtually every European state. Some of these (such as Odessa) also functioned as bacteriological research stations. Yet while many countries were content with small-scale and scattered anti-rabies dispensaries, it was in the largest German state, Prussia, that a central state research institution was established. Although he used the Pasteurian anti-rabies vaccine, Robert Koch was critical of state production of it.[17] He was not so much an imitator of Pasteur, as a rival anxious to overtake Pasteur in contributions to medical research. Since their publications on anthrax in 1876 and 1877, a feud had festered between Koch and Pasteur, caused by differing scientific aims and methods, cultural misunderstandings and personal rivalry.[18] At the time of the foundation of his institute, Pasteur was ailing and from 1887 semi-paralysed: he died in 1895. This contrasts to Koch, who was twenty-one years younger than Pasteur and at the height of his career and public influence. Like the Pasteur Institute, Koch's Institute for Infectious Diseases, founded in 1891, drew its support from an innovative therapy for a major disease – in this case, tuberculosis. When this was announced to the International Medical Congress in Berlin on 4 August 1890, Pasteur telegraphed his congratulations to Koch and refused to doubt the efficacy of the cure. Thus Pasteur's considerable reputation reinforced the belief in tuberculin as a fundamental scientific achievement.[19] Koch persuaded state officials that he needed an institute for pure research in order to develop his innovative therapy. Just as Pasteur had made exaggerated claims for the efficacy of his anti-rabies serum, so Koch's announcement of a cure for tuberculosis was also premature and open to doubt.

Personal psychology was also important in the genesis of the

[16] *L'Inauguration*, pp. 26–30.

[17] Geheimes Staatsarchiv Stiftung Preussicher Kulturbesitz Abteilung Merseburg (hereafter GStAM), Rep. 92, Althoff AI, Nr 256, Institut für Infektions-krankheiten, Koch to Althoff 26 February 1887.

[18] H. M. Mollaret, 'Contribution à la connaissance des relations entre Koch et Pasteur', *NTM: Schriftenreihe für Geschichte der Naturwissenschaften, Technik und Medizin*, 20 (1983), pp. 57–65. T. D. Brock, *Robert Koch: A Life in Medicine and Bacteriology* (Madison, Wis., 1988), pp. 169–77.

[19] B. Möllers, *Robert Koch: Persönlichkeit und Lebenswerk 1843–1910* (Hanover, 1950), pp. 187 and 197.

institutes. While the psychology underlying the Pasteur Institute was that of a prophet seeking a living memorial, Koch wished to free himself from an unhappy marriage. After his daughter married Eduard Pfuhl, an assistant, Koch's marriage began to break up. While working on tuberculin, Koch fell in love with Hedwig Freiburg, the illegitimate daughter of a Berlin worker, who was an actress in the nearby Lessingstrasse. Koch's relations with the Berlin medical faculty were also unhappy. The establishing of a new institute offered Koch a means of escape from a series of embittered relationships.[20]

Scientifically, Koch and Pasteur were very different. It is conventional to liken the microbiology of Pasteur to the bacteriology of Koch. However, in many ways Pasteur, born in 1822 and a chemist by training, had great similarities to the chemist Max Pettenkofer, born in 1818, who was also interested in processes of fermentation; Pettenkofer applied his chemistry to a range of nutritional and economic topics, and Pasteur too developed an interest in infection viewed as a chemical process of fermentation and intoxication. Koch, by contrast, worked with sophisticated microscopical staining and observational techniques, for example developing methods for the culture of bacteria and photomicroscopy. The Koch school of bacteriology can be seen as an outgrowth of an earlier generation of botanical and zoological researches into cellular morphology. Most of the major discoveries in bacteriology between 1876 and 1900 were by Germans or by German-trained researchers.[21] However, it is important to appreciate the diversity of approaches that distinguished Koch from many German bacteriologists, including some of his own disciples. Likewise, certain Pasteurians such as Roux and Yersin recognised the need to deploy the observational methods of German bacteriology. This raises the question whether the practices of Pasteurians were derived from Pasteur, or whether he merely set certain aims and provided an institutional setting.

The Pasteur Institute was a model for Koch of how to exploit a major scientific innovation. There were visits to the Pasteur Institute by German architects, as well as reports by diplomats. A file on the Pasteur Institute kept by the Prussian Medical Department provides details of a visit by a representative of the Imperial Health Office in 1890, and a further visit was made by a Prussian state architect that

[20] Möllers, *Koch*, pp. 224–5. Brock, *Koch*, pp. 214–15.
[21] W. Bulloch, *A History of Bacteriology* (London, 1938), pp. 236–8.

year.[22] Certain pieces of equipment were derived from the Pasteur Institute: one was based on Roux's method of temperature control for storage of bacteria.[23] Rivalry with French science had spurred on the founding of another institute for pure and applied scientific research – the Imperial Institute of Physics and Technology (Physikalisch-Technische Reichsanstalt), established in Berlin in 1887. This was a joint venture by Werner von Siemens, the electrical engineer, who provided much of the finance, and the Imperial government, which took responsibility for the administration and further development of the institute.[24] Koch played on the Prussian state's anxiety to assume the lead in medical research, and thus pressurised the state to provide resources to emulate the Pasteur Institute. In 1887 Friedrich Althoff was appointed as head of the Prussian Education Ministry: he supported the development of research institutes and the modernisation of clinical facilities. Althoff welcomed the opportunity of undermining the independence of university faculties, which he regarded as maintaining a vested interest often opposed to innovative researchers. A state institute provided facilities for collaborative research. Althoff justified the expenditure for this by proclaiming, 'We are on the threshold of a new therapeutic era.'[25] Koch's venture also benefited from the support of Gustav von Gossler, the minister responsible for education and the church (*Kultusminister*), who hoped that the sensational impact of a cure for tuberculosis would bolster up his politically insecure position. When the cure for tuberculosis was debated in the Reichstag on 29 November 1890, Gossler stated that Koch would be freed from teaching responsibilities in order to conduct further research into infectious diseases.[26]

Prussian state funding far exceeded the limited contributions to the Pasteur Institute made by the French state. But the initial wave of public generosity meant that Pasteur had double the resources for building, having collected nearly 2 million francs. Koch received 744,505 marks to cover building costs. Of this 593,522 marks were spent on building hospital facilities and 122,823 marks were for the conversion of an apartment block into a research institute. Pasteur's

[22] GStAM, Rep. 76VIIIB, Nr 3592, Institut Pasteur in Paris, Dez. 1890–Juni 1916. A visit to Paris was made by Paul L. Friedrich, who reported to Dr Köhler of the Imperial Health Office. A further visit was made by Böttger, the architect of Koch's institute on 18 February 1891. See Rep. 76VIIIB, Nr 2892, Bl. 186–7.

[23] Möllers, *Koch*, p. 215.

[24] D. Cahan, *An Institute for an Empire: The Physikalisch-Technische Reichsanstalt 1871–1918* (Cambridge, 1989), pp. 39–42.

[25] GStAM, Rep. 76VIIIB, Nr 2892, Bl. 189; also *Deutsche medizinische Wochenschrift*, 14 May 1891.

[26] Möllers, *Koch*, pp. 197 and 200.

problem was that the capital left after the expensive investment in buildings was inadequate to pay for annual running costs. Here Koch had the advantage with an assured annual budget of 165,000 marks.[27] Koch's substantial salary of 20,000 marks with a living allowance of 1,200 marks aroused the jealousy of other university professors.[28] Municipal support was initially beneficial for Koch. On 21 November 1890 Koch was made an honorary citizen of Berlin because of his contributions to therapy. The expectation was that the municipality would provide clinical facilities. However, the criticisms by Virchow and other radical medical reformers, who called doctors using Koch's remedy 'poisoners and murderers', meant that the Prussian assembly became sceptical of tuberculin therapy.[29] This change of heart among leading figures in the medical profession came too late to jeopardise the rapid progress of the foundation of the Institute, which was officially opened on 17 August 1891.[30]

Location and organisation of the Pasteur Institute

Pasteur's initial preference was for an out-of-town location at Garches, a public property lent to him since 1884 for rabies research, and he intended to establish a smaller rabies institute in Paris. Pasteur declined a central location offered to him by the municipality, stating that he required a site which was 'modest but independent'. There had been vigorous protests from the local population when Pasteur first established a kennel yard for experimental dogs.[31] He wished to avoid the institute becoming a municipal hygiene institute carrying out routine functions. In the event, a vast site of 11,000 square metres was obtained in the 15th arrondissement of Vaugirard, then an artisan district on the outskirts of Paris, where such products as *Eau de Javel* (a chloride bleaching water) were manufactured. The cost of the land was 420,000 francs and the construction cost came to 600,000 francs. It was this far-sighted investment which led to short-term problems with running costs,[32] and made Pasteur hope for the miracle of a rich American.

[27] 10 French francs were equivalent to 8 German marks and to 8 shillings. 20 marks were equivalent to £1 sterling.

[28] GStAM, Rep. 76VIIIB, Nr 2893, Errichtung und Verwaltung des (staatlichen) Instituts für Infektionskrankheiten in Berlin 1892–1898, Bl. 236. Rep. 76VIIIB, Nr 2899 betr. den Etat des Instituts für Infektionskrankheiten, 1890–1898.

[29] GStAM, Rep. 76VIIIB, Nr 2892, Bl. 195; also *Haus der Abgeordneten*, 9 May 1891.

[30] GStAM, Rep. 76VIIIB, Nr 2926. Die Bauten f. d. Institut f. Infektionskrankheiten, Bl. 105–17.

[31] Geison, 'Pasteur', p. 403.

[32] 'L'Institut Pasteur', *Annales de l'Institut Pasteur*, 3 (1889), pp. 1–14.

An advantage of Pasteur's site was that it had ample space for growth. This suited the institute in that it could develop a multiplicity of functions, combining research with teaching and therapy. The researchers benefited in that the residential provisions allowed for the development of a remarkable *esprit de corps*. A central focus was a restaurant, nicknamed 'Le Microbe d'Or'. Pasteur lived in, and there was accommodation for assistants above the library. There were apartments for Chamberland and Roux; despite a penchant for personal hedonism, the latter's dedication gave him an aura of monastic devotion. Later the crypt, housing Pasteur's tomb, confirmed the religious idealisation of the institute's creator. A spirit of devotion was also evident among the institute's janitors and housekeeping staff, who included two of the cases on whom rabies treatment had been used, and a family over three generations.[33]

It was not until July 1900 that a donation was made enabling a hospital pavilion to be opened, so providing clinical facilities on a scale comparable with those attached to Koch's institute. Given the initial lack of clinical facilities, the location near the Hospital for Sick Children (Hôpital des Enfants Malades) was fortuitous as this brought the Pasteur Institute in contact with the *interne* Alexandre Yersin, who alerted Roux to the problem of diphtheria.[34] This hospital also provided a convenient location for clinical trials for serum therapy. The income from research and production of sera and additional donations placed the institute's finances on a firm footing. Moreover, serum therapy for diphtheria opened up new contacts with medical practitioners. The marginal specialism of child health could make common cause with bacteriology.[35] The location near municipal stables was helpful in providing additional sources of animals. This was in marked contrast to the difficulties of the Berliners in stabling animals on their cramped site, forcing Behring and Ehrlich to resort to renting an arch of the S-Bahn, the newly constructed urban railway.

Although the Pasteur Institute was independent of the university, a central function was that of teaching a course in microbiology. The teaching laboratories provided ample space for a course organised by Roux and Metchnikoff. As Paris was a major medical centre, the institute had a ready source of recruits for the courses from among qualified physicians. The Paris location was also suitable for

[33] Delaunay, *L'Institut Pasteur*, pp. 322–31.

[34] H. H. Mollaret and J. Brossollet, *Alexandre Yersin ou le Vainquer de la Peste* (Paris, 1985), pp. 58–61.

[35] P. Huard and M. J. Imbault-Huart, 'La pédiatrie parisienne au XIXème siècle', *Episteme*, 8 (1974), pp. 231–71.

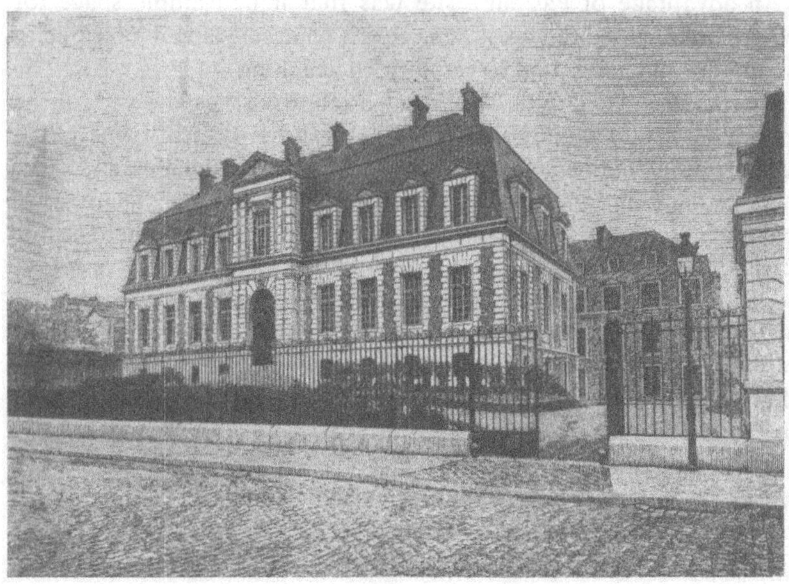

Fig. 2. Pasteur Institute, exterior.

developing contacts with military medical authorities. From the first course on microbiology commencing in March 1894, which was attended by one Russian and one American physician, numerous foreign 'élèves' flocked to the institute.[36] The institute's postgraduate teaching meant that Pasteurian microbiology began to permeate the medical profession and public health institutions.

The institute was organised as a number of departments. Pasteur planned six departments with the following heads:

Rabies	Grancher (1843–1907)
General microbiology	Duclaux (1840–1904)
Microbiological techniques	Roux (1853–1933)
Microbiology applied to hygiene	Chamberland (1851–1908)
Microbiological morphology	Metchnikoff (1845–1916)
Comparative microbiology	Gamaleia (1859–1949)

The departmental chiefs were a heterogeneous group. The staffing of the institute underlined the point that medical research was to be open to all with scientific qualifications and not to be the exclusive domain

[36] M. Faure, 'Cent années d'enseignement à l'Institut Pasteur', in M. Morange (ed.), *L'Institut Pasteur* (Paris, 1991), pp. 62–74.

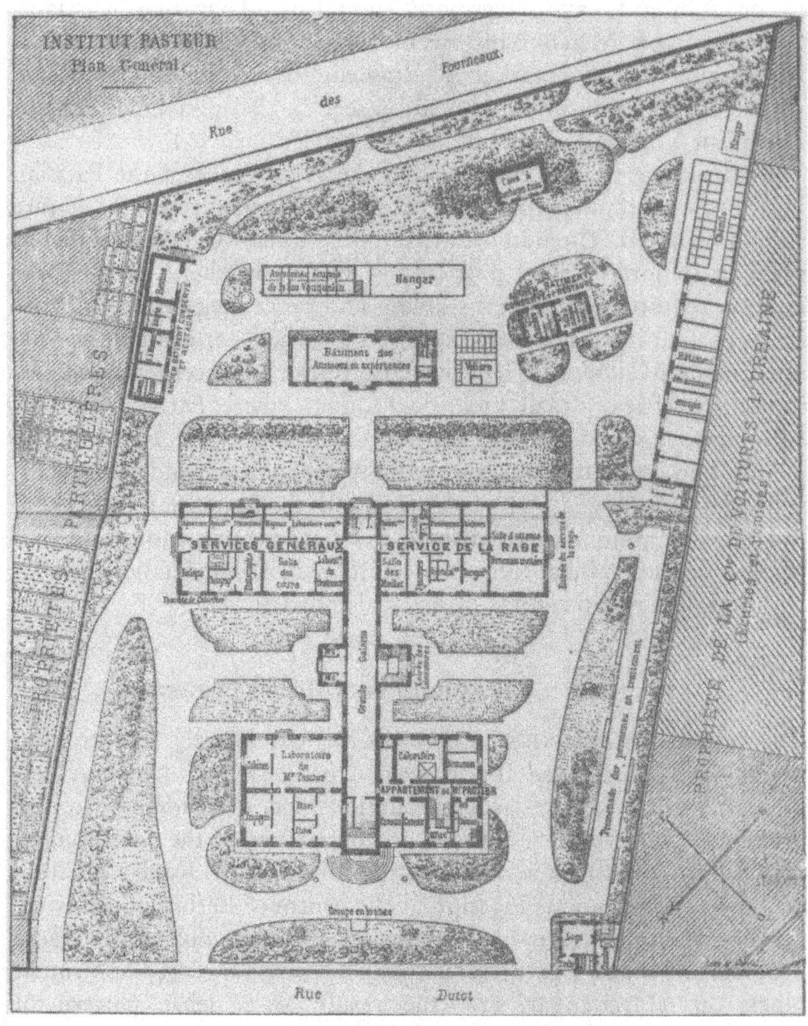

Fig. 3. Pasteur Institute, floor plan.

of doctors. Some of the doctors in the institute were primarily laboratory researchers like Roux, others like Grancher were primarily clinicians. Grancher was a distinguished physician who had first used rabies therapy.[37] Duclaux was a physicist and chemist, and there were

[37] For Roux's distinctive contribution to Pasteurism, see G. L. Geison, 'Pasteur, Roux and rabies: scientific *versus* clinical medicine', *Journal of the History of Medicine and Allied Sciences*, 45 (1990), pp. 341–66; also P. J. Weindling, 'Roux et la Diphtérie' in Morange (ed.), *L'Institut Pasteur*, pp. 137–43.

to be zoologists and veterinary specialists. That two Russians, Gamaleia and Metchnikoff, were taken under the wing of the Pasteurians was a remarkable testament to their internationalism. This cosmopolitanism could also be seen in the number of Eastern European women doctors taking courses.[38]

At the same time as appreciating the importance of the Parisian location, the rapid expansion of the Pasteurian research empire should be noted. The outpost at Garches on the Marne continued to play an important role, particularly when diphtheria serum production required substantial stabling and processing facilities. Provincial Pasteur institutes were rapidly established, for example at Lille under Albert Calmette. There were European and overseas outposts, in North Africa, Brazil and Indo-China, where Paris-trained researchers could find an outlet for their talents – as Yersin did in Indo-China. This internationalism was also typical of Koch and of German-trained bacteriologists, who competed with the Pasteurians in seeking the causes of major tropical diseases and devising preventive remedies for them. These global functions reinforced the importance of Paris and Berlin as world centres of medical research.

Location and organisation of Koch's institute

The Pasteur Institute was remarkable for its relatively decentralised structure. This allowed for internal expansion and diversity. Peripheral siting, flexible accommodation and a readiness to use provincial and overseas locations all contributed to the development of a healthy pluralism at this institute. By contrast, Koch's institute was given a prestigious location at the centre of Berlin, but prestige conflicted with efficiency and expansion. From the outset there were problems of space. The architect had to convert a rented apartment block on a triangular site – the result of a dense pattern of urbanisation in central Berlin, where the adoption of Haussmann's model of wide avenues had resulted in high density tenements.[39] The 'Triangle' was chosen because it was adjacent to vacant land near the Charité hospital and the S-Bahn. Here Koch's institute was provided with a clinical department, consisting of seven hospital barrack-type buildings which were built with 108 beds for 60 men, 36 women and 12 children, with a further three blocks for accommodation, admini-

[38] In 1909, of 102 élèves, there were five women. See Faure 'Cent années'.

[39] N. Bullock and J. Read, *The Movement for Housing Reform in Germany and France 1840–1914* (Cambridge, 1985), p. 91.

stration and disinfection facilities. The barrack style was chosen partly for reasons of economy and partly because the land could not support more substantial buildings.

The urban environment was important in the political background to Koch's institute. On 27 October 1890 a confidential letter was sent by the Prussian civil servant in charge of universities, Althoff, to the Berlin mayor Max von Forckenbeck, directing that Koch should have a new institute with 150 beds.[40] This was intended for the tuberculin therapy which Koch had been covertly developing as an answer to the Pasteurian triumph with the sensational cure for rabies. Forckenbeck was a liberal (a member of the Deutsch-Freisinnige Partei), and was keen to promote municipal improvements. Koch's therapy should be seen as equivalent to other technical innovations sponsored by Forckenbeck such as electrification, the S-Bahn and other public transportation, and parks.[41] Koch's therapy was to be used in the new municipal hospitals so that it could benefit the less well off. There were links to the central state and military hospital, the Charité, with the provision of a nearby site for experimental wards. The order of nurses chosen was the 'Sisters of the Mark Brandenburg' (Märkische Schwestern) – a non-confessional nursing order.[42] Whereas Pasteur initially only had outpatient treatment facilities, Koch's institute was original in combining a hospital with research laboratories. Whether in practice the laboratory researchers made full use of the clinical facilities is a moot point, as arrangements came to be made with a variety of hospitals.

Koch did not live in, but moved out to the suburb of Berlin-Westend after his divorce in 1893. The janitor lived in the cellar, and the ground floor contained service flats. On the first floor was the academic research department; on the second was the administrative office for the clinical department, a department for microphotography, and a library. In the attic was a photographic darkroom (a facility lacking at the Pasteur Institute). The lighting was electric. A specially important feature was the temperature control for the incubator room, using Roux's invention of electromagnetically controlled gas heating. French items of equipment included recording and electrical warning thermometers manufactured by Richard Frères.[43]

It was in keeping with the rigid hierarchical structure of Koch's

[40] GStAM, Rep. 76VIIIB, Nr 2892, Die Errichtung und Verwaltung des staatlichen Instituts für Infektionskrankheiten, Bl. 7, Althoff to Forckenbeck, 27 October 1890.

[41] W. Ribbe (ed.), *Geschichte Berlins* (Berlin, 1987), p. 761.

[42] Möllers, *Koch*, p. 214.

[43] P. Böttger, *Das Koch'sche Institut für Infektionskrankheiten in Berlin* (Berlin, 1891), p. 18.

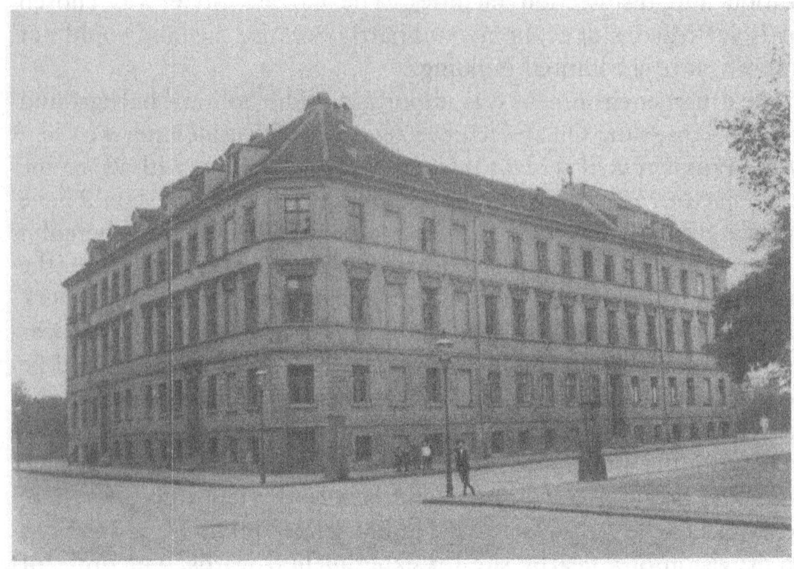

Fig. 4. Koch's Institute for Infectious Diseases, exterior.

institute that the most important of the staff were military medical officers, seconded by the army; there was also one naval medical officer. There were only two departments, the clinical under Ludwig Brieger, and the scientific under Richard Pfeiffer, a military medical officer. There were four assistants: two who were military medical officers, Behring and Pfuhl (the latter was Koch's son-in-law), and two others (Paul Frosch and Johannes Petruschky). There were three voluntary assistants (M. Beck, Hermann Kossel and August von Wassermann), and places for independent researchers including Ehrlich, Dönitz, Cornet and the visiting Japanese researcher Shibasaburo Kitasato. Between 1892 and 1900 there were a further twenty-one military medical officers stationed at the institute for up to three years.[44] In all there were twenty-five places for researchers.[45] There was greater hierarchy, uniformity and direct state and military involvement than at the Pasteur Institute. Moreover, all the German researchers held medical qualifications, which was in marked contrast to the Pasteurians. By 1904 there were six departments (for research, infectious diseases, immunology and serum therapy, tropical diseases, wound research, and biochemistry) as well as clinical facilities at the

[44] Möllers, *Koch*, p. 401.
[45] GStAM, Rep. 76VIIIB, Nr 2904, Die Beamten des Instituts für Infektionskrankheiten in Berlin.

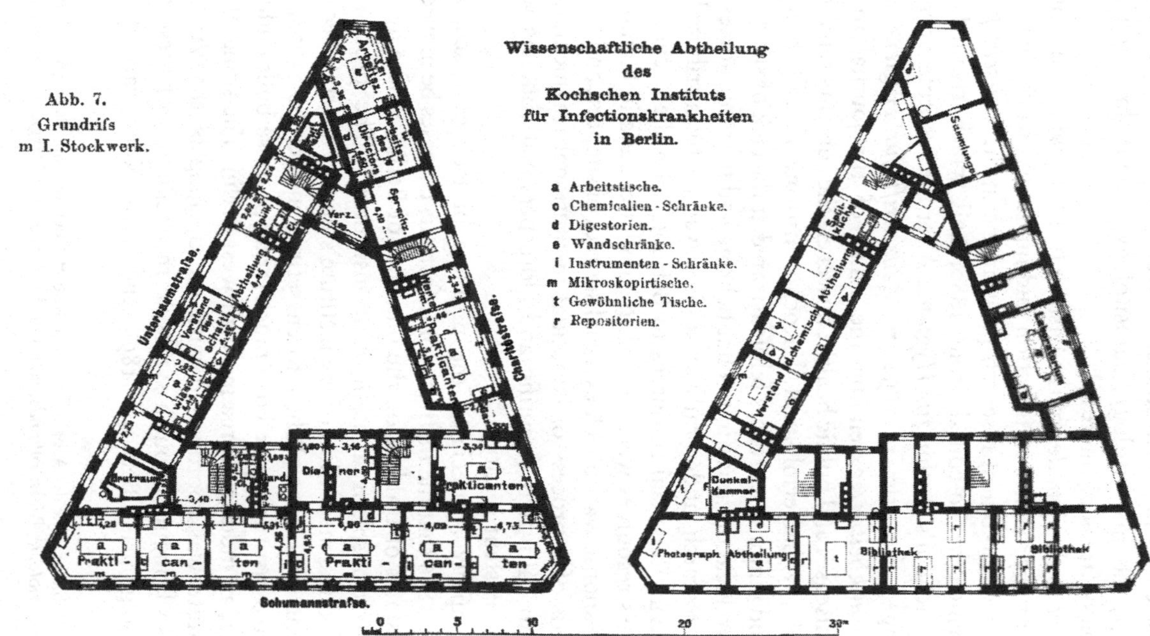

Fig. 5. Koch's Institute for Infectious Diseases, floor plan.

new municipal Virchow Hospital. The institute was tending to further diversification of microbiology on the Pasteurian model. This can be seen in the scientific papers produced between 1891 and 1915 covering bacteriology, therapy, virology, parasitology, immunology and serology as major areas of interest.[46]

In contrast to the *Annales* of the Pasteur Institute, which contained a plurality of approaches to infection and immunity, Koch remained tied to his bacteriological research programme in the *Zeitschrift für Hygiene* which he co-edited from 1880, and which rivalled the Pettenkofer school's *Archiv für Hygiene*. After the Institute opened, Koch changed the title, in 1892, to *Zeitschrift für Hygiene und Infektionskrankheiten*, extending the range of the journal to all infectious diseases and public health; however, the contents remained overwhelmingly bacteriological.[47] Koch's institute rapidly became cramped and junior researchers felt frustrated at the lack of space and at the hierarchical organisation. That Behring had to stable horses for diphtheria research under railway arches was partly attributed to Koch's denying financial resources to Behring, with the excuse that the institute's resources were needed to combat cholera in Hamburg. Behring's response was to seek external sources of support, and herein lay the seeds of a process of continual institutional fragmentation. Behring also cultivated scientific and close personal contacts with Roux at the Pasteur Institute.[48]

Althoff rapidly appreciated the problem of lack of space, and proposed in 1896 that the Institute for Infectious Diseases be moved to the royal estates of Dahlem on the outskirts of Berlin, where he was planning to transplant a number of institutes.[49] The process of dispersal and fragmentation of the institute's initial core staff became fully evident after 1900. When Koch retired in October 1904, the reconstructed institute moved to a much larger purpose-built building in Wedding, an industrial area in north-west Berlin. The siting of the Koch institute was coordinated with the opening of the Virchow Hospital, so bringing about a symbolic reconciliation of these two heroic protagonists. Between 1896 and 1905 Koch carried out

[46] K. Gerber, 'Bibliographie der Arbeiten aus dem Robert-Koch-Institut 1891–1965', *Zentralblatt für Bakteriologie, Parasitenkunde, Infektionskrankheiten und Hygiene*, 203 (1966), pp. 1–265.

[47] [Editorial Foreword], *Zeitschrift für Hygiene und Infektionskrankheiten*, 11 (1892), pp. 1–2.

[48] GStAM, Rep. 92, Althoff B, Nr 9 Bd 1, Bl. 26–7, Behring to Roux, 5 April 1896 concerning the Pasteur Institute. Behring Archives, Behring-Werk Marburg, letter from Roux to Behring, 26 December 1895.

[49] GStAM, Rep. 92, Althoff, Nr 244/1, Bl. 46, Behring to Althoff, 16 May 1896.

protracted research in Africa, and his activities should be seen in the context of German colonialism and the assertion of cultural supremacy through medical science. Backed by the powerful civil servant Althoff, the talented medical researchers Behring and Ehrlich moved to new urban sites on the peripheries of Prussia. Behring, after a brief and unsuccessful period as professor of hygiene during 1894–5 in the industrial centre of Halle, moved to the small university town of Marburg. After taking over the diphtheria serum testing station in 1896, Ehrlich moved outside Prussia to the city of Frankfurt-on-Main, a major German commercial centre, which lacked a university. Here, with support of the dynamic mayor Adickes, the financier Speyer, and Hoechst (chemical and pharmaceutical manufacturers), he established a new institute for experimental therapy.[50]

Conclusions: hierarchical and pluralistic institutional structures

Rather than providing an analysis only of the scientific research undertaken in these two institutes, it is necessary to reconstruct the course of their relations with state, municipal and public bodies, and to take account of their differing cultural values. This provides a corrective to evaluations of research from modern scientific perspectives and to quantitative sociological comparisons. It has been observed that there were many similarities between French and German universities in the later nineteenth century, for example comparable numbers of professors and students. Moreover, both countries shared bureaucratic traditions.[51] The comparison which I have made here reveals the contrasting internal structures, organisation and administrative contexts of the two institutes. The Pasteur Institute benefited from a multiplicity of sources of funding and from a pluralist internal structure that allowed contrasting lines of research to be developed. An example of this is the good relationship maintained between Roux and Metchnikoff, despite Roux's adoption of a modified version of a humoralist approach to immunity and Metchnikoff's cellular approach to immunity. The obvious German contrast is the embittered course of relations between the bacteriologists and Virchow. Pasteurians blended federalism and satellite institutes, as at Lille, with the concept of a central institute and a unity

[50] T. Lenoir, 'A magic bullet: research for profit and the growth of knowledge in Germany around 1900', *Minerva*, 26 (1988), pp. 66–88.

[51] P. Lundgreen, 'The organization of science and technology in France: a German perspective' in Fox and Weisz (eds), *Science and Technology in France*, pp. 311–32.

of common concern with microbiology. Above all, the nineteenth-century hero-worship of great men artificially concentrated attention on Pasteur. Although Pasteur played the role of hero, after a brief walk-on part when the institute was founded he was an off-stage presence, absent from the developing structures of the institute. The lack of either state or effective personal control by Pasteur contrasts to the rigidity of the central state position of Koch's Institute for Infectious Diseases, with its greater dependence on a unitary hierarchy. This was less able to accommodate the individualism of particular positions among researchers, and tensions arose as between Koch and Behring, and Behring and Ehrlich. Within a few years Koch had himself taken a final bow and departed from the stage of this institute.

The long-term record of the institutes has been problematic, particularly for the inter-war period. The Pasteur Institute tended, during the twentieth century, to fossilise under Roux's directorship, and it was only at the expense of considerable internal dissension among leading researchers that the momentum in original research was restored. The Koch institute came to assume an increasingly important role as a national research centre, but later succumbed to the racialisation of medical sciences under Nazism. Although the well-established institutional structures of the 1890s have been enduring, the maintenance of the originality that first led to the founding of such research centres has been problematic. The importance of these two institutes lies less in their scientific or therapeutic achievements, and more in the two contrasting models which they offer of institutes for pure research in the medical sciences. For whether medical research is best undertaken with the support of the state or with the popular support of charitable donations remains an open question.

6

French military epidemiology and the limits of the laboratory

The case of Louis-Félix-Achille Kelsch

MICHAEL A. OSBORNE

This history of the status of laboratory knowledge and its incorporation within the ranks of French military medicine advances along two intertwined axes, the institutional and the biographical. Our gaze falls first on that hub of French army medicine, the Val-de-Grâce hospital and its associated postgraduate medical school for army doctors. The narrative then shifts to examine how a good soldier associated with that institution, a French army physician and epidemiologist named Louis-Félix-Achille Kelsch (1841–1911), viewed laboratory medicine in the years prior to World War I. As I hope to show, it was still possible in the early years of this century to attribute an aetiological role to Pasteur's microbes and yet reject the idea that all or even most epidemic disease resulted from an invasion of microbes. A final section considers Kelsch's career against a backdrop of current historiography on the reception of Pasteurian ideas and finds that historiography overstating the completeness and rapidity of army medicine's incorporation of the Pasteurian programme.

Val-de-Grâce, like much of the Parisian hospital system, was a creation of the Revolution. In the second half of the nineteenth century, two military medical schools furnished Val-de-Grâce with students. In 1856 the newly created Ecole de Service de Santé Militaire de Strasbourg began to send its medical and pharmacy graduates to Val-de-Grâce for practical and specialised instruction in the techniques of military medicine. After the Franco-Prussian War, with

Acknowledgements: I thank the American Council of Learned Societies, the Centre National de la Recherche Scientifique, and the Centre de Recherche en Histoire des Sciences et des Techniques for financial assistance. The Editors, Andrew J. Butrica, Robert Fox, Gerald Geison and Anita Guerrini assisted with intellectual tasks at various stages. At Val-de-Grâce, it is a pleasure to record my debts to Professor Bazot, le médecin chef des services; the Conservateur en chef of the archives; and especially to M. Camille Gargar for his pleasant and skilled assistance that was always above and beyond the call of duty.

Strasburg in German hands, the military medical school at Lyons replaced the Strasburg school as the source of students for instruction at Val-de-Grâce.[1] In the journey from Empire to Third Republic the institution underwent many changes. This institutional instability could have provided opportunities for developing programmes in laboratory medicine, but no one seized the chance. The nature of military careers, which often mandated sojourns to the colonies or war zones, and Val-de-Grâce's practice of limiting a professor's tenure to ten years, made it difficult even for a committed individual to build and retain control of a laboratory. Still, instruction in laboratory medicine gained a foothold at Val-de-Grâce before the bacteriological revolution. The history of the growth of laboratories at Val-de-Grâce is one of fits and starts, and in this respect the army's experience was not so different from that of the civilian medical faculties.

Antoine-Baudoin Poggiale, a physician and military pharmacist, advocated laboratory medicine at Val-de-Grâce as early as the 1850s. The first incumbent of the chair of toxicology and chemistry created in 1852, his duties included instruction in microscopy. Primarily a chemist, Poggiale was interested in creating an analytical medical laboratory, and at the time of his promotion to pharmaceutical inspector for the army, he had completed substantial analyses of drinking water and foodstuffs, and had investigated the chemical composition of human and animal blood. His insistence that the chemical laboratory should have a place in medicine made him the target of caustic remarks by Armand Trousseau, perhaps the last great figure in the French clinical school's classical era.

After the Franco-Prussian War, Val-de-Grâce founded a number of specialised laboratories. While the founding dates of the laboratories and the names of the key personnel are known, little archival information has survived that would allow us to reconstruct how these laboratories functioned and to estimate their real impact on medical instruction. Some historians have concluded that Louis Vaillard's creation of a bacteriological laboratory in 1889 (mentioned below) had a significant impact on the education of army medical men and provided the basis for 'new programmes of teaching which

[1] I have taken general details on Val-de-Grâce from A. Fabre, *Le Val-de-Grâce* (Paris, 1975), and J. Rieux and J. Hassenforder, *Histoire du Service de Santé Militaire et du Val-de-Grâce* (Paris, 1951). Navy medical men were trained at a separate institution, the Ecole de Médecine Navale et Coloniale de Bordeaux.

resulted from the Pasteurian revolution'.[2] Still, the precise effect of the laboratory on the majority of Val-de-Grâce's student body remains enigmatic. As late as a quarter century after the founding of the Pasteur Institute, long after the emergence of medical bacteriology, Val-de-Grâce's laboratory and museum of hygiene, which had been founded around 1880 and was dedicated to the older techniques of public health, was still better endowed with instructional material than Vaillard's bacteriological laboratory.[3]

The introduction of laboratory medicine at Val-de-Grâce, particularly bacteriology, was closely associated with the history of the chair of illnesses and epidemics of armies. Léon Collin, a skilled vaccinator who took up that post in 1867, became an early convert to Pasteur's doctrines. Louis Vaillard, a friend of Roux who became the chair's fourth incumbent in 1892, had already distinguished himself as an adjunct professor at Val-de-Grâce by founding the first French military bacteriological laboratory in 1889. Jacques Léonard has identified other conduits of Pasteurian ideas as well. Both the clinical professor Charles-Pierre Godélier and the professor of hygiene, Antoine Villemin, knew Pasteur and became his enthusiastic supporters. Others associated with Val-de-Grâce, such as Emile-Arthur Vallin, are said to have carried the Pasteurian message far and wide. Vallin held Val-de-Grâce's chair of hygiene and legal medicine from 1874 to 1884, and later assumed the directorship of the Ecole de Santé Militaire de Lyon.[4] While much of this history seems to indicate that army medicine was quick to embrace Pasteurian ideas, we need to question the rapidity with which this happened; in other words we need a chronology to make sense of accounts which typify physicians as adopting the microbe theory in a 'desperately slow' fashion, or 'early on'.[5]

Even after advocates of a microbial theory of disease are identified within the ranks of Val-de-Grâce's professoriate, a semiotic question lingers. Neither all microbes nor all microbe theorists were created equal, and we need to know the nature of the messages presented to students at Val-de-Grâce. While it is true that the chair of illnesses and epidemics of armies eventually added bacteriology as one of its official responsibilities, this was not until after the new science's utility had

[2] Comité d'Histoire du Service de Santé, *Histoire de la médecine aux armées*, 3 vols. (Paris, 1984), vol. II, p. 179. [3] A. Mignon, *Ecole du Val-de-Grâce* (Paris, 1914), p. 15.

[4] Jacques Léonard, 'Comment peut-on être Pasteurien?' in Claire Salomon-Bayet (ed.), *Pasteur et la révolution pastorienne* (Paris, 1986), pp. 143–79, at p. 160.

[5] Bruno Latour, *The Pasteurization of France*, trans. Alan Sheridan and John Law (Cambridge, Mass., 1988; original French edition, 1984), pp. 133 and 52.

been proven in the heat of World War I. The message delivered to students before that time was dependent on the professor, and Collin and Vaillard must have converted some to Pasteur's ideas. But in the case of Louis-Félix-Achille Kelsch, the chair's third incumbent, the message was weakly Pasteurian at best.

Kelsch held the chair of illnesses and epidemics of armies during the formative years of medical bacteriology, from 1882 to 1892. Avoiding immediate seduction by Pasteur's ideas, he was enough of an old school epidemiologist and sanitary expert to qualify equally well as both an army doctor and a hygienist. Sandwiched between Collin and Vaillard, his personal trajectory none the less went counter to theirs, and for most of his life he sought to limit the sphere of laboratory medicine. Kelsch's biographer has tried to link his reserve towards Pasteurian ideas with his schooling and early scientific interests in pathological anatomy and histology.[6] This assessment, however, does not get at the root of Kelsch's resistance to Pasteurian doctrine, nor does it consider the evolution of Kelsch's scientific interests, which by 1900 had shifted far from pathological anatomy to include epidemiological and aetiological concerns.

Kelsch devoted considerable professional energy to laboratory medicine, even though he was not always its advocate. For ten years he lectured to Val-de-Grâce students on contagion, the germ theory of disease, and many subjects of concern to Pasteurian science. These lectures are notable both for their reserved acceptance of the germ theory of disease and for what they reveal about military medicine and the medical world of Val-de-Grâce during the Third Republic. A reflective person, Kelsch eventually fashioned a synthesis between the new bacteriology and those grand old traditions of military medicine in which he had been trained, medical geography and pathological anatomy. But during the period of his professorship at Val-de-Grâce, Kelsch's faith in the special nature of military medicine and his dissatisfaction with the theory of contagion relegated the knowledge produced by the medical laboratory to second-class status.

A young military physician just returned from duty in Algeria, Kelsch began his career in academic medicine as a professor at the Ecole du Service de Santé Militaire de Strasbourg. Alsatian by birth and a graduate of Strasburg where he had defended his medical thesis

[6] Serge Helfer, *Kelsch: sa vie, son oeuvre, 1841–1911* (Lyons, 1972), p. 40. Helfer does not cite Kelsch's article on cerebrospinal meningitis. The journal *Le Caducée* reprinted parts of it upon Kelsch's death and called it his epidemiological credo. See *Le Caducée*, no. 4 (18 February 1911) and my discussion of the article below. For biographical details of Kelsch, see Helfer and the obituary in *Revue Internationale de la Vaccine*, 1 (1911), pp. 417–23.

on dyspepsia in 1866, he did not long remain in this familiar milieu. Kelsch became an adjunct in epidemiology and general pathology at the Val-de-Grâce in 1870, and it was at the same institution in 1873 that he took charge of a ward when the cholera once again visited Paris. Kelsch, who had chosen French citizenship after his homeland fell to the Germans, developed none the less a deep familiarity with German science. He was critical of Virchow's pathology, whose descriptions of typhus lesions he disputed, and of Koch's work on tuberculosis. Like Henri Roger, professor of experimental and comparative pathology at the Paris Faculty of Medicine, Kelsch felt that German medicine's concentration on laboratory medicine limited its view.[7] A different kind of medicine, the medicine of the field, was something Kelsch knew quite well, and he refined his knowledge by leaving Val-de-Grâce in 1874 for a five-year tour of work in North Africa. Thus, it was with substantial knowledge of both Val-de-Grâce and the field conditions of military medicine that Kelsch became a full professor at Val-de-Grâce in 1882.

The course on army medicine for 1888 opened with a synopsis of the special nature of medical education at Val-de-Grâce and the goals of military medical practice. Students arrived there with a medical degree in hand, and Kelsch began with the presumption that his auditors had already mastered the basics of medicine. The class in army medicine aimed at imparting a knowledge of aetiological nosography which would lead to improved procedures of disease prevention. As medical officers in the French army, students at Val-de-Grâce were destined to treat many of the same diseases found in civilian life. However, these same men would need to practise a medicine differing from civilian medicine in both action and goal.

The civilian physician, according to Kelsch, overly 'absorbed himself in the clinical difficulties of the particular fact'.[8] This myopic view of disease, while it might lead to diagnostic precision and perhaps appropriate therapy, menaced the military physician because it slowed the development of an overview of disease causality. The military physician, unlike his civilian counterpart, was caretaker for a whole regiment. He could not afford to focus on the individual manifestations of disease and the therapy of the individual patient. Military physicians needed to be more than clinicians, said Kelsch, for

[7] Cited in Harry W. Paul, *The Sorcerer's Apprentice: The French Scientist's Image of German Science, 1840–1919* (Gainesville, Fla., 1972), p. 51.

[8] A. Kelsch, 'La médecine d'armée – les causes morbigènes', *Archives de Médecine et de Pharmacie Militaire*, 11 (1888), pp. 337–53, at p. 338.

the uniform they wore charged them with 'a much greater task than to cure illness, [and] that is to seek the cause of illness in order to impede its advance or prevent its return'.[9]

A primary goal of the military physician was to preserve the ability of the fighting force to carry out its function, and, in this medical cosmos, therapy for those who were already sick-listed was a secondary task. Military medical practice also required the physician to act with greater speed than was usually necessary in civilian settings. It mandated a rapid analysis of disease signs and encouraged a quick leap to a synthetic view of aetiology. The men were not to linger over clinical signs, for diagnosis was only the first step from whence they began 'to trace back from the effect to the cause, to connect together manifestations disparate in appearance'.[10] The very nature of military life required that the epidemiological question be posed and posed anew at each examination. For example, a civilian physician might encounter two cases of diarrhoea in three days and treat them as isolated incidents. Soldiers, on the other hand, shared common living quarters, ate the same food, and were often similar in age. These men formed a homogeneous group which provided fertile ground for epidemic disease. Thus even a minor affliction such as diarrhoea – which if allowed to become generalised in a regiment would compromise its ability to fight – required quick containment so it would not reach the epidemic stage. The military physician, counselled Kelsch, was under an 'obligation to discover the cause of every morbid manifestation as soon as possible'.[11] In matters medical, they were to seek the synthetic view, and in time, he hoped, they would 'get accustomed to see things from the high ground and from a distance'.[12]

The great achievements of the medical laboratory, particularly the discovery of the causes of anthrax and fowl cholera, and the development of methods to combat them, loomed large in Kelsch's concept of disease and in his vision of military medicine. He considered disease a specific entity with a specific cause, and Pasteur's research on germs confirmed these ideas. By applying ammonia to the intestines of healthy dogs, Kelsch had produced lesions like those associated with dysentery.[13] He was also aware that arsenic, potassium and other substances each produced their own characteristic lesions when applied to healthy human tissue.[14] From the

[9] *Ibid.* [10] *Ibid.*, p. 339. [11] *Ibid.* [12] *Ibid.*

[13] Helfer, *Kelsch*, p. 13; and Kelsch, 'Les causes morbigènes', pp. 347–9.

[14] *Ibid.*, p. 348.

specificity of the pathological effects these substances provoked in the anatomical laboratory, Kelsch reasoned that diseases in nature must also have a specific action which would imply a specific cause.

Kelsch's lectures reveal a highly selective appropriation of laboratory knowledge. While he enthusiastically endorsed the idea that a specific germ, one of those 'active agents that vegetate silently around us or even within our organism', lay behind nearly all diseases, the discovery of microbes had solved only part of the aetiological riddle.[15] Smallpox excepted, germs in and of themselves were not sufficient engines of disease. Moreover, Pasteur had shown that the virulence of germs fluctuated within very wide boundaries as they passed through different animals and encountered different environments. For example, why was it, asked Kelsch, that widely separated cases of cerebrospinal meningitis should suddenly appear, and why did the disease only strike some members of a family and not others?[16] The answers, it seemed, which revealed the limitations of Pasteur's bacteriology for Kelsch, could only be determined by detailed study of what he called secondary causes: those factors of individual and public hygiene such as meteorological influences, diet and vices which contributed to the genesis of disease but were powerless to cause it in and of themselves. Indeed, recent laboratory research on the duration of immunity conferred by vaccino-therapy, debate over the role of carrier germs, and the realisation that the experimental culture of bacteria required careful control of the media, had revealed a dynamic dimension of disease which could only be seized by a pluralistic approach to aetiology. In Kelsch's medical world, microbes were crucial elements in the development of disease; but they were not the only elements, merely the most powerful actors in the aetiological process.

The image of laboratory medicine provided Kelsch with a rather loose model for epidemiological method. The strategy was resolutely conservative, for Kelsch was less interested in controlling society through laboratory methods than in using laboratory science to support a continuation of the kind of medicine so decried by Claude Bernard, the medicine of observation.[17] 'Applying the language and

[15] *Ibid.*, p. 349.

[16] A. Kelsch, 'De la méningite cérébro-spinale épidémique, étude critique de sa pathogénie', *Revue d'Hygiène et de Police Sanitaire*, 33 (1911), pp. 1–53, at pp. 4 and 12.

[17] The difficulty in demarcating between the laboratory and society is well told by Bruno Latour. My point is that Kelsch delimits a restricted sphere for the laboratory and uses laboratory knowledge in a conservative manner. See Bruno Latour, 'Give me a laboratory and I will raise the world' in Karin D. Knorr-Cetina and Michael Mulkay (eds), *Science Observed: Perspectives on the Social Study of Science* (London, 1983), pp. 141–70.

notions of the laboratory to acts of nature,' Kelsch instructed his students, 'we will say that these cosmic and hygienic influences, by their contingent disruption, achieve the environment of extra- and intra-organic culture appropriate to the cultivation of a germ.'[18] The philologist and physician Emile Littré had completed his translation of Hippocrates in 1861, and Kelsch's message here should be read as part of a widely felt enthusiasm in French medicine for the objects studied by the physician of Cos. Read in this manner, Kelsch calls not for an extension of the laboratory but for continued scrutiny of the environmental factors in the disease process. In case some auditors might have interpreted these remarks as a call to enlarge the laboratory's sphere through the extension of a research programme on media and the conditions of culture, Kelsch quickly disabused them of the notion. Whatever the future progress of bacteriology might be, Kelsch continued, it could never substitute for 'the observation of the pathogenic conditions of epidemic illness, [or] for the study of the environment of cultivation in that great laboratory of nature'.[19] It was not coincidental that the study of the secondary factors had a long tradition in French military medicine, especially among physicians such as Kelsch who had served in North Africa and in the febrile regions of the Mediterranean Basin.

Medical geography provided the necessary complement to laboratory science in aetiological matters. The study of secondary factors in the disease process by historical medical geography is a recurring theme in Kelsch's work, and it assumed 'a practical importance of the first order for the military physician'.[20] In contrast to the civilian physician, the medical officer was likely to practise in several different provinces and countries during his career, and the unique disease ecologies of these locations would each require different strategies of disease avoidance. While there had been pre-Revolutionary calls for a medical geography which would provide the military with a catalogue of the predominant diseases in each region of France, this task proved formidable.[21] By the middle third of the nineteenth century, urban and industrial hygienists such as René Villermé were using proto-statistical methods to correlate civilian patterns of mortality with geographical location and occupation.[22] Military medical officers of the same era

[18] Kelsch, 'Les causes morbigènes', p. 350.
[19] *Ibid.* [20] *Ibid.*, p. 344.
[21] 'Projet d'une géographie médicale de la France à l'usage des troupes', *Journal de Médecine Militaire* (1786), p. 137.
[22] William Coleman, *Death is a Social Disease: Public Health and Political Economy in Early Industrial France* (Madison, Wis., 1982).

filled the pages of reviews such as the *Annales d'Hygiène Publique* with medical geographical studies of their stations of duty, and a bold few of their number attempted the grand synthesis.

A watershed of sorts in French military medical geography occurred in the 1830s. Only a few years earlier, Antoine-Barthèlmy Clot, who had accepted a contract from the Egyptian government to reorganise its health services, had begun to describe the health conditions of the Nile Valley.[23] The French Army captured the city of Algiers in the summer of 1830 and, except for a few months in the period 1858 to 1860, military governments ran the colony for the next forty years. After 1834, medical geographers could support their investigations with a growing body of vital statistics collected on the African Army. The military medical literature of this era reflects a growing concern with the infectious diseases encountered in North Africa by settlers and soldiers. This efflorescence of literature on the fevers and ocular diseases of North Africa was not due solely to the fact that military medical men were encountering a new disease environment. Service in Algeria provided a quicker route to advancement than metropolitan duty, and perhaps a number of ambitious physicians who published more than their peers went there. Kelsch wrote frequently on the problems of colonial medicine, especially on the pathological anatomy of typhoid and paludine fevers of Algeria, but also on more general topics such as the diseases of Indo-China, as well as on hygienic matters such as the establishment of health services in Martinique, Guadeloupe and Réunion.[24] Thus Kelsch looked both to the laboratory bench and to the world at large for models of military medicine. He especially hoped that some of his students would emulate such great medical geographers of the day as Jean Boudin, author of the massive *Traité de géographie et de statistique médicales et des maladies endémiques*.[25]

As the subtitle of Boudin's study noted, it was a compilation of

[23] The panorama of French medical activity in Egypt is covered in Serge Jagailloux, *La médicalisation de l'Egypte au XIXe siècle* (Paris, 1986); LaVerne Kuhnke, *Lives at Risk: Public Health in Nineteenth-Century Egypt* (Berkeley, 1990).

[24] The scope of Kelsch's research up to 1890 is available in *Exposé des titres et des travaux scientifiques du Dr A. Kelsch* (Paris, 1890). Helfer's incomplete bibliography lists 108 items. See Helfer, *Kelsch*, pp. 54–62. Philip D. Curtin provides an excellent synthesis of French and British vital statistics and tropical medicine in *Death by Migration: Europe's Encounter with the Tropical World in the Nineteenth Century* (Cambridge, 1989).

[25] J.-C.-M.-F.-J. Boudin, *Traité de géographie et de statistique médicales et des maladies endémiques*, 2 vols. (Paris, 1857); Michael A. Osborne, 'The medicine of the hot countries, philology, and European settlement in Algeria', seminar paper at the Shelby Cullom Davis Center for Historical Studies, Princeton University, April 1992.

what was known about medical meteorology, medical geology, the geographical distribution of diseases, and the comparative pathology of the human races. The book presented Boudin's findings in the form of maps and charts which displayed seasonal and geographical variations in morbidity and mortality patterns. The maps were quite specific in content and they covered topics ranging from the epidemiology of lightning strike injuries to the distribution of hernia and goitre among men exempted from military service. In short, it contained detailed information on Kelsch's secondary factors and their role in the disease process. Like Kelsch, Boudin wrote from a firsthand knowledge of the disease ecology of military life. He had familiarised himself with the geography of the Mediterranean Basin during tours of duty in Spain, Greece and Algeria. Kelsch admired Boudin's methods, and some thirty years later he sought to combine the findings of the medical laboratory with those of medical geography.

Kelsch produced two works of synthetic scope: the *Traité des maladies des pays chauds, région prétropical* of 1889, and the *Traité des maladies épidémiques, étiologie et pathologie des maladies infectieuses*, the two volumes of which appeared in 1894 and 1905.[26] The *Traité des maladies des pays chauds* became a handbook for French physicians in North Africa. It was accomplished with the collaboration of Kelsch's friend Paul-Louis André Kiener, an adjunct professor at Val-de-Grâce before accepting a chair at the Montpellier Faculty of Medicine. The two men had similar scientific interests, and they shared common roots both as Alsatians and as fellow graduates of Strasburg and Val-de-Grâce's Ecole d'Application. Their book on pathological anatomy and histology utilised Val-de-Grâce's histological collection and won the Académie de Médecine's Godart prize for 1890.

Although Kelsch remained interested in macroscopic and cellular pathological anatomy, the *Traité des maladies des pays chauds* looked back to observations he had collected in North Africa, notably during his extended sojourn there between 1874 and 1879. By the time of the Godart prize, Kelsch's research activities had expanded well beyond pathological anatomy. With Louis Vaillard, his successor as Val-de-Grâce's professor of epidemiology, Kelsch published an inquiry into the microbiology of leukaemia in the *Annales* of the Pasteur

[26] L.-F.-A. Kelsch and P.-L.-A. Keiner, *Traité des maladies des pays chauds, région prétropical* (Paris, 1889, new edn, 1890); L.-F.-A. Kelsch, *Traité des maladies épidémiques* 2 vols. (Paris, 1894 and 1905).

Institute.[27] In this entry into the proper domain of bacteriology, the two men produced *in vitro* a pure culture of bacteria isolated from the blood and lymphatic tumours of a young soldier. Although a rabbit and white mouse inoculated with the material died and were found to be contaminated with the bacteria, the authors stopped short of claiming to have isolated the causal organism of leukaemia. While Kelsch did not become a bacteriologist, his publications after 1890 covered a range of topics where he considered germs, contagion and, especially, the aetiology and prophylaxis of epidemic disease. He also turned towards problems of medical administration upon his election to the Académie de Médecine in 1893.

By the time the first volume of the *Traité des maladies épidémiques* appeared in 1894, Kelsch had been promoted to the directorship of the Ecole de Service de Santé Militaire in Lyons. Léonard, basing his account largely on the presence at Lyons of the Pasteurian Emile-Arthur Vallin, portrays the students there as breathing in the Pasteurian concepts which would revolutionise both medical-surgical practice and public and private hygiene.[28] Kelsch's message, however, cannot have radicalised many students. It stressed both the continuity of epidemiological practice and the limits of bacteriology. The preface to the *Traité des maladies épidémiques* provided an opportunity to reflect on the state of epidemiology during the period of his professorship at Val-de-Grâce. It had been in that decade, he wrote

> that the immortal discoveries of Pasteur and his school had opened new horizons to medicine and changed the orientation of its efforts. One could believe at first that microbiology would surely modify the objective of epidemiology by substituting the search for first causes for that of secondary causes: nothing of the kind. The search for secondary causes of illnesses, that is to say the whole group of cosmic, telluric and hygienic circumstances which are necessary for microbes to live and exert their pathogenic functions, that search which is the essential goal of epidemiology will always force itself on the physician as a vital problem, whatever might be the progress of bacteriology. It is in acting on these secondary factors of infection that hygiene has the greatest chance to fight against the invisible enemies which surround us; to seek to reach them directly would be a vain or at least inadequate endeavour in the majority of cases.[29]

In the early 1890s, then, Kelsch held fast to the view that the utility of laboratory medicine was limited. Apparently, his opinions did not impede his advancement within the military hierarchy, for the post at

[27] A. Kelsch and L. Vaillard, 'Tumeurs lymphadémiques multiples avec leucémie, constation d'un microbe dans le sang pedant la vie et dans les tumeurs enlevées aussitôt après la mort', *Annales de l'Institut Pasteur*, 4 (1890), pp. 276–84.

[28] Léonard, 'Comment peut-on être Pasteurien?', p. 160.

[29] Kelsch, *Traité des maladies épidémiques*, vol. 1, p. i.

Lyons was only a prelude to the call back to Paris and the directorship of the Ecole d'Application at Val-de-Grâce.

After his return to Paris Kelsch produced a series of articles critical of the concept of contagion, and it was in pointing out the inadequacies of contagion as an explanatory model for epidemics that he refined his concept of the autogenesis of disease. Gerald Geison has noted how Pasteur fought tenaciously against the doctrines of the interiority and spontaneity of disease. Although Kelsch's theory of disease autogenesis employed microbes as causal agents it embraced a notion of the interiority of disease which distanced Kelsch from Pasteur and his school.[30]

Kelsch's Val-de-Grâce lecture of 1889 on seasonal catarrhal afflictions predates his use of the term autogenesis.[31] None the less, the lecture, later recycled as a chapter of the *Traité des maladies épidémiques*, contained many of the points which he later combined into his theory of autogenesis. The class of seasonal catarrhal illnesses contained a number of little-studied, acute complaints – afflictions such as colds, sore throats and bronchitis common in winter, and diarrhoea and intestinal complaints which struck in summer. By marshalling a number of geographical studies on the low frequency of bronchitis in the polar regions, Kelsch criticised the notion that meteorological factors acting alone could provoke bronchitis. At base, he argued, the seasonal pattern of catarrhs did not hold up. The term seasonal illness now applied to an ill-defined class of disease, a sort of artifact of Hippocratic thinking that had weathered the development of the modern concepts of contagion and infection. The real power of meteorological factors in the aetiological process lay in their ability to stimulate 'the number and activity of germs, to favour their entry into the organism, and finally, to render the organism more receptive to [germs]'.[32] Kelsch supported this contention by citing laboratory studies by Rosenthal and Quinquaud which showed that cold temperatures disrupted the physiology of warm-blooded animals. Such a state, he supposed, left the animals particularly vulnerable to invasion by germs. If further proof were needed, even the great Pasteur had shown that hens resistant to anthrax developed the disease when cooled.[33]

30 Gerald Geison, 'Pasteur, Louis' in *Dictionary of Scientific Biography* vol. x, pp. 350–416, at p. 384.

31 A. Kelsch, *Des catarrhales saisonnières* (Paris, 1889).

32 *Ibid.*, pp. 58–9.

33 *Ibid.* pp. 59–60. Kelsch realised that Pasteur's hens seemed to return to a state of health when warmed. His point was that cooling influenced an organism's receptivity to microbial activity. This agrees quite well with Latour's account of how Pasteur's explanation for the variation of virulence hooked the hygienists. See Latour, *Pasteurization*, pp. 62–5.

Kelsch deployed a twofold strategy to associate bronchitis, sore throat, diarrhoea and other catarrhal ills with germs. He did not approach the problem with flasks, cultures and a programme of laboratory research. Instead, he began with the presumption that humans lived in a sea of microbes. Some existed around us where they remained poised to invade the organism, whereas others – the ones crucial for autogenesis – were beyond any sanitary cordon or Listerian strategy, for they resided within the body. Military physicians had to be aware that disease could arise from within the body, 'especially the latent microbism of the buccal cavity'.[34] His second tack was to associate catarrhal afflictions with epidemic diseases already linked to bacteriological origins, diseases such as cholera, diphtheria and dysentery. By tracing the histories of various influenza, diphtheria and cholera epidemics and making comparisons with (respectively) bronchitis, sore throat and diarrhoea, Kelsch demonstrated to his own satisfaction that the acute illnesses were merely mild forms of the epidemic diseases. From his perspective as a military epidemiologist, sensitised as he was to find and prevent nascent epidemics, Kelsch concluded that diarrhoea was merely a non-epidemic form of cholera, and that in several instances diarrhoea had also presented itself as aborted epidemics of typhoid fever and dysentery.

Kelsch's ideas found their 'theoretical consecration in the works of Pasteur and his school on attenuated illnesses. Nature certainly commands processes of attenuation for the morbid grains which live freely in the environment [just] as the bacteriologist has his [processes] for those that he keeps captive in his flasks.'[35] To be sure, not all catarrhal illnesses could be linked with other endemic or epidemic diseases. But the general image of the disease that arises from within, from a germ inhabiting a body that suddenly responds to environmental stimuli and increases in virulence, became a major preoccupation for Kelsch.

Kelsch's final version of his autogenesis theory appeared in a study of cerebrospinal meningitis.[36] This disease had flared up in Upper Silesia in 1905, had become generalised among the miners of the Ruhr Valley in 1907, and had attacked Paris, the French countryside, and no fewer than forty-five garrisons of the French Army during the winter of 1909–10. In investigating the role of contagion in the epidemic's genesis and extension, Kelsch began with the historical medical

[34] Kelsch, *Des catarrhales saisonnières*, p. 62.
[35] *Ibid.*, p. 56.
[36] Kelsch, 'De la méningite cérébro-spinal épidémique'.

geography of past epidemics. Four discernible periods had marked the development of the disease in the previous century. From 1805 to 1837, meningitis had flared up in the United States and manifested itself in Europe as a series of sporadic, isolated incidents. From 1837 to 1850, simultaneous cases had appeared with great frequency throughout the United States, France, Algeria, Italy and Denmark. In the third period, from 1854 to 1875, the plague seemed to peak as it raged anew in the countries visited in the previous period and extended to Latin America. The final quarter of the century had witnessed the disease's return to a more limited, sporadic mode of behaviour.

The most striking feature of this history was the simultaneous appearance of the disease in widely separated locations. Invasion by microbes could not explain the origins of the 1837 outbreaks, nor could it, in the strict formulation he attributed to a diffusely defined German school, cast light on the different patterns of morbidity and mortality assumed by the disease. Kelsch was unwilling to let the laboratory mediate all of medicine. He felt he had 'found in the lessons of observation protection against the ill-conceived practices of experimentation', and he accused the Germans of misconstruing or ignoring the variability of the germ.[37] Their fault had been to focus on the means of propagation of the epidemic after it had begun to blossom. Both the carrier germs of apparently healthy subjects and the immediately virulent diplococci passed from the ill to others had a role in the extension of the epidemic, but the transmission of these contagious elements was 'only an insignificant factor in the forces which create[d] the epidemic impulse'.[38] Belief in the incessant variability of the motor of disease formed the pivot upon which Kelsch's epidemiology turned, and on this point he was unambiguously Pasteurian. Confirmation of the variability of the meningitis diplococcus could be found even across the Rhine, and Kelsch was quick to employ this research to criticise contagion theory and promote his own theory of autogenesis.

The German school was of course not unanimous in its opinions, and studies of the 1907 meningitis epidemic in the Ruhr by two physicians working at the Gelsenkirchen laboratory of hygiene and bacteriology, Joseph Hohn and Hayo Bruns, had produced evidence that the frequency of carrier germs in the pharyngeal mucus of healthy subjects rose and fell in tandem with the reported frequency of

[37] *Ibid.*, pp. 52 and 6.

[38] *Ibid.*, p. 21.

subjects who developed meningitis.[39] The discovery indicated that variations in the population of carrier germs, many of which had been detected in subjects having no apparent contact with meningitis victims, were 'subordinated to a law, or at least a general influence, and not a fortuitous circumstance such as [transmission] by a fit of coughing or by a bout of sneezing'.[40] By Kelsch's account, Bruns and Hohn had suggested that the Ruhr meningitis epidemic had become manifest only after causes of a cosmic order had created a pool of carrier germs sufficient to start an epidemic. The suggestion presumed that carrier germs existed prior to the outbreak of the epidemic, and Kelsch seized the idea as an implicit expression of the theory of autogenesis.

The theory of autogenesis was not in the exact sense a theory of the spontaneous generation of disease, for illness always arose from pre-existing germs. Of the two great modes of disease propagation, autogenesis and contagion by invading germs, autogenesis was clearly the most important for epidemiology and military medicine. The invading germs, wrote Kelsch, those passed from the ill to the healthy, were 'only an insignificant factor in the forces which create the epidemic impulse'.[41] In autogenesis a whole fund of environmental secondary factors sparked harmlessly saphrophytic germs to fiery virulence. Although Kelsch could not specify the precise mechanisms which created such an increase in pathogenic potential, he felt confident of their existence, for the discovery of radioactivity and its effects on life had shown the ability of environmental forces to disrupt vital processes. He did not consider in print the possibility that factors internal to the germs themselves might effect such a transformation.

The value of a theory of autogenesis for epidemiology was clear. It explained, in a way contagion could not, the apparent spontaneity and geographically dispersed patterns of epidemic disease. Epidemics grew from a core of *in situ* germs, and 'autogenesis preceded and subsequently reinforced contagion in all phases of the evolution of the epidemic'.[42] The sorts of germs most closely associated with the Pasteurian programme – those invaders transmitted to healthy individuals from the infected – were to Kelsch secondary elements in epidemic propagation. These germs of contagion caused sporadic cases of disease, but were 'powerless to create an epidemic'.[43]

[39] *Ibid.*, pp. 16–23. The study cited is Hayo Bruns and Joseph Hohn, 'Ueber den Nachweis und Vorkommen des Meningokok im Nasenrachenraum', *Klinisches Jahrbuch*, 18 (1908), pp. 285–310.
[40] Kelsch, 'De la méningite cérébro-spinal épidémique', p. 18.
[41] *Ibid.*, p. 21.
[42] *Ibid.*, p. 26.
[43] *Ibid.*, p. 42.

The meningitis study appeared in 1911, the year of Kelsch's death. Its conciliatory tone towards bacteriology demonstrates that its author had reconceptualised the relationship between laboratory medicine and epidemiology. Some two decades earlier in the *Traité des maladies épidémiques* and his Val-de-Grâce lectures, Kelsch had stressed the limited value of bacteriology for epidemiological investigation. Although he had been willing then to concede to the laboratory the study of first causes, and to use the model of laboratory investigation in some phases of epidemiological field studies, his intent was to reserve for epidemiology the study of the all-important secondary factors. By 1911, however, Kelsch no longer wrote about bacteriology and epidemiology as separate spheres, or of epidemiology as an area of medicine which bacteriology had failed to reform. He continued to practise historical medical geography, and at certain junctures he still charged epidemiology with the responsibility for the study of secondary factors. The formulation of the theory of autogenesis, however, marked a rise in the status of the laboratory for Kelsch, for when he published his last statement on the study of secondary factors, he left it to 'the bacteriologist to determine the mode of action of cosmic and cosmo-telluric agents on the germs which they hold under their dependency'.[44]

Army doctor and epidemiologist/hygienist though he was, Kelsch was neither an immediate nor a complete convert to the Pasteurian programme. Chronology, that meagre tool of the historian, has a certain value for this narrative. We should not read Kelsch's position of 1911 back into the lectures he had given at Val-de-Grâce in the 1880s or retrospectively impose it upon his thinking of the middle 1890s during his time at the Ecole de Service de Santé at Lyons. In the years of his professorships at Val-de-Grâce and Lyons, the discoveries of laboratory medicine had led him to a conservative defence of medical geography and military epidemiology. His message of the 1880s and early 1890s was not that of a convinced Pasteurian; he had at that time called for continued reliance on observational medicine. Laboratory medicine was called upon to play only a secondary role in the major task of the military physician, preventive epidemiology. Germs were important in the study of aetiology, but Pasteur's science had seemed incapable of bringing about a complete reform of medicine.

The medical laboratory and the disciples of Pasteur and Koch could

[44] *Ibid.*, p. 44.

do much for preventive medicine, but to this military epidemiologist they seemed to have little or no application to the problems he encountered daily. A key problem of army medicine had been to identify rapidly the disease and then prevent its spread. In other words, quarantine those on the sick-list and devote most attention towards the health of the other members of the battalion so they would always be poised to enter battle.

The case of Kelsch gains broader significance when viewed in the light of Bruno Latour's study of Pasteur.[45] Central to this account is the selective adoption of Pasteurian ideas by three groups of practitioners – civilian doctors, hygienists and army physicians. Kelsch, of course, would fall squarely in Latour's last category by virtue of his profession, and perhaps too in the second category by virtue of his Val-de-Grâce teaching duties. Latour, who writes as an epistemologist, has little use for chronology and claims that historical time is reversible. Be that as it may, time does apparently vary in speed, for civil physicians, as viewed through the editorial pages of the *Concours Médical*, are characterised as 'desperately slow' in accepting the concept of the microbe in 1895.[46] Following Jacques Léonard, Latour portrays the civil medical corps as sceptical towards medical microbiology. Here he is on firm ground. The reasons offered by civilian physicians for rejecting Pasteur were manifold: traditional medicine was working; anti-septic surgery was effective and should not be jettisoned for the aseptic technique. Worst of all, the findings of the microbiological laboratory threatened to intervene in the mainstay of the medical encounter, the physician–patient relationship.[47] Civilian medicine made some attempts to unite clinics with medical laboratories in the 1870s and 1880s, but the proud, empiric heritage of the French clinical school as well as professional associations militated against the union of clinic and laboratory. The separation of clinic and laboratory endured in civilian medical education as well. George Weisz, in his study of the civilian medical faculties of *fin-de-siècle* France, notes that reforms in medical education in the decade or so before World War I tended to emphasise 'clinical training at the expense of laboratory medicine'.[48] The reform

[45] Latour, *Pasteurization*.
[46] *Ibid.*, p. 133.
[47] Jacques Léonard, *Les médecins de l'ouest au XIXème siècle* (Paris, 1978), esp. pp. 924–34; Léonard, 'Comment peut-on être Pasteurien?'.
[48] George Weisz, 'Reform and conflict in French medical education' in R. Fox and G. Weisz (eds), *The Organization of Science and Technology in France, 1808–1914* (Cambridge, 1980), pp. 61–94 at p. 94. On the general insufficiency of French laboratory science, see

of 31 July 1893, for example, which mandated examinations in those Pasteurian bastions, microbiology and parasitology, did so only for pre-medical students, not for students enrolled in a medical faculty. Thus at the institutional level the foundation disciplines of laboratory medicine tended to be dispersed throughout the pre-medical curriculum rather than taught as a unit within the medical schools.

The hygienists, that group of statisticians, medical geographers, public health investigators, sewer pipe designers and swamp-drainers, provide Latour with a counterpoint to the sceptical physicians. The hygienists, with their miasms and concern with the localised and spontaneous character of epidemic disease, seized upon 'any argument about microbes to emerge from the microbiological laboratories'.[49] In contrast to the 'desperately slow' physicians, this group 'considered early on that microbiology was a complete and definitive science and that *all that remained* [Latour's emphasis] was to apply it'.[50] By this argument, Pasteur's microbes, which varied in their virulence according to environmental conditions and could be attenuated *in vitro*, gave the hygienists a focus, and reordered epidemiological problems.[51]

To be sure, many French hygienists disputed the contagion models of disease production; but Latour postulates that as a body the hygienists emerged from their clouded iatro-environmentalism to embrace a kind of *microbe* theory of contagion by invasion. As we have seen, Kelsch emphatically opposed this version of contagion theory. Latour further argues that a parallel shift in the strategy of disease prevention focused hygienic activities on the extermination of microbes. This new strategy attempted to head the microbes off at the pass: 'Either the microbe gets through and *all the precautions are useless*, or hygienists can stop it getting through and *all other precautions are superfluous* [Latour's emphasis].'[52] Latour's ideas are influential, and others such as Anne Marcovich have applied them to the history of medical practices in the French colonies. While her research shows that French medicine in Indo-China continued to use swamp-draining and other old stand-bys of disease prevention after Pasteur, she none the less concludes that 'the only factor which concerned medical authorities "after Pasteur" was the existence (or absence) of the micro-organisms which cause diseases and the

Fernand Papillon, 'Les laboratoires en France et à l'étranger', *Revue des Deux Mondes*, 94 (8), 1 August 1871 pp. 594–609.

[49] Latour, *Pasteurization*, p. 43.

[50] *Ibid.*, pp. 133 and 52.

[51] *Ibid.*, pp. 45 and 62–5.

[52] *Ibid.*, p. 48.

implementation of the means (preventive vaccinations and curative serums) to cope with them'.[53]

Latour's third group, army medicine, also underwent a comparatively rapid conversion, for it 'seized upon Pasteurism with the same avidity as hygienists'.[54] According to Latour two circumstances hastened the acceptance of Pasteurian ideas within the military: army doctors did not have a physician–patient relationship to protect, and the military discipline imposed on a largely homogeneous population of men had caused barracks life to mimic the highly controlled conditions of Pasteur's laboratory. In other words, military medical practice easily admitted Pasteur's microbes because it was in a certain sense already 'pasteurized institutionally'.[55] The army doctors provide something of a control group within the population of physicians, for unlike civilian medicine, Latour writes, army medicine 'converted to Pasteurism without putting up the slightest resistance'.[56]

This account of Kelsch, however, has been a chronicle of selective appropriation, conservative incorporation and long-sustained resistance to certain bacteriological canons. As such it is a cautionary tale which calls into question Latour's account of events. Kelsch's message at both Val-de-Grâce and Lyons was not so revolutionary, nor was it 'pasteurized' in great degree. His incorporation of Pasteurian ideas emerged as part of a progressive and dynamic dialectic between anatomical pathology and medical geography on the one hand, and bacteriology on the other. Additionally, Kelsch's equivocal position on Pasteurian laboratory medicine in the 1890s raises concerns about the appropriateness of Léonard's image of Lyons as a military medical school engaged in the transmission of Pasteur's revolutionary science.[57]

Kelsch's reserve towards an all-sufficient microbial theory of disease was certainly not unique, and reverberations of similar views can be found in other national contexts among the key figures of scientific hygiene such as Sir Arthur Newsholme in England and Max von Pettenkofer in Germany.[58] Kelsch used Pasteur's microbes in a

[53] Anne Marcovich, 'French colonial medicine and colonial rule: Algeria and Indochina' in Roy MacLeod and Milton Lewis (eds), *Disease, Medicine and Empire: Perspectives on Western Medicine and the Experience of European Expansion* (London, 1988), pp. 103–17, at p. 114. [54] Latour, *Pasteurization*, p. 114. [55] *Ibid.* [56] *Ibid.*, p. 116.

[57] Léonard, 'Comment peut-on être Pasteurien?', p. 160.

[58] Professor John Eyler of the University of Minnesota is completing a book-length study of Newsholme. C.-E. A. Winslow, *The Conquest of Epidemic Disease* (1943; reprint edn, Madison, Wis., 1980), pp. 311–36, provides an accessible summary of Pettenkofer's views.

conservative manner to defend medical geography and military epidemiology, and by accepting microbial explanations Kelsch came just within the outermost orbit of the Pasteurian programme. But labels are misleading, for Kelsch was not totally, or even mostly, in step with the standard Latourian Pasteurians of French army medicine, for he did not embrace Pasteurism 'with the same avidity as [the] hygienists', nor did he convert to 'Pasteurism without putting up the slightest resistance'.[59] An influential figure in French military medical education, Kelsch put up considerable resistance, and his message may have influenced others to adopt similar views. In the medical world of Val-de-Grâce, and more generally in French army medical education, the celebration of nuptials between clinic and bacteriological laboratory would await the end of the war to end all wars.

[59] Latour, *Pasteurization*, pp. 114 and 116.

7

Transforming plague

The laboratory and the identity of infectious disease

ANDREW CUNNINGHAM

Introduction

The coming of the laboratory radically transformed the identity of infectious disease. This is one of the least appreciated – and, indeed, least obvious – of the changes of thinking and practice brought about in medicine by the coming of the laboratory. To show what this transformation comprised and how it happened, I shall take as my example the traditionally most feared, and in that sense the most important, of all infectious diseases: plague. These are the things I hope to show: one, that following the advent of laboratory medicine, infectious diseases are now necessarily and exclusively defined by the laboratory and thus receive their identity from the laboratory; two, that the laboratory concept of disease – with each disease having a single unique material cause, a cause which is identifiable in, and only in, the laboratory – is different from previous concepts of disease (and not merely a development of previous concepts); and three, that the dominance of the laboratory concept of disease has had a significant effect on our understanding of many *pre*-laboratory diseases – leading us to read them as if they were laboratory diseases; hence the coming of the laboratory has led to the *past* of medicine being rewritten to accord with the laboratory model of disease, and it has thereby been misunderstood.

The history of medicine as conventionally written is based on the assumption of a simple continuity in the identity of diseases, and thus tends to make invisible the issues which are actually involved in speaking of the 'identity' of a disease. For instance, a demographic historian has recently written that

Acknowledgements: My thanks to Dr Yoko Mitsui and Dr Perry Williams for their most helpful and sympathetic criticisms and guidance.

The most obviously difficult task for the historian is to identify the diseases at work in periods of high mortality and hence to try to form reliable hypotheses about the way in which they spread and the effects they might be expected to produce. He wants to be able to name the epidemic and to use modern experience of it as an aid to interpreting the partial evidence which survives for past outbreaks.[1]

This desire to name past diseases is quite common amongst historians of medicine as well as historical demographers, and it underlies much work in both disciplines. It is a claim about *identity*: that disease X in the past *was the same as* (or was identical to) disease Y in the present. The success of the venture of identifying past diseases depends on us having authentic means to make this claim of sameness, this claim of identity, about diseases. In pursuit of a more refined and reliable means of making such identifications, demographic and medical historians have increasingly turned to refining their own understanding of the modern disease: if they have a full and proper understanding of disease Y in the present then, they believe, they will be on the firmest ground possible in saying that disease X in the past was (or was not) the same as disease Y in the present. That is, they have moved to acquiring greater technical medical knowledge. But this assumes that the making of such claims about sameness is in principle non-problematic, and simply a matter of having sufficient technical information at one's command. What really needs to be asked, however, is this: *what conditions would need to be satisfied* for the claim of sameness, of identity, to stick? And this is a philosophical and historiographical question, not a technical medical one. The historian of demography or of medicine customarily takes the familiar (modern medicine) and then applies it to the unfamiliar (past disease), seeking thereby to convert the unfamiliar into the familiar; hence, he feels, he can explain what a particular past disease 'really' was, how it was 'really' transmitted, what the past people 'really' saw, and what they 'missed'. What I shall be doing here, by contrast, is seeking to make an aspect of *modern* medicine look unfamiliar, and thereby explore how it was *constructed*; with respect to plague this will involve looking at the role of the laboratory in transforming the identity of plague. Then we should be able to see how *pre*-laboratory plague thereby became alien and unfamiliar to us.

Before proceeding with the argument, however, it will be useful to have some image of plague in our minds. In our world, the laboratory world, the 'medical facts' about it are usually taken, in brief, to be as

[1] Paul Slack, 'Introduction', in *The Plague Reconsidered: A New Look at its Origins and Effects in 16th and 17th Century England*, supplement to *Local Population Studies* (Matlock, Derbyshire), 1977, p. 6.

follows.[2] Plague is caused by a micro-organism, a bacillus, usually known as *Pasteurella pestis*. Plague is a disease of the rat. It is endemic in rat populations and periodically appears in a more virulent form and then becomes epidemic. The vector of the causative micro-organism of plague is the rat flea, whose proventriculus becomes 'blocked' with large quantities of the bacillus which it therefore cannot avoid regurgitating into rats as it tries to suck their blood. The rats thereby get plague. As the rats begin to die in great numbers from the plague so their fleas have to look for new hosts and hence they land on humans and transmit the bacillus into the bloodstreams of their human hosts. The humans are thereby given plague. There are three major forms of plague in the human, all of which have an extremely high mortality rate: (1) 'bubonic', spread directly by the rat flea, and whose typical lesions are 'buboes' which appear in the groin, armpit and neck; (2) the even more lethal variation of this, 'septicaemic', where the patient dies of sudden blood-poisoning before the buboes have time to appear; and (3) 'pneumonic', a complication of the bubonic and which can spread from person to person by infected droplets in the breath, and which does not therefore need the assistance of the rat flea in order to spread. These are the basic 'medical facts' about plague, as currently accepted.

Identifying disease

What constitutes the identity of a disease? This is not a topic which has received much discussion from doctors or philosophers or even medical historians, so there is little in the current literature to help us.[3]

[2] I have chosen to take this account from Leslie Bradley, 'Some medical aspects of plague' and Jean-Noel Biraben, 'Current medical and epidemiological views on plague', in *The Plague Reconsidered*, pp. 11–23 and 25–36, respectively, where the expression 'medical facts' is used, though without inverted commas. The accounts given in this work are completely conventional in modern terms, and the definition given in the text could have been derived from any modern handbook on plague or infectious diseases.

[3] There seem to be only two kinds of recent concern with it. The question has arisen over whether certain conditions are 'real' diseases, and in particular whether madness is one. The model of somatic disease against which comparison is often made is infectious disease, for here, it is assumed, the criteria of identity are the strictest. The other kind of discussion seems to be restricted to those who want medicine to continue to be treated as an art as well as a science. Here the treatment of the historical concept of disease has been unsatisfactory, being built around a supposed eternal dichotomy between 'ontological' and 'physiological' approaches. Yet this applies very poorly to the pre-laboratory age and anyway, as a dichotomy, seems to date from the emergence of laboratory medicine itself. Those historians who have chosen to write on the history of the concept of disease seem to be concerned to deny the validity of a strict 'ontological' concept, and to promote a form of 'physiological' concept. This is true even for Owsei Temkin; see his articles 'The scientific approach to

But we can certainly say that disease does not seem to be a 'natural kind'. Rather, a 'disease-entity' is a mental construct made up of experiences of pain, distress and debilitation, the outward visible appearances that accompany these experiences, the succession of all these over time together with the outcome (recovery, disablement death), the changes that the pathologist can find in the parts of the body, together with peoples' thoughts about the origin and reasons for what is happening and why it turns out as it does. A 'disease' is constituted by all these taken together. Two people undergoing the same set of these are usually judged to be undergoing the same (identical) disease.

Such mental groupings of experiences and natural phenomena, these 'disease-entities', do not necessarily correspond from one culture to another, and they have not necessarily been constant over time even within one particular culture. For instance, for a very long period in the history of our own western medical tradition it was the case that each 'disease' was thought of as being unique to each sufferer. Equally, the way a disease-entity is built up – the set of elements constituting its identity – may be changed over time. With the advent of French hospital medicine in the years round 1800, for instance, the localised pathological changes which happen within the body during the course of diseases came to be thought of as essential elements of the identity of those diseases, and disease nomenclature came to reflect this.[4] Again, some diseases in the past – diseases which were experienced, suffered from, treated, cured – ceased to be regarded as diseases at all; the most celebrated such ex-disease is perhaps chlorosis, from which thousands of young women suffered, especially in the nineteenth century, but which it is impossible to

disease: specific entity and individual sickness' (1963), and 'Health and disease' (1973), both reprinted in his *Double Face of Janus* (Baltimore, 1977), pp. 441–55 and 419–40; see also Sir Henry Cohen, 'The evolution of the concept of disease', *Proceedings of the Royal Society of Medicine*, 48 (1955), pp. 155–60. For a brief historical account of objections to the 'ontological' views of the bacteriologists, see Knud Faber, *Nosography in Modern Internal Medicine* (Oxford, 1923), pp. 186–94. For a recent example of the second type of concern, see Eric J. Cassell, 'Ideas in conflict: the rise and fall (and rise and fall) of new views of disease', *Daedalus* 1986 (= *Proceedings of the American Academy of Arts and Sciences*, 115), pp. 19–41. For examples of both types of concern see the entries by Guenter B. Risse and H. Tristram Engelhardt, Jr, under 'Health and Disease' in *Encyclopaedia of Bioethics*, ed. Warren T. Reich, 4 vols. (New York, 1978), vol. II. F. Kräupl Taylor, *The Concepts of Illness, Disease and Morbus* (Cambridge, 1979), gives a sophisticated philosophical treatment of the issues, but again assumes a long historical lineage for the 'ontological' concept.

[4] See Erwin H. Ackerknecht, *Medicine at the Paris Hospital, 1794–1848* (Baltimore, 1967); Michel Foucault, *The Birth of the Clinic: An Archaeology of Medical Perception* (London, 1973; original French edition, 1963); on the change in nomenclature see Faber, *Nosography*.

suffer from today, not because it has been eliminated but because people have ceased making identifications of it as a disease.[5]

Our actual concept of any disease, on the basis of which we may make claims that disease X is 'the same as' (identical to) disease Y, is constituted by what we may call its 'operational definition'. That is to say, by the questions people ask and the operations people actually engage in when finding or checking the 'identity' of any disease. It all comes down to the answers people give to certain questions – 'Is so-and-so ill?', 'What disease is it?', 'Is it cholera (or whatever)?' – and to the procedures people apply in reaching answers that satisfy at any given moment in history.[6]

Plague too is like this: it is defined by – that is, its identity derives from – the questions we ask and the activities we undertake in making the identification. How then do we today answer, to our own satisfaction, the question 'Is this a case of plague?' A modern expert at plague diagnosis explains how one starts:

> The essential first step in the diagnosis of plague is to suspect the diagnosis of any person with a fever who lives in a known endemic area of the world or who has visited a known endemic area within the last few days. The diagnosis should be more strongly suspected if the patient with fever also has a painful bubo, cough, or signs of meningitis. Once the diagnosis is suspected, a physician should proceed to establish the diagnosis by bacteriological methods.[7]

That is the 'clinical diagnosis'. But all it can do is *suspect*. The only way a suspicion of plague can be confirmed or *established* is 'by bacteriological methods'; in other words, by a laboratory. The staff of the laboratory make this authentication by running tests to discover whether the pertinent bacterium is present or not: 'The absolute confirmation of plague infection in human beings, rodents, or fleas requires the isolation and identification of the plague bacillus,

[5] On chlorosis see Karl Figlio, 'Chlorosis and chronic disease in nineteenth-century Britain: the social constitution of somatic illness in a capitalist society', *Social History*, 3 (1978), pp. 167–197; but compare Irvin Loudon, 'The disease called chlorosis', *Psychological Medicine*, 14 (1984), pp. 27–36. For another instance, this time of the twentieth century, see Robert P. Hudson, 'Theory and therapy: ptosis, stasis, and autointoxication', *Bulletin of the History of Medicine*, 63 (1989), pp. 392–413.

[6] Although this particular formulation seems to be original with me, Charles Rosenberg has recently written 'In some ways disease does not exist until we have agreed that it does – by perceiving, naming, and responding to it', 'Disease in history: frames and framers', in *Framing Disease: The Creation and Negotiation of Explanatory Schemes*, Supplement 1 to *Milbank Quarterly*, 67 (1989) guest-edited by Charles Rosenberg and Janet Golden, pp. 1–16, at pp. 1–2. Similarly, though he is primarily concerned with the involvement of value judgements in the act of ascribing disease-status, Lawrie Reznek argues that disease-status 'is a division that is invented by our adoption of one descriptive definition of disease rather than another', and concludes that 'disease judgements, like moral judgements, are not factual ones', *The Nature of Disease* (London, 1987), pp. 80 and 213.

[7] Thomas Butler, *Plague and Other Yersinia Infections* (New York, *c.* 1983), pp. 163–4.

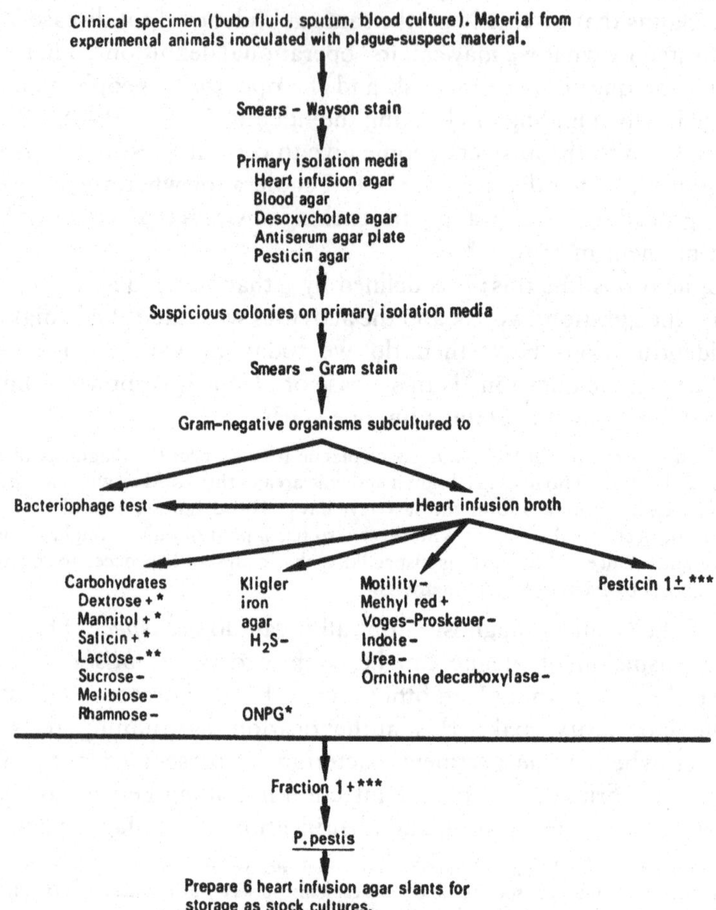

Fig. 6. How plague is identified today, according to laboratory criteria. This flowchart comes from the *Plague Manual* of the World Health Organisation. It should be noted that the internationally accepted name of the plague bacillus is now *Yersinia pestis*.

Yersinia (*Pasteurella*) *pestis*.'[8] The necessary procedure to do this is detailed in Fig. 6. Clinical specimens are brought into the laboratory; they are then put through various treatments and tests, in a sequence

[8] M. Bahmanyar and D. C. Cavanaugh (eds.), *Plague Manual* (Geneva, 1976), p. 14.

shown by the arrows. If they pass all these tests (that is, if a particular, predictable result is obtained in each test), then we have identified *P. pestis*. These conditions must be satisfied, for they reveal either the presence or the absence of the plague bacillus. And if the bacillus is present, then this disease *is* plague.

It can be seen from this sequence of operations which we use today to identify plague that conclusive identification of plague can be made only by finding the bacillus. For we see this as the *cause* of the disease. Indeed we commonly refer to the bacillus as 'the causative micro-organism of plague'. Every modern account of plague that we might read today starts from this: from the bacillus as the *cause* of plague. But this is not only the case in medical texts, where we might expect it, but also in historical writings about plague, right at the beginning when the writer is about to make the identification of past plague with modern plague.[9] This seems so natural today that it scarcely bears remark. We simply take it for granted that the plague bacillus is the cause of plague, and that therefore the specification of the identity of plague, whether in the present or in the past, must start from the bacillus, the cause. Indeed, this is what I did above, when asking what are the 'medical facts' about plague today. But, as we shall see, this identity of plague derives from the laboratory, and was new with the introduction of the laboratory.

The term 'cause' is being used here in a specific sense. The sense in which we mean that this bacillus, *P. pestis*, is the cause of plague is specified by what are known as 'Koch's postulates'. In discussing the necessary and sufficient conditions that would have to be satisfied for a micro-organism to be accepted as the direct cause of a particular disease, Robert Koch wrote that

> complete proof of the causal relationship demands, not merely a demonstration of the coincidence of the parasites with the disease, but, beyond this, it must be shown that the parasites directly produce the disease. To obtain this proof, it is necessary to isolate the parasites completely from the diseased organism, and from all the products of the disease to which any pathogenic influence could be ascribed; then to excite anew the disease with all its special characteristics by the introduction of the parasites alone into a healthy organism.[10]

[9] See, for instance, *The Plague Reconsidered*, or Folke Henschen, *The History of Diseases*, translated by Joan Tate (London, 1966; original Swedish edition, 1962), who treats every disease like this.

[10] Robert Koch, 'Die Aetiologie der Tuberkulose', *Mittheilungen aus dem Kaiserlichen Gesundheitsamte*, 2 (1884), pp. 1–88, at pp. 3–4. The translation is by Stanley Boyd, as given in W. Watson Cheyne (ed.), *Recent Essays by Various Authors on Bacteria in Relation to Disease* (London, 1886), pp. 70–1. There is, unfortunately, no one final statement of these postulates by Koch. For the development of Koch's arguments on the causal relationship, see the important recent series of articles by K. Codell Carter: 'Koch's postulates in relation to

These criteria date from 1884. The micro-organism must be constantly present in cases of the disease; it must be absent from other diseases (i.e. it must be unique to this disease); it must be possible to experimentally induce the disease in a healthy susceptible animal (if one exists) using *just* the micro-organism; and the micro-organism must then be found to have multiplied in that now-sick animal. After giving an example in the case of anthrax, Koch had concluded that

> in the face of these facts, it is impossible to come to any other conclusion than that the splenic fever [= anthrax] bacillus is *the cause* of the disease, and not merely an accompaniment of it... These conclusions are so unanswerable that no one now opposes them, and science universally accepts the bacillus anthraxis as the cause both of the common typical splenic fever we are familiar with in our domestic animals, and also of the clinically different forms of the disease which occur in man.[11]

These are the criteria of 'cause' that we are applying to *P. pestis* when referring to it as the cause of plague. It follows from this that for infectious diseases in general, without the pertinent micro-organism present there can be no instance of the disease! For the micro-organism initiates, produces, brings into existence the whole sequence of inner changes in the body which constitute the disease. For instance the micro-organism might produce a toxin, which in turn damages certain cells, which leads in turn to malfunction, pain or death. In the case of plague the bacillus *P. pestis* is the cause which originates and produces all the bodily and mental experiences which constitute the disease of plague, right through to the production of buboes, and beyond to death. In this sense the micro-organism *P. pestis* is the essential initiator and cause of all the pathology, all the symptoms, all the experience of the disease of plague. Although today plague may be clinically *suspected* it is never *proved* (that is, never identified) without isolating its *cause*, the micro-organism. For a hundred years now this has been the case, and every outbreak of suspected plague in that hundred years which has been conclusively diagnosed as being plague has been diagnosed (identified) as plague only by finding the micro-organism *P. pestis* present.

What is more, because we take a particular micro-organism to be the *cause* of the disease, all the other features of the modern disease-entity of plague – that is, all the other features of its identity – follow from this 'cause'. Our understanding of how plague *spreads* depends

the work of Jacob Henle and Edwin Klebs', *Medical History*, 29 (1985), pp. 353–74; 'Edwin Klebs' criteria for disease causality', *Medizinhistorisches Journal*, 22 (1987), pp. 80–9; 'The Koch–Pasteur dispute on establishing the cause of anthrax', *Bulletin of the History of Medicine*, 62 (1988), pp. 42–57; see also William Coleman, 'Koch's comma bacillus: the first year', *Bulletin of the History of Medicine*, 61 (1987), pp. 315–42.

11 Cheyne (ed.), *Recent Essays*, p. 72; emphasis as in Boyd's translation.

on seeing the micro-organism as the cause, for it is the micro-organism itself of which the rat flea (and, under the flea, the rat) are the vectors: the very cause is transmitted from one creature to another. Similarly our understanding of the different *forms* that plague takes comes from seeing the micro-organism as the cause: bubonic, septicaemic and pneumonic plague, although they present clinically in such different ways are, for us, all forms of the *same* disease because we find they all have the same micro-organism present as cause. As a modern expert has written:

Clinically, the two chief types [bubonic and pneumonic] are so distinct that they would rank as different diseases if they were not known to have a common origin and to be linked by intermediate types. At the bedside, nothing could be more unlike than cases of true pneumonic and uncomplicated bubonic plague; in the one the brunt of the infection falls upon the lungs, in the other on the lymphatic system.[12]

Again, our understanding of the *epidemiology* of plague is built on seeing the micro-organism as the cause: properly-identified cases of plague (i.e. identified in a laboratory) have a large-scale incidence of a certain distinctive form; thus if a yet-unidentified disease has this particular incidence, then it must be plague (and the bacillus will be there as its cause). The same is true of the *symptoms* of plague, and of its *pathology*: the 'true' symptoms and the pathological changes typical of plague are those regularly seen in cases where the 'causal micro-organism of plague' has been established as present. This way of working outwards *from* the cause *to* the symptoms and pathology (rather than in the other direction) has had significant effects on the classification of diseases – that is, on what conditions count as what disease. As a recent commentator has pointed out, the search for and discovery of causal micro-organisms of diseases has

led to the redefinition and reclassification of many disease entities... With the discovery of the tubercle bacillus and its role in disease, for instance, what had been designated phthisis was reordered into a number of conditions, only some forms of which were tuberculosis. The forms assigned as tuberculosis were those in which the bacillus could be demonstrated by staining and grown in culture...[13]

[12] L. F. Hirst, *The Conquest of Plague: A Study of the Evolution of Epidemiology* (Oxford, 1953), p. 28.

[13] Mervyn Susser, *Causal Thinking in the Health Sciences: Concepts and Strategies of Epidemiology* (New York, 1973), p. 23. For another instance, concerning the discovery of the bacillus of diphtheria in 1891, see Charles-Edward Amory Winslow, *The Conquest of Epidemic Disease: A Chapter in the History of Ideas* (Madison, Wis., 1971; original edition, 1943), p. 341: 'Thus, it appeared that between one-quarter and one-third of the cases of "clinical diphtheria" were not the true disease. On the other hand, 80 per cent of a series of cases of "membraneous croup" proved on culture to be true laryngeal diphtheria. The value of the bacteriological criterion was further demonstrated by epidemiological studies, which showed the fatality of culturally-proved diphtheria to be 27 per cent, of "false diphtheria" to be less than 3 per cent.'

By seeing specific micro-organisms as the 'causes' of certain diseases, it has thus become possible to think in terms of *specific* infectious diseases: each such specific disease has a specific cause, a particular micro-organism. This sense of 'cause', as a specific causal agent which alone brings about the disease, is fundamental to our modern meaning for the term 'aetiology', the discipline where we discuss the causes of diseases.

The role of the laboratory in all this is absolutely crucial. The laboratory today holds total authority on the authentication of plague, for the final diagnosis – the identification – is impossible without the laboratory. So much so is this the case that even if a patient appears to have all the symptoms of plague, yet they cannot be said to have plague until the laboratory has spoken. As the eminent bacteriologist E. E. Klein wrote in 1906:

> It is admitted on all sides that the *Bacillus pestis* is the real and essential cause of Oriental or bubonic plague, and consequently that the presence of this microbe in any material derived from a human or an animal being denotes the disease plague in such a being. It is likewise admitted that a patient, although exhibiting one or more symptoms suspicious of the disease plague – e.g. fever with swollen and inflamed subcutaneous lymph glands in one or other region of the body, cervical, axillary, inguinal, or femoral, – need not necessarily be affected with bubonic plague, notwithstanding that such person might have been indirectly exposed to plague infection. Should, however, in such swollen inflamed glands the *B. pestis* be demonstrated, epidemiologists and physicians would accept such a case unquestionably as true plague...[14]

And of course the presence of *B. pestis* can only be established in the laboratory, using all the proper tests. That tests of this kind are conducted in the laboratory is not a matter of mere convenience and coincidence – it is not the case that the laboratory just happens to be the best or most convenient and well-equipped place in which to make such tests – for such tests ***are what constitute the central, the defining, activities of a medical microbiological laboratory.*** Without it they are, quite literally, unthinkable. The laboratory makes the tests, but equally the tests make the laboratory.

The laboratory has this same role as the unique authenticator in the case of all laboratory-defined diseases, all those diseases where we now believe a micro-organism to be the unique cause; and therefore in all these cases too the laboratory has transformed the identity of disease. Indeed it is the laboratory which defines which diseases count as members of the category of 'infectious diseases', for infectious

[14] E. E. Klein, *Studies in the Bacteriology and Etiology of Oriental Plague* (London, 1906), p. xiii. On Klein see the extensive obituary by William Bulloch in *Journal of Pathology*, 28 (1925), pp. 684–97.

diseases today are those which have transmittable micro-organisms as their cause, whether a bacterium, a virus or other tiny parasite. This is a considerable proportion of all conditions known as 'disease' (even in the loosest formulation of the category of 'disease'), since infectious diseases constitute about half of all the cases that present to a general doctor. To this total we can add all those diseases where a micro-organism is believed to be the causative agent but which is still being hunted down in the laboratory. In most cases, of course, the doctor does not in practice invoke the laboratory before he offers a diagnosis of, for instance, influenza or chicken-pox, for he has been trained to trust in his skills in recognising and correlating symptoms and signs. But if the doctor has any doubt about his diagnosis in any particular case, then he does indeed send specimens and samples along to the laboratory for inspection so that a proper diagnosis can be made. Such behaviour on the doctor's part shows that all his diagnoses of infectious disease are only provisional until they have laboratory confirmation. This does not mean his diagnoses are necessarily inaccurate if he has not first consulted the laboratory, but it does mean that the laboratory is the final arbiter of the accuracy of the diagnoses the physician offers. It also shows that his diagnosis is based on a micro-organism as being the cause.

Old plague

How was plague identified – what was its identity – before the advent of the laboratory? While it would be misleading to claim that there was just a single picture of plague before the lab, since every outbreak revealed much disagreement and conflict amongst practitioners over the nature and treatment of plague,[15] yet the pre-lab identity of plague differed radically from its post-lab identity in a number of striking ways, which can be considered under two main heads.

In the first place, like all other diseases, plague before the laboratory was always identified by its *symptoms* and its course. Primarily this means it was identified by the presence of buboes. But pre-lab symptoms were many and complex, and even the buboes were not necessarily evident, nor were they even always taken to be the most important symptoms. Generally, as a late eighteenth-century investigator noted, buboes and carbuncles 'are equally diagnostics of

[15] On the complexities and varieties of concepts of plague before the lab see for instance Jon Arrizabalaga, 'Facing the Black Death: perceptions and reactions of university medical practitioners' in L. Garcia-Ballester *et al.* (eds.), *Practical Medicine from Salerno to the Black Death* (Cambridge, in press).

the true plague; their presence, separately or in conjunction, leaves the nature of the distemper unequivocal; but fatal has been the error of rashly, from their absence, pronouncing a distemper not to be the plague'.[16] If the buboes are present, then the disease is definitely plague; but if they are absent, it still might be plague. Dr Andrew White, a military surgeon with the British army, had to contain an outbreak of plague on the island of Corfu, and his account of the symptoms of plague (first published in 1845) hardly touches on the buboes:

> The symptoms of the plague in Corfu, as collected from the medical officers employed on that occasion, were as follows:-
>
> More or less fever, sometimes of a *remittent*, sometimes of an *intermittent* type; great prostration of strength; staggering like a drunken man; often violent headache; tremors; derangement of the stomach, with a sensation of burning heat; vomiting, sometimes of a yellow, at others of a blackish matter, like coffee-grounds; involuntary evacuations, both of urine and faeces at times, when the patients did not appear to be very ill, and which seemed the effect of fear, stupor, coma; often violent and sudden exacerbations of fever, which could not be said to belong to any type; a white, glossy tongue, the edges of which were generally clean, with a streak in the middle. The countenance exhibited an appearance of terror mixed with anxiety, and, as it were, claiming pity, which is difficult to describe, but which is well known to those who see plague patients, and is very characteristic of the disease. Sometimes the disease was ushered in with furious *delirium*, approaching to a state of *phrenitis*, with the eyes, as it were, ready to start from their sockets, and the face flushed, as if mad with the effects of drink and passion, so that for a time they became quite unmanageable. The duration of the paroxysm sometimes lasted for hours, after which they became calm and composed, and in some instances appeared to be quite rational. In some cases, these violent exacerbations were succeeded by cold *rigors*; these alternated, and the unhappy sufferer was carried off by them, sometimes without exhibiting those eruptions [i.e. the buboes] which are supposed necessary to form the character of plague.
>
> Buboes and carbuncles were very common symptoms, particularly after the first ebullition of the disease was over...[17]

The buboes are very common, but not universal, symptoms, and other symptoms have to be recognised in order to be able to identify plague. Indeed, so important were these other symptoms that one night during this Corfu outbreak White himself 'went to bed with all the horrors of plague about me' because he believed his servant was showing severe symptoms of plague. What had happened in fact was that the servant had, quite untypically, got very drunk and was staggering around – and staggering was (as White's own report above shows) one of the prime symptoms of plague!

[16] Patrick Russell, *A Treatise of the Plague: Containing an Historical Journal, and a Medical Account, of the Plague, at Aleppo, in the Years 1760, 1761, and 1762* (London, 1791), p. 112.

[17] Andrew White, *A Treatise on the Plague, More Especially on the Police Management of That Disease* (London, 1846), p. 141.

This symptom-based identity of pre-lab plague meant that although medical men might claim to have supreme authority in making the identification, yet in practice theirs was neither the first nor the last word. Pre-lab plague could, in practice, be identified by anyone. If people thought there was an outbreak of plague amongst them, those who could afford to usually fled. They rarely waited for the doctors to tell them what they already knew about the identity of the disease. In the case of post-lab plague, by contrast, the identification of the disease cannot be made by lay-persons. Indeed it cannot even be made by clinical practitioners. It can only be made by the workers in a bacteriological laboratory.

The second major way in which pre-lab plague differed from post-lab plague, was with respect to *cause*. The term 'cause' was used in a different sense by pre-lab doctors, and had been for at least two millenia. 'Aetiology' also therefore meant something different. There was a whole hierarchy of causes, with many items at each level of the causal hierarchy.[18] These still prevailed in the nineteenth century, when generally there were taken to be four inter-related types of cause operative. There were *predisposing* causes, such as the particular constitution of the patient, the weather, the season of the year and the state of the soil. There were *external* (procatarctic or preceding) causes, such as the six 'non-naturals': the state of the air around a patient, and the nature, quality and quantity of his food and drink, his sleep and watch, his inanition and repletion, his movement and rest, and the passions of his mind. There were *antecedent* causes, such as some obstruction within the body. And there were *immediate* causes, such as a particular state of the blood. In plague, as in every other illness, these causes were operative. Some, such as the 'non-naturals', the physician could regulate to ward off or repel the disease; others he could not. Such causes were obviously not necessarily unique to a particular disease.

Moreover, pre-lab plague did not have a *specific causal agent*. As Vivian Nutton has written, about the concept of 'the seeds of disease' in the Ancient and Medieval periods:

> A disease did not have an existence in its own right, but as a deviation from the norm within the patient, and although these authors accepted and wrote of such disease entities as fever and phthisis, they insisted on always taking into account 'the peculiar nature of each individual'. The nature of disease was to be found in man's temperament, the structure of his parts, his physiological and psychological dynamism, and could be defined very much in terms of impeded function. Set against

[18] See for instance the listings and explanations of them under 'Aetiology' in Robert Hooper, *Lexicon Medicum; or Medical Dictionary*, 6th edn (London, 1831).

this background, the seeds of disease act only as an initial cause: they are not the disease, any more than a blow to the head or a poisonous mushroom. They merely trigger a situation which eventually may lead to a humoral disorder and a bodily malfunction, and it is the latter which for Galen constituted disease and illness.[19]

These same attitudes described by Nutton for the Ancient and Medieval periods can still be seen in that great pre-laboratory work on plague in English, the 1791 *Treatise of the Plague* by Dr Patrick Russell, FRS, built on his experience of outbreaks of plague in Aleppo in the 1760s. In this Russell defines plague only by its symptoms. Of *cause*, in the sense in which the micro-organism is today seen as the cause of plague, as a unique material entity, specific to the disease, he naturally says nothing. Admittedly for Russell, as for many people of earlier centuries, there is indeed some invisible material entity present and active, a 'contagion': 'The plague is a contagious disease; that is, an emanation from a body diseased, passing into one which is sound, produces, in time, the same disease; and the person thus infected becomes in like manner capable of communicating the plague to others.'[20] But this 'contagion' is not the cause, but merely the *means of transmission* of the plague, acting only (as Nutton expresses it) to 'trigger' the disease. And this specific 'contagion' exists only under certain atmospheric conditions: it is brought into existence by a certain state of the air, and spreads only with an appropriate state of the air, and it has an effect on any given individual only if that individual is personally susceptible. As Russell wrote,

In what this particular constitution of the air consists, which in one case favours the spreading of the distemper, and in the other checks or extinguishes it; whether it operates by heightening the powers of the infectious effluvia, or by inducing an epidemical change on the human body, whereby it is rendered more or less susceptible of, or enabled to resist their influence, the effluvia remaining the same; are points involved in much obscurity. It seems in the mean while incontestible that without a concurrent state of the air, the plague will not become epidemical; and without a certain state of the body, the infection will not take effect.[21]

This 'contagion', originating in a particular state of the air, and spreading as a consequence of the state of the air, is quite different from the post-laboratory concept of a causative micro-organism which exists independently of any 'epidemic constitution'.

However, even though the pre-lab concept of 'cause' differed from the post-lab concept, it was nevertheless possible, as William Coleman has pointed out, for medical men in the early to mid nineteenth

[19] Vivian Nutton, 'The seeds of disease: an explanation of contagion and infection from the Greeks to the Renaissance', *Medical History*, 27 (1983), pp. 1–34, at p. 15.

[20] Russell, *Treatise*, p. 296.

[21] *Ibid.*, p. 261.

century to develop a science of epidemiology. They simply did not invoke aetiology. Coleman's study of work on yellow fever shows that clinicians could and did build pictures of the large-scale (epidemic) behaviour of yellow fever, without feeling the need to discuss the issue of cause at all.[22] Our modern-day discipline of epidemiology, by contrast, depends crucially upon the identification of the 'cause' of epidemic diseases: epidemic spread leads us in the first place to seek out a causal agent, and if we find a micro-organism candidate then thereafter our understanding of what is being spread epidemically is built on our view of the micro-organism which we have identified as the cause.

Not only did a pre-lab disease not have a specific causal agent, but it was possible to have 'mixed' diseases. It was also the case that diseases were considered capable of transforming into other diseases during their course, and that the 'morbific matter' could move around within the body, thus altering the locus of disease ('metastasis') and hence the form and nature of it.[23] This applied to plague as much as any other disease: a fever of one kind could, perhaps, turn into plague through a change in climatic conditions. Pre-lab diseases were simply not as fixed or constant as those post-lab ones whose identity is built on the isolation of a specific material causal agent.

All the differences between the identity of pre-lab plague and post-lab plague are encapsulated in one word: 'pathogen'. Although it is classical Greek in form, this word was new in the late nineteenth century. In the *Oxford English Dictionary*, which is a historical dictionary, the first recorded occurrence of 'pathogen' in English is dated as 1880, and defined as 'a micrococcus or bacterium that produces disease'.[24] 'Pathogenic', 'pathogenetic' and other forms are recorded as occurring before this date, but not the substantive 'pathogen': 'disease-causing entity'. A 'pathogen' is a specific material agent, which is itself the cause of the disease.

[22] William Coleman, *Yellow Fever in the North: The Methods of Early Epidemiology* (Madison, Wis., 1977). He writes, 'It is an untoward result of the triumph of the germ theory of disease that the development of epidemiology has come to be viewed primarily through the spectacles of that theory and of etiological reasoning in general. This is misleading, even false', p. xiii.

[23] See, for example, Malcolm Nicolson, 'The metastatic theory of pathogenesis and the professional interests of the eighteenth-century physician', *Medical History*, 32 (1988), pp. 277–300.

[24] The term does not appear, for instance, in the 1874 edition of Robley Dunglison's *Medical Lexicon: A Dictionary of Medical Science* (Philadelphia).

The transformation of plague

How was plague transformed from a disease whose identity was symptom-based into one whose identity was cause-based? The transformation of the identity of plague took place in the laboratory, and from that moment on plague would only be identifiable in the laboratory. It is common to see this event as a simple 'unmasking' or a 'drawing back the veil' on what had been known all along to be there but which had hitherto simply evaded the light of science, and that is the language that was also used by many contemporaries about the event just after it had happened, and which has been regularly used since. But it was not a simple 'unmasking'. Instead, the new view of the disease, its new identity, was a *construction* since it involved, and depended totally on, a new way of thinking and seeing, the laboratory way of thinking and seeing. As we have seen, post-lab plague is defined by and from its *cause*, and as Bruno Latour has correctly remarked, 'a cause is always the *consequence* of a long work of composition and a long struggle to attribute responsibility to some actors'.[25] The laboratory was the instrument used to attribute responsibility to micro-organisms. Yet the laboratory is never a mere instrument: it is also a *practice* which defines, limits and governs ways of thinking and seeing. Plague acquired its new identity from this new activity, this new practice. Therefore the laboratory had to precede, both in time and conceptually, the 'causative micro-organism' identity of the disease. It was necessary to take the laboratory to the disease, and then to take the disease through the laboratory.

The transformation of the identity of plague happened in Hong Kong in the summer of 1894. Plague broke out in early May, being immediately identified by the native population, who at once took to flight. The outbreak was of especial interest to those colonial powers with major interests in the region: Britain (the 'lessee' of Hong Kong), France and Japan. The first telegram report of it in *The Times* of London on 13 June expresses very clearly the precise nature of Britain's interests as the colonial master of this showpiece of Victorian commercial values:

> Half native population Hong Kong left, numbering 100,000. Leaving by thousands daily; 1,500 deaths; several Europeans seized [by the disease], one died. Labour market paralyzed. Deaths nearly one hundred daily. Government anticipating failure of opium revenue; proposes taking over and destroying all unhealthy native quarters.

[25] Bruno Latour, *The Pasteurization of France*, translated by Alan Sheridan and John Law (Cambridge, Mass., 1988; original French edition, 1984), p. 258.

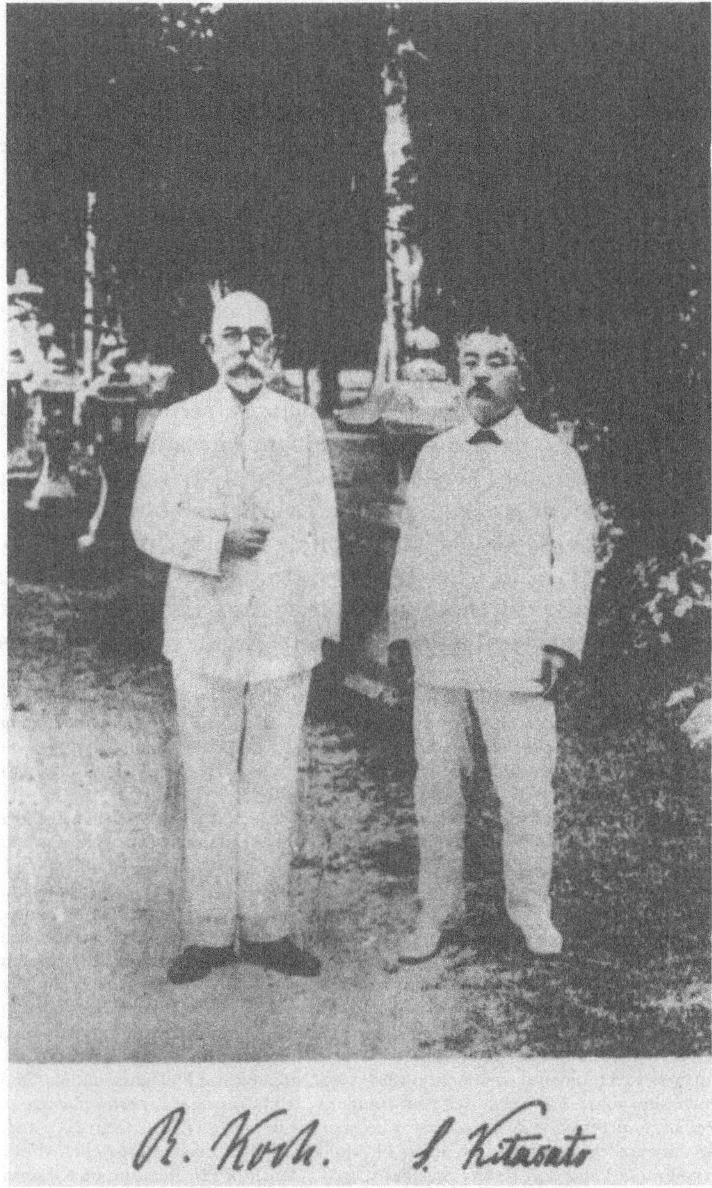

Fig. 7. Shibasaburo Kitasato and his teacher Robert Koch in Japan in 1908. According to his biographer, 'Kitasato was a man of filial affection toward his parents and a devoted follower of his teacher. While Koch was in Japan, Kitasato always attended his teacher with the utmost care as though serving his own father.' (Mikinosuke Miyajima, *British Medical Journal* (1939, 1), pp. 1141–2). Kitasato was said to be Koch's favourite pupil.

The disease continued to rage over the summer. By 4 September, when Hong Kong was formally declared to be free from the plague, the official British government figure for those who had died was over 2,500, almost all of them Chinese, while unofficial reports put the figure at 'over 3,000, out of a normal native population of 150,000, reduced certainly to 100,000 by panic and flight'.[26]

The two investigators who (to use the customary phrase) 'discovered' the plague bacillus in Hong Kong in 1894 were Shibasaburo Kitasato and Alexandre Yersin.[27] The rivalry between Koch and Pasteur in Europe, on nationalist and scientific grounds, was continued here in Hong Kong by their volunteer champions: the German school of Koch was represented by Kitasato (Fig. 7), a Japanese, and the French school of Pasteur by Yersin (Fig. 8), a Swiss who had become a naturalised Frenchman. Kitasato was sent by the Japanese government, Yersin by the French Ministry of Colonies. They arrived within days of each other, they tried to work within the territory of the same plague hospital and they struggled for a monopoly of investigative facilities. In the event they worked separately, with Yersin choosing to follow Pasteur's advice on what to do when trying to defeat a Kochian rival: 'As much as possible, work

[26] The unofficial figure is from *The Times* of 28 August 1894, p. 6, col. 2. For the official figures, and the British Government's information on the epidemic, see *Correspondence Relative To the Outbreak of Bubonic Plague at Hong Kong*, and *Further Correspondence*, presented to both Houses of Parliament in July and August 1894 respectively (Command Papers 7461 and 7545).

[27] I have chosen to treat Kitasato's name in western style, that is with the given name first and the family name second. For information in English on the life and works of Kitasato see the obituaries of him in the *Proceedings of the Royal Society*, series B, 109 (1931–2), pp. xi–xvi, by William Bulloch, and in the *British Medical Journal* (1931, 1), pp. 1141–2 by Mikinosuke Miyajima; the article in the *Dictionary of Scientific Biography* by Tsunesaburo Fujino. Both on Kitasato in particular and the general issue of Japanese involvement in late nineteenth century science in general, see the indispensable writings of James R. Bartholomew: 'Japanese culture and the problem of modern science' in Arnold Thackray and Everett Mendelsohn (eds), *Science and Values: Patterns of Tradition and Change* (New York, 1974), pp. 109–55; *The Formation of Science in Japan: Building a Research Tradition* (New Haven, 1989); and 'The acculturation of science in Japan: Kitasato Shibasaburo and the Japanese bacteriological community, 1885–1920', unpublished Ph.D dissertation (Stanford University, 1971). For Yersin see Paul Hauduroy (ed.), *Yersin et la peste: ouvrage publié pour la cinquantenaire de la découverte du microbe de la peste* (Lausanne, 1944); and now see the excellent biography by Henri H. Mollaret and Jacqueline Brossollet, *Alexandre Yersin ou le Vainqueur de la Peste* (Paris, 1985). Much of the literature on Kitasato and Yersin deals with the question of whether they in fact discovered the 'same' bacillus, and which of them therefore has the right to the credit for its discovery. This is not a concern of my paper, but on it see E. Lagrange, 'Concerning the discovery of the plague bacillus', *Journal of Tropical Medicine and Hygiene*, 29 (1926), pp. 299–303; Norman Howard-Jones, 'Kitasato, Yersin, and the plague bacillus', *Clio Medica*, 10 (1975), pp. 23–7; and David J. Bibel and T. H. Chen, 'Diagnosis of plague: an analysis of the Yersin–Kitasato controversy', *Bacteriological Reviews*, 40 (1976), pp. 633–51.

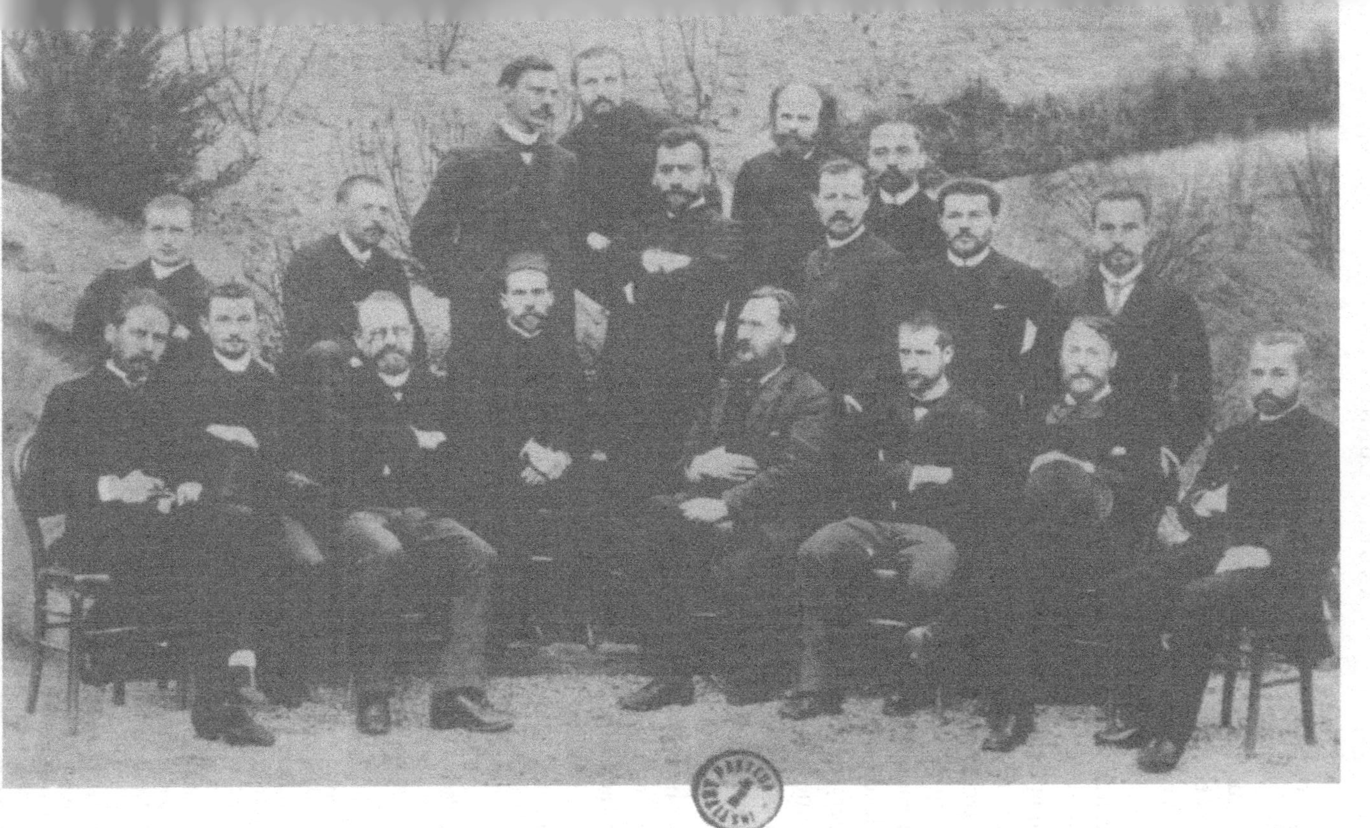

Fig. 8. Yersin in the first course of microbiological technique at the Pasteur Institute; the class was run by Dr Roux and Yersin was his *préparateur*. Yersin is seated in the front row, third from right, and to the left of him (on his right) sit Metchnikoff, Roux and Laveran.

by yourself. Keep your cadavers to yourself.'[28] Yet their roles in 'discovering' the plague bacillus and transforming the identity of plague, had a great deal in common. Let us see how the transformation was effected by their activities.

As Kitasato was a bacteriologist and Yersin was a microbiologist (these were the preferred terms used in their respective German and French schools), on the very first day that they could, they each *looked for* a micro-organism. As Yersin wrote, 'It was obvious that the first thing to do was to see whether there was a microbe in the blood of the patients and in the pulp of the buboes.'[29] And in order for them to search for a causative micro-organism it was necessary for each of them to have available to them a *laboratory*: that is, a dedicated space (a room) with special equipment in it. Kitasato, arriving first, made friends with Dr Lowson of the Colonial Medical Service, who 'put everything needful at our disposal in the most friendly spirit. A room in the Kennedy Town Hospital (one of the plague establishments) was given to us, and there we began our work on June 14th.'[30] Yersin, however, was denied space in the Kennedy Town Hospital, apart from a little space on a gallery. But he made friends with a long-established Catholic priest, and was thus able to build a laboratory of his own. As he wrote to his mother on 24 June, 'After having stayed at the hotel for some days, I have built myself a straw hut near the hospital for the plague victims and there I have set up my living quarters and my laboratory.'[31] This straw hut (Fig. 9), in the grounds

[28] On this rivalry see Yersin's letter to his mother of 24 June 1894, as translated by Ingrid Ebner in Butler, *Plague*, pp. 15–16; and the account by Mollaret and Brossollet, *Yersin*, pp. 133–8. Pasteur's advice, 'Autant que possible, travaillez seuls. Ayez vos cadavres à vous', was given in a letter to Straus and Roux in 1884; see *Correspondance de Pasteur, 1840–1895*, ed. Pasteur Vallery-Radot, 4 vols. (Paris, 1940–51), vol. III, p. 430; translated in Thomas D. Brock, *Robert Koch: A Life in Medicine and Bacteriology* (Madison, Wis., 1988), p. 176.

[29] 'Il était tout indiqué de rechercher tout d'abord s'il existe un microbe dans le sang des malades et dans la pulpe des bubons'; Alexandre Yersin, 'La peste bubonique à Hong-Kong', *Annales de l'Institut Pasteur*, 8 (1894), pp. 662–7, my translation. Translated in Hubert A. Lechevalier and Morris Solotorovsky, *Three Centuries of Microbiology* (New York, 1974; 1st edn, 1965), pp. 152–6; all subsequent quotations from Yersin are from here, unless otherwise noted. This translation is reprinted in Butler, *Plague*, pp. 17–22.

[30] S. Kitasato, 'The bacillus of bubonic plague', *Lancet*, 25 August 1894, pp. 428–30. All subsequent quotations from Kitasato are from here. Kitasato wrote his paper in German, and this was translated into English by Dr Lowson; this English form, as published in the *Lancet*, is the definitive version. See Bartholomew 'The acculturation of science in Japan', p. 174.

[31] Letter to his mother, 24 June 1894, as translated in Butler, *Plague*, pp. 15–16; the French original is published by H. H. Mollaret, 'Alexandre Yersin tel qu'en lui même enfin... Les révélations d'une correspondance inédite échelonnée de 1884 à 1926', *La Nouvelle Presse Médicale*, 2 (1973), pp. 2575–80, at p. 2577, and reproduced in facsimile on p. 2578: 'Après être resté quelques jours à l'hôtel, je me suis fait construire une paillotte à la côté de l'hôpital des pestiférés et j'ai établi là mon domicile et mon laboratoire'.

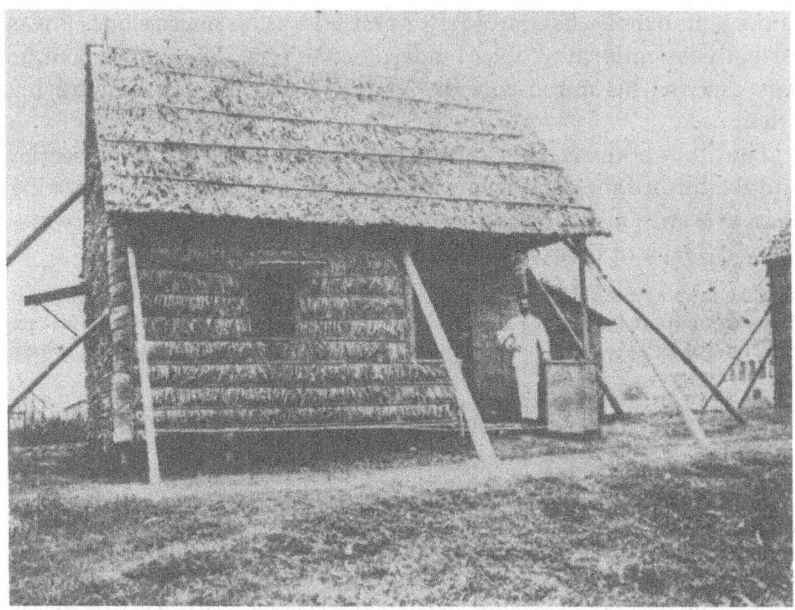

Fig. 9. Yersin outside his straw-hut laboratory in Hong Kong, 1894. He took this photograph himself to send home to his mother.

of the Alice Memorial Hospital, was Yersin's laboratory, within which he discovered his plague bacillus, and he constantly referred to it as such. To make these enclosed areas into laboratories proper, it was necessary to install in them certain equipment. 'I settled with my laboratory equipment in a straw hut that I had built with the permission of the English government, in the grounds of the main hospital', as Yersin wrote.[32] This equipment to transform inner space

[32] 'Je m'installai avec mon materiel de laboratoire dans une cabane en paillotte que je fis construire', Yersin, 'La peste bubonique', p. 662; translation as printed in Butler, *Plague*, p. 17. The set of items which constitute the essential equipment of a microbiological laboratory for the investigation of plague could be carried in three hands, as is shown in the opening passage of the autobiography of a slightly later 'plague fighter' (as he called himself), Wu Lien-Teh: 'Late in the bitterly cold afternoon of December 24, 1910, there arrived at the large railway station of Harbin in North Manchuria a young Chinese doctor... accompanied by his assistant... The doctor had in his right hand a compact, medium-sized British-made Beck microscope fitted with all necessaries for bacteriological work, while the assistant carried a handy-sized rattan basket containing various stains, glass slides, cover-glasses, small bottles of alcohol, test-tubes, platinum loops, needles, dissecting forceps, scissors and such other paraphernalia as are needed for laboratory investigation. Another but smaller basket held three dozen tubes of agar media packed in an upright position and held in place by packets of cotton wool; these media were most important for the routine growth of bacteria, particularly plague bacteria.' Wu Lien-Teh, *Plague Fighter: The Autobiography of a Modern Chinese Physician* (Cambridge, 1959), p. 1.

into a laboratory each investigator had brought with him. The most important item in a bacteriologist's arsenal was his microscope; it was virtually his emblem of office: indeed when Yersin got off the boat he was carrying his microscope in one hand and his autoclave in the other.

Thus they both arrived, transformed certain areas into laboratories and established themselves inside them, and they both started looking for a causative micro-organism. On the very first day, at the very first autopsy, each of them found one. Kitasato reported:

> On that day we were able to see a post-mortem examination performed by Professor Aoyama [one of the Japanese team]. I found numerous bacilli in the bubo (in this case a swelling of the inguinal glands), in the blood of the heart, in the lungs, liver, spleen, &c.

When Yersin eventually got started with his investigations he too immediately found a candidate micro-organism:

> With the help of Father Vigano, I try to persuade some English sailors, whose duty it is to bury the dead from the city and the other hospitals, to let me take the buboes from the dead, before they are buried. A few dollars conveniently distributed and the promise of a good tip for every case have a striking effect. The bodies before they are carried to the cemetery are deposed for one or two hours in a cellar. They are already in their coffins in a bed of lime. The coffin is opened, I move the lime to clear the crural region. The bubo is exposed, within less than a minute I cut it away and run to my laboratory. A film is prepared and put under the microscope; at the first glance, I see a real mass of bacilli, all identical. They are very small rods, thick with rounded ends and lightly coloured.[33]

It was never a problem for Yersin to see the bacillus: 'I always find it; for me there is no doubt.'[34]

Looking down his microscope each man could see a micro-organism of a particular known form (rod-like, i.e. a bacillus) but

[33] 'J'essaye, avec le père Vigano, d'obtenir de quelques matelots anglais qui ont pour mission de faire enterrer les cadavres de la ville et des autres hôpitaux qu'ils me laissent enlever les bubons des morts, avant qu'on ne les porte en terre. Quelques piastres judicieusement distribuées et la promesse d'un bon pourboire pour chaque bubon que je pourrai enlever ont un effet immédiat. Les morts, avant d'être enterrés au cimetière, sont déposés pendant une heure ou deux dans une sorte de cave. Ils sont déjà dans leur cercueil et recouverts de chaux. On ouvre un des cercueils et j'enlève un peu de la chaux pour découvrir la région crurale. Le bubon est bien net, je l'enlève en moins d'une minute et je monte à mon laboratoire. Je fais rapidement une préparation et la mets sous le microscope. Au premier coup d'oeuil je reconnais une véritable purée de microbes, tous semblables. Ce sont de très petits bâtonnets trapus, à extremités arrondies et assez mal colorés'. Yersin's diary for 20 June 1894; reproduced in facsimile in Hauduroy (ed.) *Yersin et la peste*, and in Lagrange, 'Discovery of the plague bacillus'; as translated by Lagrange.

[34] Yersin's letter to his mother of 24 June 1894, as translated in N. Howard-Jones, *The Scientific Background of the International Sanitary Conferences, 1851–1938* (Geneva, 1975), p. 79; the French original is 'Je le retrouve toujours; pour moi, il n'y a pas de doute', see Mollaret, 'Alexandre Yersin tel qu'en lui-même enfin', p. 2577.

with its own unusual and distinctive properties. It could be uniquely characterised in the laboratory according to its motility, staining reactions and behaviour when cultivated, and these characteristics gave it its unique identity, making it distinguishable from all other micro-organisms. This unique identity was described by each investigator. Kitasato's micro-organisms

are rods with rounded ends, which are readily stained by the ordinary analine dyes, the poles being stained darker than the middle part, especially in blood preparations, and presenting a capsule sometimes well marked, sometimes indistinct... I am at present unable to say whether or not 'Gram's double-staining method' can be employed... The bacilli show very little movement, and those grown in the incubator, in beef-tea, make the medium somewhat cloudy.

Yersin's micro-organisms were

short, stubby bacilli which are rather easy to stain with analine dyes and are not stained by the method of Gram. The ends of the bacilli are colored more strongly than the center. Sometimes the bacilli seem to be surrounded by a capsule... In broth, the bacillus has a very characteristic appearance resembling that of the erysipelas culture: clear liquid with lumps depositing on the walls and bottom of the tube.

Both investigators thought that the bacillus they had found was the causative agent of plague that they had come to Hong Kong to find. But before their rod-shaped micro-organisms, their bacilli, could be determined to be the causative agent of plague, they had to be put to and pass certain other tests, which both investigators employed. These were the tests to fulfil 'Koch's postulates'. Kitasato wrote, 'I still had doubts about the true significance of what I found; I therefore made a cultivation...'. This was the first test he applied: could his bacillus be cultivated artificially, would it grow in a pure form outside the human body? Kitasato found that it would:

The growth of the bacilli is strongest on blood serum at the normal temperature of the human body (37 °C): under these conditions they develop luxuriantly and are moist in consistence and of a yellowish grey colour; they do not liquefy the serum. On agar-agar jelly (the best is good glycerine agar) they also grow freely. The different colonies are of a whitish-grey colour and by a reflected light have a bluish appearance; under the microscope they appear moist and in rounded patches with uneven edges... If a cover-glass preparation is made from a cultivation on agar-agar, and, after having been stained, is observed under the microscope long threads of bacilli are seen.

Yersin too had success in making his bacillus grow in pure cultures outside the body:

The pulp of buboes, seeded on agar, gives rise to transparent, white colonies, with margins that are iridescent when examined with reflected light. Growth is even better if glycerol is incorporated into the agar. The bacillus also grows on coagulated serum... Microscopical examination of the cultures reveals true chains of short bacilli interspersed with larger spherical bodies.

Once each bacillus had been successfully cultivated there was a second test to be made, the test on live animals. Kitasato mainly used the experimental animal which Koch had made indispensable, the white mouse:

The mice, which were inoculated on the first day with a piece of spleen and some blood from the finger-tips [of the first corpse post-mortemed by Professor Aoyama], died in two days' time, and at the post-mortem examination upon them I found oedema round the place of inoculation, and the same bacilli in the blood, in the internal organs, and in the oedematous part around the place of inoculation. All animals which had been inoculated with the cultivations (pigeons excepted) died after periods extending from one to four days, according to the size of the animal. The same state of the organs after death and the same bacteriological observations always obtained as in the case of the mice.

Yersin too turned to animals to test whether his bacillus was the true causative micro-organism of plague. He found it was.

If one inoculates mice, rats or guinea pigs with the pulp from buboes, they die, and at autopsy one can note the characteristic lesions as well as numerous bacilli in the lymph nodes, spleen and blood. Guinea pigs die in 2 to 5 days, mice in 1 to 3 days.

So when the bacillus was inoculated into healthy animals it produced 'the characteristic lesions'; it killed the animals in a few days; it produced 'the same state of organs after death', and 'the same bacilli' were found in the blood and in the internal organs of the dead animals.

The third test each bacillus had to pass was whether it was present in all cases of the disease. Kitasato found that his bacillus was indeed always present (well, almost always):

Every day I took blood from many plague patients and examined it, and almost every time I found the bacilli as above described, sometimes in great numbers, sometimes only few in number... On the other hand, these same bacilli were to be found at every post-mortem examination (of which we had upwards of fifteen) in great quantity in the bubonic swellings, in the spleen, the lungs, the liver, in the blood contained in the heart, in the brain, intestines – in fact, in all internal organs without exception – and every cultivation from any particle of these parts invariably produced the same bacilli.

Yersin too found his bacillus everywhere present in the body of humans or animals suffering from the plague: 'The pulp of the buboes always contains masses of short, stubby, bacilli... One can find them in large numbers in the buboes and the lymph nodes of the diseased persons', and in inoculated animals 'at autopsy, one recovers the bacillus from the blood, the liver, the spleen and the lymph nodes'.

Yersin, as a true Pasteurian, subjected his bacillus to one further question: did it exist naturally in, or could it be cultivated into, forms

THE LANCET,] THE PLAGUE AT HONG-KONG. [AUGUST 11, 1894. 325

Madeira; rainless and cloudless days are more frequent, and the temptations to invalids to overdo their strength are consequently greater. There is also more wind and more dust." Regarding Puerto Orotava, the author says: "In a good winter there is but little cold weather, but what cold there may be is felt, as it is accompanied by damp. From the middle of January to the end of February is the worst time, and in a bad year may be disagreeable, the sky being overcast day after day, and the sun being obscured by the thick mantle of clouds which will then envelop the island. Such winters are, however, the exception ...... a day when there is no sunshine, or when one cannot be out of doors for at least three or four hours, is almost unknown."

THE PLAGUE AT HONG-KONG.

We have received the following notes from Dr. J. A. Lowson of Hong-Kong, who has forwarded a number of preparations of the plague bacillus, some of them prepared for him by Professor Kitasato, others prepared by himself, of which we give several representations. The organism—which is a bacterium resembling the bacilli found in the hæmorrhagic septicæmias, except that the ends are somewhat more rounded—when stained lightly appears almost like an encapsuled diplococcus, but when more deeply stained it has the appearance of an ovoid bacillus, with a somewhat lighter centre, especially when not accurately focussed. When, however, it is focussed more accurately it is still possible to make out the diplococcus form. It is quite possible that the capsule has been produced artificially,

FIG. 1.

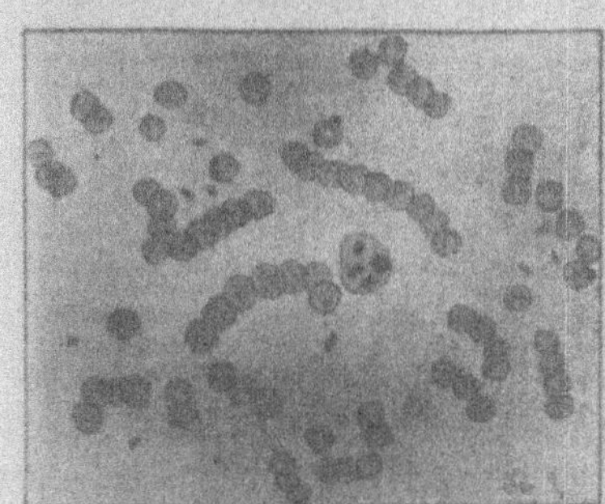

Ob. 1/12 homog. + oc. 8 compens.; length of tube 140 mm. Bacilli and blood from case of plague. Illustration of preparation made by Professor Kitasato and forwarded by Dr. Lowson.

though in Fig. 3 this does not appear to be the case. The positions in which it is most frequently met with—sometimes apparently in almost pure cultures—are the glandular enlargements which occur in the groin, in the axilla, and in the neck, though these enlargements are not always met with in the rapidly fatal cases. These enlarged glands are intensely congested, or rather they appear to be infiltrated with blood. In this blood, which is in a state of disintegration, mixed with the elements of the glandular tissue which are also broken down, the organisms are exceedingly numerous. They are also met with in considerable numbers in the spleen and in the other organs in those positions where there is a slowing of the circulation as it passes through capillary networks or sinuses. The organisms are also found even in the blood in the heart and large bloodvessels, as seen in Fig. 1. Dr. Lowson hopes shortly to be able to send an account of the disease and also

FIG. 2.

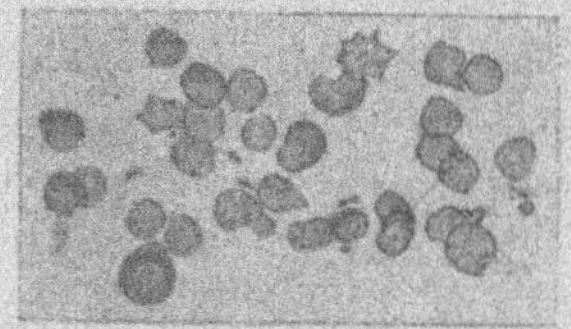

Ob. 1/12 homog. + oc. 8 compens.; length of tube 180 mm. Bacilli in blood of mouse. Illustration of preparation made by Professor Kitasato and forwarded by Dr. Lowson.

of the appearance of the micro-organisms when cultivated outside the body; but he says: "I have recently been so

FIG. 3.

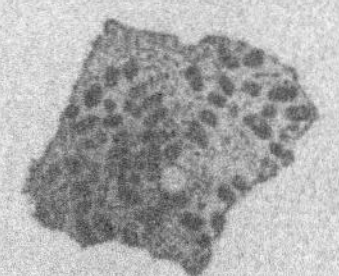

Ob. 1/12 homog. + oc. 8 compens.; length of tube 150 mm. Illustration of preparation of splenic pulp in case of plague made by Dr. Lowson.

engaged in looking after the sick, organising hospital work, inspecting insanitary houses, and looking after the disposal

FIG. 4.

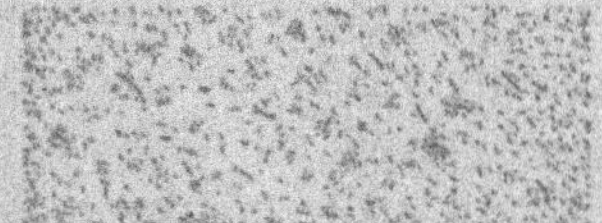

Ob. 1/12 homog. + oc. 8 compens.; length of tube 140 mm. Illustration of plague bacillus prepared by Professor Kitasato and sent by Dr. Lowson.

of the dead that I have been unable to find time to do more than send you these few notes and specimens, which, however, I thought might be of interest to some of your readers."

EXHIBITION OF AMBULANCE WORK AT CHUDLEIGH.—On July 28th the annual exhibition of the Chudleigh Cottage Garden Society was held in a field close to Chudleigh Rocks. In the evening the Ambulance and Field Stretcher Bearer Company, under the direction of Surgeon-Captain C. L. Cunningham, gave an excellent exhibition, in which they showed that they had fully availed themselves of the lessons in ambulance work received from their director. A sham fight was organised between a supposed party of Arabs and a company of Engineers; the wounded were brought out of action and were promptly attended to with all proper detail. The men in the course of the sham fight availed themselves for signalling purposes of an ingenious method of signalling invented by Surgeon-Captain Cunningham for use in the Soudan campaign.

Fig. 10. Plague as identified by Kitasato. Note that most of the article announcing Kitasato's discovery is taken up by reproductions of the microscopic image of the plague bacillus.

with lesser virulence, and which could thus be used to give animals and humans immunity against the plague? Kitasato, as a true Kochian, asked and answered a different final question: 'What means are to be employed against the plague? – preventive measures, general hygiene, good drainage, perfect water-supply, cleanliness in dwelling-houses, and cleanliness in the streets.'[35]

The bacillus that Kitasato found and the bacillus that Yersin found passed all the tests of Koch. 'From this evidence', wrote Kitasato, 'we must come to the conclusion that this bacillus is the cause of the disease known as the bubonic plague; therefore the bubonic plague is an infectious disease produced by a specific bacillus'. Yersin concluded similarly that 'Plague is thus a contagious and transmissible disease', whose cause is the bacillus he had found.

As soon as they were each certain that they had discovered the causal micro-organism of plague, each of them got into print as quickly as possible. Yersin, typically for a Pasteurian, placed his report in the *Annales de l'Institut Pasteur*. Kitasato, however, had been befriended by the British Dr Lowson, who encouraged him to let him translate his original German text into English and to send it to London to be published in *The Lancet*. Yersin and Kitasato sent not just descriptions of their successful hunt for 'the causative micro-organism' of plague but, most importantly, pictures (Fig. 10 and 11). What was portrayed in these pictures was not the *symptoms* – the patients suffering the disease – but the *microbe*, a thing which could only be seen down the microscope. And the message of these pictures is this: 'here is the micro-organism = here is the disease (plague)'. They had taken into their laboratories a disease whose identity was constituted by symptoms; they had emerged with a disease whose identity was constituted by its causal agent.

After Kitasato and Yersin had each found their plague bacillus, the tiny micro-organism was given its new scientific name. That name was in Latin. Hitherto what had been named in Latin or Greek was the disease (*pestis*); henceforth it was the micro-organism. The name given to the micro-organism directly expresses its causal relation to the disease. Its first name was *Bacterium pestis*, the bacterium of the plague. In 1900 it was renamed *Bacillus pestis* the bacillus of the plague. From 1923 it was called *Pasteurella pestis*, which is short for 'the Pasteur-genus causative micro-organism of the plague'. A new genus, *Yersinia*, was proposed in 1954, and today the bacillus is

[35] For this contrast between the styles of Pasteurians and Kochians, see Brock, *Robert Koch*, p. 177.

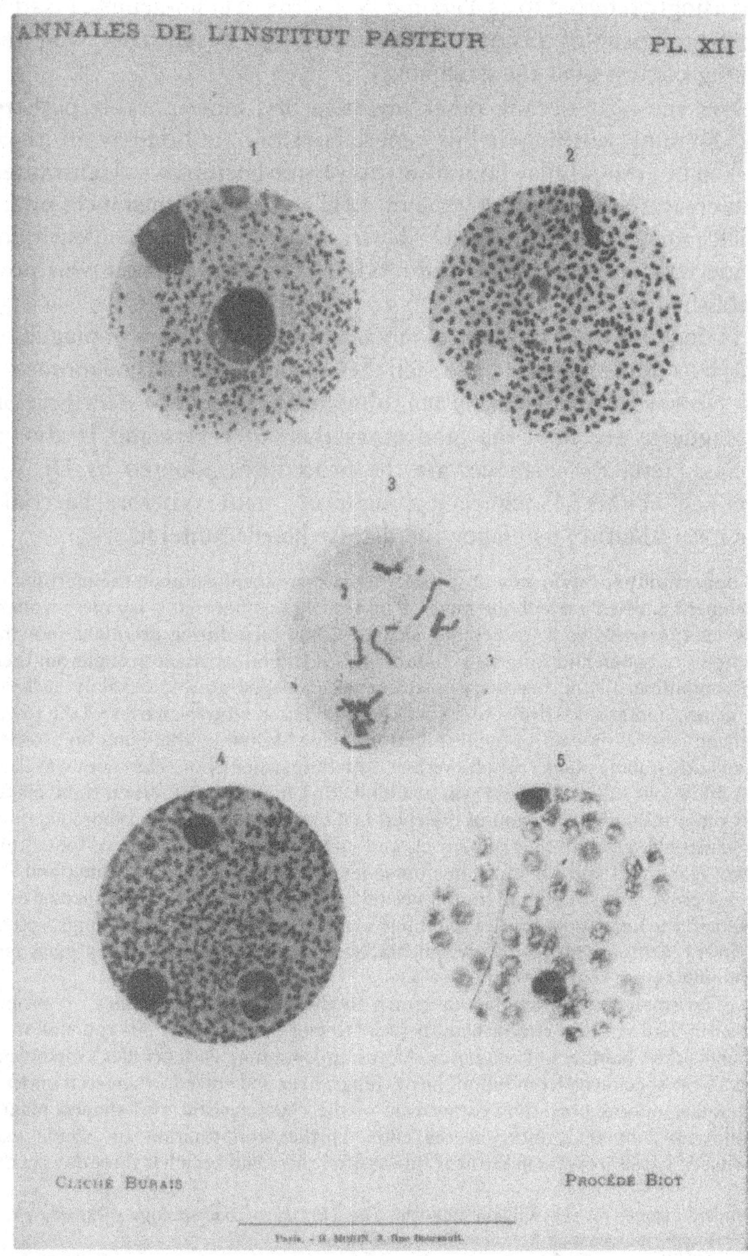

Fig. 11. Plague as identified by Yersin. These were the pictures which accompanied his announcement of his discovery of a plague bacillus in the *Annales* of the Pasteur Institute.

increasingly referred to as *Yersinia pestis*, the 'Yersin-genus causative micro-organism of plague'.[36] (Evidently the Pasteurians won the naming contest over the Kochians.)

Over the next decade other investigators, most notably perhaps P.-L. Simond working in his tent laboratory in Bombay in 1897, worked out the details about how this plague bacillus was transmitted from creature to creature by the rat flea, and the circumstances under which man becomes affected. The transformation of the identity of plague was now complete: the modern identity of plague was now established.[37]

Having looked at the central moment of identification of plague by Kitasato and Yersin, we have seen the essential role of the laboratory in it. Now we can look briefly at a subsequent moment of identification of plague to see how the laboratory thereafter was and is always crucial. Here, for instance, are the procedures adopted by Dr Wu Lien-Teh in the Manchuria epidemic of 1910–11 before he could diagnose (identify) as plague the disease he encountered:

> The opportunity to perform a post-mortem upon a patient came on the morning of December 27, when a telephone message informed the office that a Japanese woman inn-keeper, married to a Chinese at Fuchiaten, had died during the night showing symptoms of cough and spitting of blood. Dr Wu and his assistant brought out their case containing all the necessary instruments and apparatus for exactly such an emergency, and at once drove to a small house lying in a poor quarter of the town. A female corpse, dressed in a cheap cotton-padded kimono, was lying on a soiled *tatami* laid on some planks raised two feet from the earthen floor. The room was dark and untidy, but sufficient water was available for a limited postmortem to be made. After the cartilaginous portion of the chest had been removed, a thick-bored syringe needle was plunged into the right auricle and sufficient blood was removed for culture in two agar tubes and for thin films on slides. Next, the surface of a lung and the spleen were scarified, and a platinum needle was inserted into the substance of each organ and the necessary cultures and films made. Pieces of the affected lungs, spleen and liver, each two inches by two inches, were removed and placed in glass jars containing 10 per cent formalin...
>
> ... The small party was glad to return to their quarters, and since no proper laboratory had yet been established, they had to work temporarily in a room allotted to them in the Chamber of Commerce. After simple staining with Loeffler's methylene blue, all the specimens from blood, heart, lungs, liver and spleen, when seen under a high-power microscope, showed swarms of the characteristic oval-shaped plague bacilli with bipolar staining at the ends. Further confirmation of plague was established in the growths in the agar tubes. After these had been left three days in the

[36] Butler, *Plague*, p. 25; William Bulloch, *The History of Bacteriology* (Oxford, 1938; reprinted 1960), chapter 8, 'Classification of bacteria'.

[37] Establishing the role of the rat and of the rat flea as the vector of the plague bacillus was not done without opposition; for the stories see Hirst, *Conquest of Plague*, pp. 130–74. For the key works in the medical literature, see Arthur L. Bloomfield, *A Bibliography of Internal Medicine: Communicable Diseases* (Chicago, 1958), pp. 47–60.

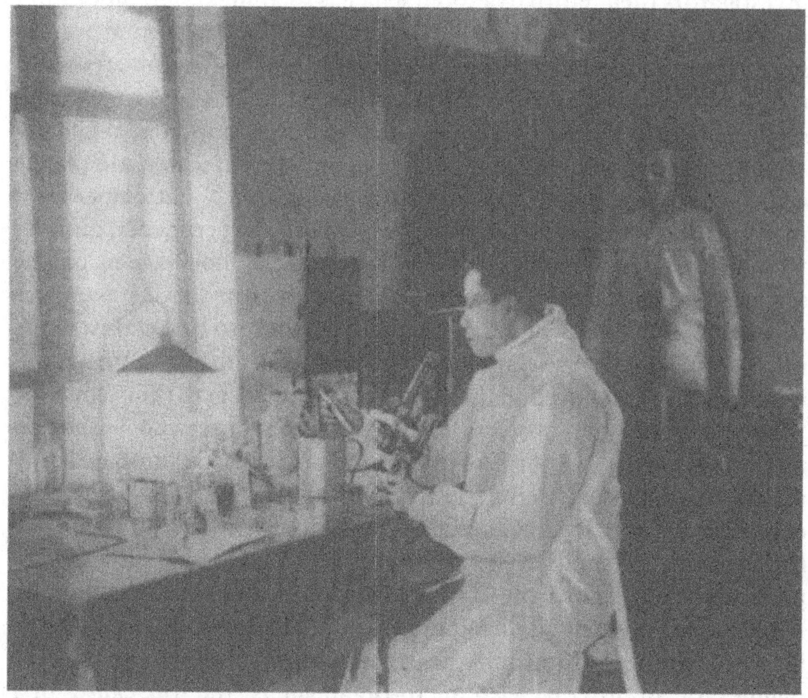

Fig. 12. Wu Lien-Teh in his temporary plague laboratory, Harbin 1911, photographed by himself.

ordinary temperature of the living room, small pin-point translucent colonies appeared in profusion. Films taken from one of these colonies showed the characteristic plague organisms. The cultures from the heart-blood and the spleen were quite pure, that is, they were not contaminated with other organisms; only the lung cultures showed slight contamination. This discovery was announced both to the local officials and the higher ones in Peking. The Taotai, the magistrate and the Chief of Police – all laymen – were invited to look down the microscope and be convinced, if possible, of the true cause of the suspicious deaths, but it was not always easy to convince persons who lack the foundations of modern knowledge and of science ...[38]

The patient showed certain symptoms (including that most striking one of all, sudden death); these symptoms lead the investigators to suspect plague. 'But is it plague?', they ask. These are the procedures that Dr Wu follows in order to answer this question with certainty, either in the affirmative or the negative. He carries out a post-mortem in order to acquire samples of some of the deceased's organs and blood, 'and the necessary cultures and films' are made. The

[38] Wu, *Plague Fighter*, pp. 11–12.

investigators then return to a room which is their makeshift *laboratory* (Fig. 12). First confirmation that the disease is plague comes from staining the specimens and then inspecting them under a microscope: the characteristic plague bacilli are observed to be present. 'Further confirmation of plague was established' by inspecting some time later the growths in the agar tubes, where again the characteristic plague organisms were readily seen in artificial culture. No attempts were made on this occasion by Dr Wu to test whether experimental animals would show the symptoms of the disease after inoculation, but he seems to have thought that the evidence in front of his eyes was sufficient, for he invited the laymen present to look down the microscope at 'the true cause of the suspicious deaths'; but they could not readily be convinced that this microscopically small thing could be 'the true cause' of a disease. Wu was one of those who wished to modernise (that is, westernise) traditional China, as his autobiography makes clear. He was right to attribute the unwillingness to believe exhibited by the local Chinese officials to their ignorance of the foundations of modern (= western) knowledge and science. In particular they lacked the laboratory way of looking and thinking. Indeed this moment of incomprehension in Manchuria, this clash between cultures, sums up the transformation of the identity of plague; for, in order to see a micro-organism as 'the true cause' of a disease one needs to be already in the laboratory thought-world. To be able to see 'the true cause' of a disease down a microscope, one needs to bring to it eyes and mind familiar with the laboratory way of seeing.

Plague transformed

Thus, as we can see here in the case of plague, the coming of the laboratory created a watershed in the identity of infectious diseases. Indeed, one could be even more precise, and actually specify the date on which they acquired their new identities: for plague it was 14–24 June 1894.[39] But in speaking of 1894 as the watershed in the definition and identity of plague, I do not mean to imply that everyone immediately in 1894 adopted this new 'bacteriologic' (as I call it) understanding. We have already seen how difficult a way of thinking this was for Chinese officials to adopt. But it was also very difficult for western medical men. There was a long battle between on the one hand the bacteriologists, and on the other the 'epidemiologists' or

[39] Kitasato found his bacillus on 14 June, Yersin his on 24 June; there is continuing debate over whether they were the same one; see note 27.

'localists' who believed some 'epidemic constitution' or special state of the soil was necessary before an epidemic could occur.[40] This battle between Kochians and Pettenkoferians, between as it were Berlin and Munich, between bacteriologists and hygienists, continued a long time. Pettenkofer's great challenge to the germ theory is famous: in 1892 he drank a culture of the cholera vibrio and did not get cholera! Indeed, one might say that it was his stubborn resistance to the germ theory both in mind and in body which obliged him ultimately to commit suicide. Similarly a long resistance was put up by clinicians, epitomised by Professor Rosenbach and his book *Physician versus Bacteriologist* of 1903.[41] For a long time it was possible to say, with the eminent British abdominal surgeon Lawson Tait in the late 1890s, that the true *causa causans* of typhus fever was not a microbe but the terrible living conditions of the poor, and that 'the laboratory fails utterly': 'Human beings alive differ in their individual results from exactly similar conditions and in ways altogether irreconcilable with the laboratory facts of bacteriology.'[42]

The fight was probably not finally over until the 1930s.[43] But eventually the bacteriologists won. We are all bacteriologists now, and none of us would attempt to identify plague today without a laboratory. To oppose the claims of bacteriology is now not a rival view, nor an alternative view, nor even a dissident view. It is now a lunatic view. That indicates how comprehensive the victory of the bacteriologists has turned out to be. But while the fight was still on – while the bacteriologists were for the first time promoting their new

[40] See Winslow, *Conquest of Epidemic Disease*, chapter 15, 'Pettenkofer – the last stand'; Richard J. Evans, *Death in Hamburg: Society and Politics in the Cholera Years 1830–1910* (Oxford, 1987), esp. pp. 237–43 and 490–507.

[41] First published as *Artz contra Bakteriologe*. See Russell C. Maulitz, '"Physician versus Bacteriologist": the ideology of science in clinical medicine' in Morris J. Vogel and Charles E. Rosenberg (eds.), *The Therapeutic Revolution: Essays in the Social History of American Medicine* (Philadelphia, 1979), pp. 91–107.

[42] Tait talked of the true 'causa causans' of typhus fever in a letter to the *British Medical Journal* (1899, 1), p. 879. The other two quotations from him are from 'The evolution of the aseptic method in surgery', *Medical Press and Circular* (1898, 1), pp. 427–30, at p. 427, where he writes also: 'this mysterious "life" is the most perfect antiseptic we have, and this prime fact is that which makes all "cultures" and all laboratory experiments fail absolutely in giving results which can safely be applied to the living body, particularly to man... When we come to consider man we find all our facts at sixes and sevens, and all theories of no avail. The laboratory fails utterly; and whilst in the processes of his body we may see verisimilitudes with those of the lower animals, we are met at once by facts which show they are not...'. On this issue in general see also Lloyd G. Stevenson, 'Science down the drain: on the hostility of certain sanitarians to animal experimentation, bacteriology and immunology', *Bulletin of the History of Medicine*, 29 (1955), pp. 1–26.

[43] See Howard-Jones, *The Scientific Background of the International Sanitary Conferences*, p. 89.

way of seeing, their laboratory way of seeing, and claiming total truth for it – at that time it was an essential (and spontaneous) part of their strategy to claim that they, and only they, had mastered the causal secrets of the age-old scourges of mankind. This is also of course the way they experienced it. And this view – that theirs was the first *successful* understanding of plague and other terrible diseases, which replaced the old, unsuccessful and *misguided* attempts – was the basis of the way they now rewrote the history of man's life with disease. The bacteriologists presented the laboratory as the glorious weapon giving men victory at last in an age-old battle between men and microbes, hitherto fruitlessly fought with the wrong weapons by their enemies – the Pettenkofers of the past and the present. They now had new heroes whom they exhumed from old books to be early microbiologists and bacteriologists, men such as Fracastoro, Leeuwenhoek, Redi, Spallanzani and Semmelweis. They themselves were the successors to these far-sighted men whose fate had inevitably been not to have been appreciated in their own day.[44] This bacteriologic account of the history was presented as the story of the fight of evidence and common sense over theory and stupidity. And this is why, in writing their histories of the triumphs of laboratory medicine, bacteriologic historians have usually applauded Kitasato and Yersin as having correctly *focused on* the essential thing about plague, its causative bacillus, and not noticed that by deploying the laboratory in investigating plague, Kitasato and Yersin were *making* the bacillus the essential thing about plague.

This bacteriologic view of the past is still shaping our accounts of infectious diseases in the long past before the laboratory. To take just

[44] For instance, nowadays we tend to see Ignaz Semmelweis (1818–65) as an early worker in the cause of the germ theory, because of his views on childbed fever. But formal recognition of the supposed 'contribution' of Semmelweis to bacteriology and antisepsis was first made only in the 1880s, by Joseph Lister – that is, after Lister himself had received widespread praise and acceptance for his introduction of antisepsis. And even then the claims of Semmelweis to 'credit' were only recognised through the insistence of the Hungarian nationalist, Dr Duka, in virtually forcing Semmelweis on Lister's attention. As Lister's biographer wrote: '[Semmelweis'] work and almost his name were forgotten until this festival at Pesth was held in Lister's honour… The history and fate of this great and unhappy man [Semmelweis] excited the liveliest interest in Lister. Here, at the completion of his antiseptic triumph, quite unexpectedly he came across a true but almost forgotten forerunner, who owing to the happy deduction of an original mind fought the unseen enemies of disease with weapons similar to Lister's, though unsupported by the scientific evidence which Pasteur had given to Lister', G. T. Wrench, *Lord Lister: His Life and Work* (London, 1913), pp. 347 and 342. Semmelweis was constructed as two heroes at once by Duka: as a Hungarian patriot and as a microbiological 'predecessor', and each facet received lustre from the other; see Liza H. Gold, 'Ignaz Philip Semmelweis and the reception of his work on puerperal fever in 19th century Britain', unpublished M.Phil. thesis (Wellcome Unit for the History of Medicine, Cambridge University, 1982).

one instance, it underlies Carlo Cipolla's account of the plague in Prato in 1629–30, such that Cipolla can write that the medical officers of Prato 'fought against an invisible enemy. They did not know what the enemy was, or how it struck. Medical knowledge was of no help and medical treatment was of no value.'[45] The only kind of knowledge about the 'enemy' that matters in Cipolla's eyes is knowledge about the bacillus! This attitude is completely typical of most historians' accounts and assumptions today. Yet these people in the past *did* know what plague was and how it struck: they just knew these things differently from how we know them, because the laboratory way of thinking did not exist.

In its co-option of the history of infectious diseases, this bacteriologic view is also the reason why the transformation in the identity of plague has gone unnoticed, not only by the historians but also by the very bacteriologists who made these new identities for infectious diseases. For Kitasato and Yersin themselves were at pains to point out that the disease whose cause they had discovered was indeed the same disease which had been a scourge for centuries. They both said (and, indeed, so did the newspapers at the time) that the disease whose cause they had discovered was 'ancient bubonic plague'. Kitasato, for instance, writes in his report:

> History shows us that plague epidemics existed in the fourteenth century both in Asia and Europe, and thousands of human beings perished. Since then from time to time, now here, now there, an epidemic has appeared, and until lately the disease almost seemed to have vanished from the face of the earth. This, however, was not so. In China it has existed to this day... The recent outbreak has given us opportunity for studying this disease – a cause of mystery for centuries – with the means which modern science places in our hand...

And indeed they were right. But only at that moment. For at the moment Kitasato and Yersin decided to go into their respective laboratories carrying their blood and tissue specimens, they were working with ancient bubonic plague. But by the time they came out of their laboratories, they had given plague a new identity. From this moment onwards plague would never – *could* never – again be identified by symptoms alone, but by its causal agent. It is this detour through the laboratory which means that pre-laboratory plague and post-laboratory plague do not have one consistent and continuous identity.[46]

[45] Carlo N. Cipolla, *Cristofano and the Plague: A Study in the History of Public Health in the Age of Galileo* (London, 1973), p. 120.

[46] On the importance and significance of the detour through the laboratory for plague see Latour, *Pasteurization of France*, pp. 94–100.

The laboratory construction of plague means that there is an unbridgeable gap between past 'plague' and our plague. The identities of pre-1894 plague and post-1894 plague have become incommensurable. We are simply unable to say whether they were the same, since the criteria of 'sameness' have been changed. As I have been arguing, this is not a technical medical issue but a logical, philosophical and historiographic one. Nevertheless, historians and bacteriologists regularly put themselves through intellectual contortions in their determination to make identifications across this divide, and presumably will continue to do so, bizarre as their assertions sometimes are by their own usual standards of evidence and proof.[47]

The laboratory identity of modern plague and other infectious diseases is now such a great truth that it has become enshrined in that higher truth, modern fiction. Fictionalised plague pre-1894 can be seen in Daniel Defoe's *Journal of the Plague Year*, written in 1722 and posing as an account of the London plague of 1665. While Defoe himself, in the voice of the narrator, asserted his belief that the disease was spread by infection, 'that is to say, by some certain steams or fumes, which the physicians call effluvia... immediately penetrating

[47] What is typically done by such enthusiasts is to identify the disease in the past on the basis of symptoms alone, working from past descriptions of 'plague' – and despite the fact that the symptoms mentioned do not tally with the modern set of symptoms. Then an unconscious logical leap is taken to identify this symptom-identified disease with our modern cause-identified plague. Hence one infers the presence of the plague bacillus in these past diseases (and treats it as the cause of the disease) from an ill-fitting set of symptoms which had been recorded by people with a pre-lab way of seeing and a pre-lab set of diagnostic categories! For instance, Dr Wu claimed that 'It is undeniable that some of the symptoms of the Black Death [of 1348] are not frequently encountered in modern outbreaks of plague, while others are altogether absent... The fact that the Black Death does not quite correspond to the form of infection as it is known today cannot eliminate the ample evidence that it was plague. The description of both the bubonic and the pneumonic types, as given by contemporary observers, leave no room for doubt', *A Treatise on Pneumonic Plague* (Geneva, 1926), p. 3. But, apart from anything else, the bubonic/pneumonic distinction had not in fact been available to those 'contemporaries', since it derives from seeing the bacillus as the cause of both of these clinically different conditions (as discussed earlier). Again, it has been written by modern historians of medicine that 'Considering the extent of the disaster, we know surprisingly little of the Black Death; for instance, the very scanty descriptions of signs and symptoms do not so much as mention blood-stained sputum (though *vomiting* of blood is described), yet this is one of the cardinal signs of a virulent pneumonia. Nevertheless, the widespread and high mortality of the plague indicate that it must have been predominantly of the pneumonic type...', F. R. Cartwright in collaboration with M. D. Biddis, *Disease and History* (London, 1973), p. 38. Similarly, Hirst, discussing Emile Rocher's 1871 account of the Yunnan epidemic, writes: 'The detailed clinical description of the human cases leaves no room for doubt that the disease was bubonic plague. Rocher also states, however, that a number of domestic animals were affected, including cattle, sheep, and goats, and sometimes even farmyard birds. We now know that none of these animals is subject to true plague', Hirst, *Conquest of Plague*, pp. 101–2. Identifications like this require something of the eye of hope.

the vital parts' of sound persons, 'putting their blood into an immediate ferment', yet he looked 'with contempt' on the opinion of those

> who talk of infection being carried on by the air only, by carrying with it vast numbers of insects and invisible creatures, who enter into the body with the breath, or even at the pores with the air, and there generate or emit most acute poisons, or poisonous ovae or eggs, which mingle themselves with the blood, and so infect the body.[48]

He condemned this as 'a discourse full of learned simplicity, and manifested to be so by universal experience'. So it is clear that Defoe's plague was transmitted by the 'seeds of disease' but not by a unique and specific material cause. We may contrast this with H. G. Wells' famous story, 'The stolen bacillus'.[49] This was published on 21 June 1894, which was by extraordinary chance in the few days interval between Kitasato's (14 June) and Yersin's (24 June) discoveries of their plague bacilli in Hong Kong. In this story, the absent-minded Bacteriologist shows round his laboratory a mysterious and evil visitor ('Certainly the man was not a Teutonic type nor a common Latin one. "A morbid product, anyhow, I'm afraid", said the Bacteriologist to himself'). The Bacteriologist takes up a sealed tube, saying 'Here is the living thing. This is a cultivation of the actual living disease bacteria ... Bottled cholera, so to speak.' His visitor, as is obvious from the description of him, is an Anarchist, who steals the tube and with it intends to poison the whole city and thus advance his nefarious political aims. Wells' story begins that popular view of the mighty power of the microbe in the laboratory tube: the deadly single material cause of untold misery. Just tip it into the water supply and the cholera is abroad: 'those little particles, those mere atomies, might multiply and devastate a city! Wonderful!', as the Bacteriologist exults.

The power of the laboratory in controlling the identification of infectious disease is perhaps best shown in the most famous appearance of plague in modern fiction, Camus' *La Peste*, about a fictional outbreak in an Algerian town in the 1940s.[50] Part of the early drama revolves around the identification of the disease. The laboratory is therefore at the centre of things, but it has not yet spoken. Castel, an older practitioner, comes to see the hero Dr Rieux.

[48] Daniel Defoe, *A Journal of the Plague Year* (first published 1722; Harmondsworth, 1966), pp. 92–3.
[49] First published in the *Pall Mall Budget*; quoted from *Selected Short Stories* (Harmondsworth, 1958; reprinted 1981), pp. 149 and 145.
[50] Albert Camus, *La Peste* (first published 1947; Paris, 1972; reprinted 1988), pp. 39–41 and 45; my translation.

'Naturally', he says, 'you know what this is, Rieux?'

'I am awaiting the result of the analyses.'

'Well, I know what it is. And I don't need any analyses. I spent part of my career in China, and I saw some cases in Paris twenty years ago. It was just that one didn't dare give it a name at that moment. Public opinion is sacred: no panic, above all no panic. And, then, as a colleague said, "It's impossible, everyone knows that it has disappeared in the West." Yes, everyone knew it, except the corpses. Come on, Rieux, you know as well as I do what it is.'

There is a pause while Rieux reflects and looks out of the window.

'Yes, Castel', he said, 'it's hardly believable. But it really appears as if it could be plague'

...

The word 'plague' had just been uttered for the first time.

A little later Rieux is presented with the mortality statistics by a clerk. 'We ought to make up our mind to call this disease by its name', Rieux says. 'Up to now we have just been shilly-shallying'. But Rieux cannot in fact bring himself to mention the name to the clerk. Not yet. For the analyses have not been completed – the laboratory has not yet spoken. Instead he turns to the clerk and says, 'But come with me. I must go to the laboratory.'

8

The laboratory as business

Sir Almroth Wright's vaccine programme and the construction of penicillin

WAI CHEN

The story of the discovery of penicillin is one of the classic discovery stories in the history of science. Its essence is simple: Alexander Fleming sees a culture plate with a patch of mould, around which bacteria have vanished. The presence of a new substance and its chief characteristic, that of killing bacteria, are evident with a single glance; it is as clear as if the spores were to stand up on the agar and say, 'I produce an antibiotic, you know.' The career of Alexander Fleming prior to this incident, and the fact that it happened in Sir Almroth Wright's laboratory at St Mary's Hospital, London in 1928, are circumstantial details in the story; it is essential to the existence of penicillin as an objective fact that it can be in principle observed by anybody anywhere. What the story describes is a process of discovering, of 'uncovering and revealing something which had been there all along'.[1]

Sociologists of science such as Gooding, Woolgar and Latour[2] have

Acknowledgements: I am grateful to the Editors for their time, energy, patience and encouragement. I am also grateful to Dr R. Iliffe and Dr T. Hochstrausser for their stimulating discussions. Finally, I would like to express my profound gratitude to my parents, without whose unfailing support none of this would have been possible.

[1] Steve Woolgar, *Science: The Very Idea* (Chichester, 1988), p. 55.

[2] David Gooding, '"In Nature's School": Faraday as an experimentalist' in David Gooding and Frank A. J. L. James (eds), *Faraday Rediscovered: Essays on the Life and Work of Michael Faraday, 1791–1867* (Basingstoke, 1985), pp. 105–35; Woolgar, *Science: The Very Idea*; S. W. Woolgar, 'Writing an intellectual history of scientific development: the use of discovery accounts', *Social Studies of Science*, 6 (1976), pp. 395–422; Bruno Latour, 'Give me a laboratory and I will raise the world' in Karin D. Knorr-Cetina and Michael Mulkay (eds), *Science Observed: Perspectives on the Social Study of Science* (London, 1983), pp. 141–70; Bruno Latour and Steve Woolgar, *Laboratory Life: The Construction of Scientific Facts*, 2nd edn (Princeton, 1986); Bruno Latour, *Science in Action: How to Follow Scientists and Engineers Through Society* (Milton Keynes, 1987). I have also derived important insights from Ludwik Fleck, *Genesis and Development of a Scientific Fact*, trans. Fred Bradley and Thaddeus J. Trenn (Chicago, 1979; first published in German, 1935).

pointed out that discovery stories of this kind only make sense once all the science has been done – when the controversy has ended, and agreement has been reached that the new object exists and what its properties are. Before that point, there is a complex social process in which the would-be discoverer assigns properties to the putative new object and tries to convince others of these claims. Only if this is successfully accomplished does this object become a scientific fact, its existence being projected back in time to allow one to speak of a discoverer. When this happens, all the work originally necessary to make the claim stand firm begins to be ignored; as Latour says, it is as if it is hidden inside a black box, so that only the certain characteristics are visible.[3] Of course, it is always possible that some new dissenter will reopen the black box and try to reconstruct its contents in a different form, just as Columbus's voyage of 1492, originally black-boxed as the discovery of a new route to India, was ten years later reboxed as the discovery of America.[4] The fact that such black boxes can be and are reopened is a powerful reason for describing the appearance of new objects not as discovery but as construction.

This chapter is about the construction of penicillin. Alexander Fleming's work has of course been much studied already, in particular by Ronald Hare and Gwyn Macfarlane;[5] yet even so, two major puzzles remain. First, although it is now clear that Fleming's penicillin work was a development of the work which he did on lysozyme, there is no explanation of why he did the original experiments which led to lysozyme's discovery (or rather, construction). The answer, I will be suggesting, lies in the nature of the laboratory where Fleming was working. Its foundation had been inspired by Sir Almroth Wright's belief in immunisation by means of vaccines, and the commercial production of vaccines was its chief source of funding. What I shall argue in the first section is that all the research undertaken by Wright's team on vaccines, bacteria, infectious diseases, and even that on antiseptics and defence mechanisms of the body, was related to the vaccine programme which provided the laboratory's financial sup-

3 Latour, *Science in Action*, pp. 2–3. See also Woolgar, *Science: The Very Idea*, pp. 39–41.

4 Augustine Brannigan, *The Social Basis of Scientific Discoveries* (Cambridge, 1981), pp. 120–9.

5 André Maurois, *The Life of Sir Alexander Fleming*, trans. Gerard Hopkins (London, 1959); Ronald Hare, *The Birth of Penicillin: And the Disarming of Microbes* (London, 1970); Ronald Hare, 'New light on the history of penicillin', *Medical History*, 26 (1982), pp. 1–24; Ronald Hare, 'The scientific activities of Alexander Fleming, other than the discovery of penicillin', *Medical History*, 27 (1983), 347–72. Gwyn Macfarlane, *Alexander Fleming: The Man and the Myth* (London, 1984).

port; what was not directly concerned with vaccine production was concerned with the extension of vaccine therapy or its defence against 'dissidents' (in Latour's terms): keeping the facts of vaccine therapy firm and its black boxes closed. In the second section, I will argue that Fleming's work on lysozyme and penicillin was also part of this vaccine programme.

The other puzzle still surrounding the story of penicillin is that neither Fleming nor anyone else at Wright's laboratory showed much interest in its therapeutic possibilities, so that it was not until fourteen years later that the use of penicillin as an antibiotic was first promoted by a quite different team of researchers at Oxford. Several historians have tried to explain this lack of interest by the poor results of the initial laboratory and therapeutic trials, yet even so, Macfarlane, the most recent, still finds it 'strange' that Fleming did not pursue such success as he had, and sees it as 'an opportunity let slip'.[6] My answer to this puzzle, in short, is that Fleming did not discover penicillin-the-antibiotic, in the same sense that Columbus did not discover America. More precisely, what I shall argue is that the identity which Fleming constructed for penicillin was not that of an antibiotic, but that of a weedkiller for bacterial farming. If this sounds rather a dull identity by comparison with the one with which we are familiar, that is because we no longer subscribe to Wright's vaccine programme. Within that laboratory, within the vaccine programme, penicillin's weedkiller identity was exciting and important, and it was the antibiotic identity which was dull and of low importance. In other words, rather than *failing* to realise the antibiotic potential of penicillin, within his own context Fleming *succeeded* in developing it into a vaccine laboratory agent. The construction of penicillin was not, as the classic discovery story implies, independent of place and person; it mattered very much that penicillin was a product of this particular laboratory, one dominated by the vaccine business.

[6] Macfarlane, *Fleming*, p. 140. See also, for example, pp. 128–30 and Hare, 'New light'.

I: ALMROTH WRIGHT'S LABORATORY AND THE VACCINE PROGRAMME

The Physician of the Future will be an Immunisator.[7]
(Almroth Wright)

The growth of Wright's laboratory

Fleming encountered penicillin while working in Sir Almroth Wright's laboratory at St Mary's Hospital. This was a self-financing laboratory single-handedly built up by Wright from a small poky room in the basement of the hospital to a grand enterprise occupying two storeys of a spacious modern building. The expansion of Wright's self-financing research empire was closely intertwined with the growing success of vaccines during this period, and was, moreover, dependent on the fortune he amassed from the sale of vaccines. Vaccines and their application in both the treatment and the prevention of disease was unquestionably Wright's most specialised and also most prized subject in medical science. Indeed, the efficacy of vaccines was the very 'scientific fact' that he sought to establish, uphold, promote, propagate and relentlessly defend in his research throughout his career.

Wright was born in 1861 in an Anglo-Irish family, his father being an evangelical vicar. In 1882, Wright graduated at Trinity College Dublin with first class honours and the Gold Medal, reading, surprisingly, English, French, German, Spanish and Italian literature. Even more surprisingly, he managed to read medicine at the same time and qualified as a doctor one year later. He then decided to pursue a career in the legal profession and promptly won a scholarship to read law. Later, his career orientation shifted yet again and he embarked on several research projects when travelling on the Continent and at Cambridge, working in many famous laboratories. After his marriage, he settled down in the Netley Army Hospital where he first invented the typhoid vaccine. But his invention was met with considerable opposition in the Army. His overbearing self-confidence marred the progress of his career within the Army. In 1902, he left when he accepted the chair in pathology and bacteriology in St Mary's Hospital, taking a considerable drop in salary. But in St Mary's, he

[7] A. E. Wright, *Studies on Immunisation: And Their Application to the Diagnosis and Treatment of Bacterial Infections* (London, 1909), title page. See also Leonard Colebrook, *Almroth Wright: Provocative Doctor and Thinker* (London, 1954), p. 47; Maurois, *Fleming*, p. 47; Macfarlane, *Fleming*, p. 58.

had a free rein: he founded his vaccine empire where he worked, and prospered; and he continued to dominate it for the rest of his life.[8]

When Wright arrived at St Mary's in 1902, his laboratory was merely a small room in the basement of the hospital. A year later, the board of governors was persuaded to give him two rooms on the second floor. Wright also persuaded them to give him £100 for equipment and another £100 for structural alterations.[9] At the beginning Wright had three assistants; he had expanded this to a team of ten around the time when Fleming joined the laboratory in 1907. In other words, within the short space of less than five years, Wright's laboratory expanded from one room in the basement to a laboratory with ten assistants.

In 1905, Lord Haldane, a friend of Wright's, became the War Minister in the Cabinet. At that time Haldane was engaged in a radical reform of the Territorial Army,[10] and he was attracted by Wright's advocacy of making anti-typhoid vaccination compulsory in the British Army. The conservative part of the Army medical establishment was dubious about Wright's typhoid vaccines and had previously barred and obstructed his proposal. At that time, the Victorian anti-vivisection and anti-vaccination campaign spirit was still running high.[11] Haldane decided to 'build up' Wright's reputation and credibility in order to promote anti-typhoid vaccination in the Army.[12] He wrote him a letter which, according to one of Wright's colleagues who saw it, went more or less as follows:

> Dear Wright, we must have your Typhoid Prophylactic for the Army, but I have failed to convince the head man in the Army Medical Service of this. I have therefore got to build you up as a Public Figure, and the first step is to make you a knight. You won't like it, but it has to be... Haldane.[13]

In 1906, Wright was knighted. In the same year, he was also elected a Fellow of the Royal Society.

Another very influential man whom Wright met around that time was Rupert Guinness, the son of the first Earl of Iveagh and the heir to the Guinness empire and the enormous Elveden estate. Rupert

[8] L. Colebrook, 'Almroth Edward Wright, 1861–1947', *Obituary Notices of Fellows of the Royal Society*, 6 (1948–9), pp. 297–314; Colebrook, *Wright*. See also Maurois, *Fleming*; Hare, 'Scientific activities'; and Macfarlane, *Fleming*.

[9] Colebrook, *Wright*, p. 173.

[10] Charles Harris, 'Lord Haldane at the War Office', *Public Administration*, 6 (1928), pp. 337–49; M. E. Howard, *Lord Haldane and the Territorial Army* (London, 1967).

[11] Dorothy Porter and Roy Porter, 'The politics of prevention: anti-vaccinationism and public health in nineteenth-century England', *Medical History*, 32 (1988), pp. 231–52; R. M. MacLeod, 'Law, medicine and public opinion: the resistance to compulsory health legislation 1870–1907', *Public Law* (1967), pp. 106–28 and 188–211.

[12] Colebrook, *Wright*, p. 40.

[13] Maurois, *Fleming*, p. 51.

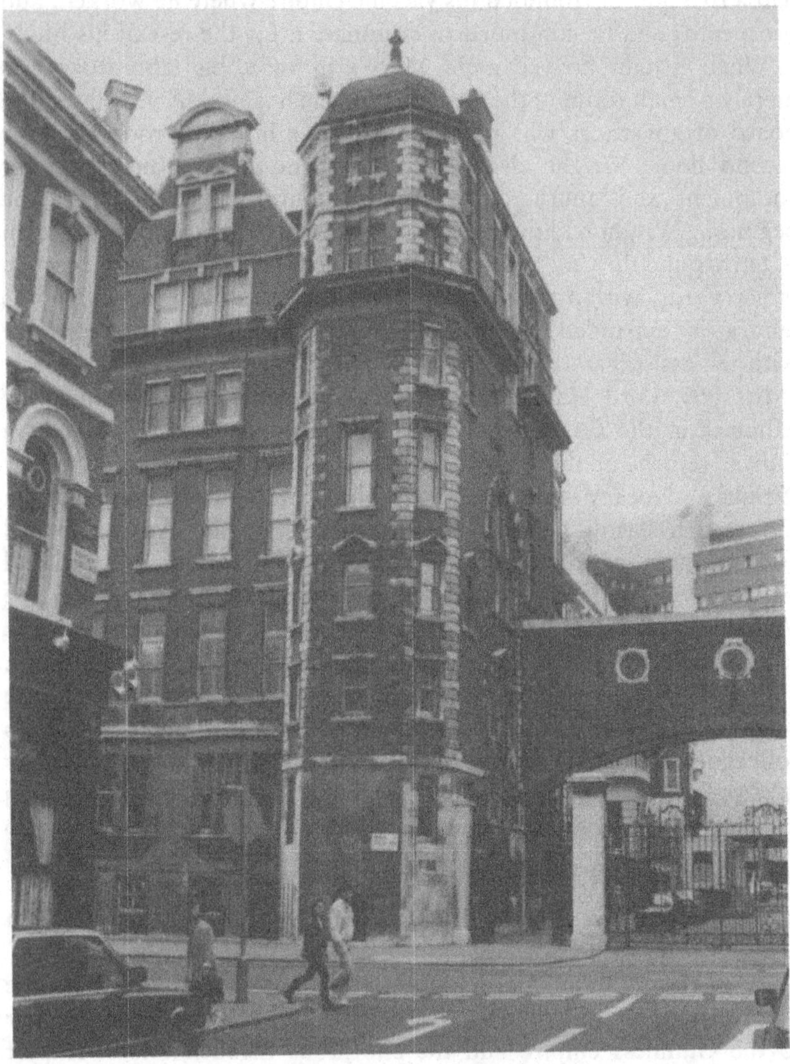

Fig. 13. Wright's Inoculation Unit, 1908–33, in St Mary's Hospital, Clarence Wing: the turret at the south-east corner.

Guinness went to consult Wright for a minor physical complaint, and they later became friends through their common interest in the prevention of typhoid infection. Guinness was already a well-known public figure who had persuaded his father to give £250,000 to the Lister Institute for research on preventive medicine. Like his father,

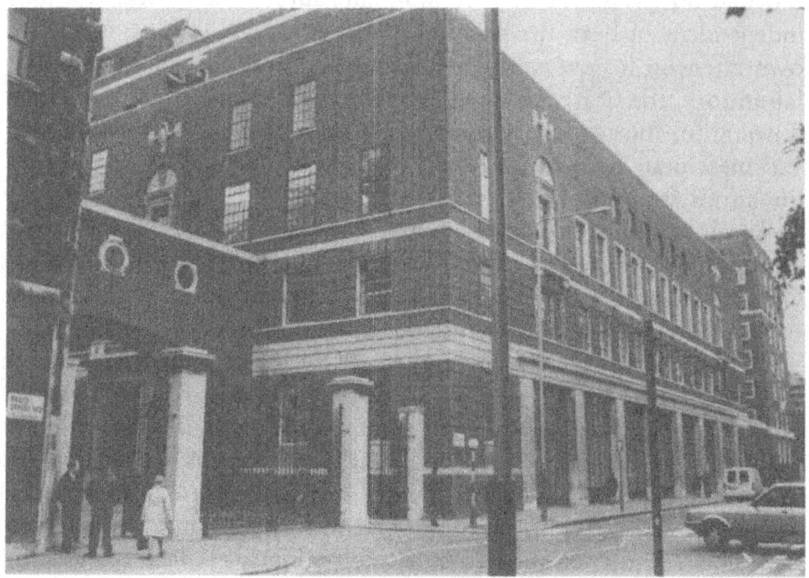

Fig. 14. Wright's Inoculation Unit from 1933, in the top two floors of the new building of St Mary's Hospital Medical School. The Inoculation Unit was the single largest donor towards the cost of the building, thanks to its great profits from the sale of vaccines.

Guinness was a great believer in the progress of science and also in applying science and technological advances in their family business, in industry as well as in medicine. During the Boer War, he went to South Africa to manage the Irish hospital which his father endowed for the war servicemen; and Guinness had become interested in typhoid when involved in helping soldiers wounded in the war. Around the time he met Wright, he was elected as a Conservative MP. With his powerful connections in society and in politics, Guinness became an influential recruiting force for Wright: he got together an impressive committee, under the chairmanship of Lord Arthur Balfour (Prime Minister 1902–5) to assist Wright and raise money.[14]

Through the help of Guinness, Wright got a complete new laboratory with in-patient wards – the first in-patient research wards attached to a laboratory in Britain. The St Mary's Hospital governors offered to accommodate the new laboratory in the Clarence Wing of the hospital (see Fig. 13). The new laboratory was named 'The

[14] H. D. Kay, 'Rupert Edward Cecil Lee Guinness, Second Earl of Iveagh, 1874–1967', *Biographical Memoirs of Fellows of the Royal Society*, 14 (1968), pp. 287–307; *Nature*, 175 (1955), pp. 975.

Inoculation Department'. It was an autonomous organisation, independent of both the hospital and the medical school: it had its own finances. It now paid ten full-time staff, the cost of running the laboratory, the Clarence Wing and its patients, and also a rent to the hospital for the accommodation. Its income derived from the sales of vaccines that it manufactured, fees from patients and private donations from informal patrons.[15]

Wright continued to maintain his close ties with the War Office. At the outbreak of the First World War, Wright knew that the Franco-German frontier was 'thickly sown with typhoid fever' and he went to Lord Kitchener to offer to turn the entire resources of his laboratory at St Mary's Hospital to the high-speed production of anti-typhoid vaccine.[16] The total quantity of vaccines produced in Wright's laboratory by October 1914 for the British Forces was as much as 2,000 gallons. The sum paid by the War Office for this was, of course, never divulged, but has been estimated by Ronald Hare (a member of Wright's team and a historian of penicillin) to have been as much as £500,000.[17] Later Wright also undertook military medical research in France during the First World War.

Apart from maintaining its existence, the financial strength of the laboratory was important in defining its relation to the medical school of St Mary's during the 1920s, when the school's new Dean, Dr Charles McMoran Wilson (later Lord Moran and physician to Winston Churchill), was trying to build up the school. The grandest part of Wilson's programme was the construction of a modern five-storey building. The cost of this was £160,000, which Wilson raised with the help of his millionaire friends and wealthy patients. But Wright himself raised the staggering sum of £105,000 just in order to furnish his unit on the top two floors of this building. There he was to acquire some twenty-seven laboratories, a lecture theatre, a library and access to an adequate out-patient department (see Fig. 14). The unit now employed seven doctors and fifteen technicians, and it paid scholarships to visiting research workers and graduates who wanted to do research. Of that £105,000, £40,000 came from Rupert Guinness (now Lord Iveagh), and £22,000 from other private donations (including Wright's own money). But the largest sum, £43,000 – a considerable sum of money in 1929 – came from the surplus of the laboratory in Clarence Wing![18]

[15] Macfarlane, *Fleming*, p. 65.
[16] Colebrook, *Wright*, p. 41.
[17] Hare, 'Scientific activities', p. 349.
[18] Colebrook, *Wright*, p. 173; Macfarlane, *Fleming*, p. 146.

Thus a main source of this fund was the profit derived from the sale of vaccines. These vaccines were manufactured in Wright's laboratory and were then distributed for sale through Parke, Davis and Company, a large and well-known pharmaceutical firm. In other words, Wright's laboratory was a vaccine factory – and a highly profitable one too. Or more correctly, the vaccine industry was central to the existence of Wright's laboratory. Because of its autonomous self-financing status and its dependence on the sale of vaccines as its main source of income, there was a strong interest in Wright's laboratory to maintain, if not to actively promote, the use of vaccine in medicine. If the sale of the vaccine went down, the income of the laboratory fell and the existence of the laboratory and its research activities became threatened.

The principles of the vaccine programme

It is necessary to stress the specific claims about vaccines made by Wright's laboratory. Wright believed that vaccines could be used not only to prevent but to cure infectious diseases. This may appear very strange to a modern reader. A vaccine nowadays usually means a kind of injection or oral preparation which is given to a person before contracting a particular disease; having been vaccinated prevents the person from contracting the disease when he or she later becomes exposed to it. This is known as prophylactic vaccination. But in the days of Wright's laboratory, vaccines were believed to have a further important function. Apart from being a form of prevention (as in prophylaxis), vaccines were thought to be a form of therapy, i.e. they cured the disease *after* the person had contracted it.

This belief was inspired by Pasteur's development of a rabies vaccine that could be given to a patient after he had been bitten by a rabid animal, and which had been shown to be effective. This led Wright to postulate that vaccine in general could be given after the patient had contracted a disease and could still stimulate the defence mechanism of the body to combat the disease and hence accelerate recovery. He believed that this applied to all transmittable diseases rather than just particular ones like rabies. For instance, if a patient suffered from boils, Wright believed that the patient could be cured by an inoculation with the same bacteria which caused them, once killed. The theory behind this was that the patient's defence mechanism was sensitised by the killed bacteria of the vaccine to fight the live ones more effectively; and hence vaccine made of killed bacteria could cure

ii. *Advertisements.*

VACCINES

for Respiratory Infections

PROPHYLACTIC inoculation against the common "cold," influenza and catarrhal conditions of the respiratory tract generally, has given a high degree of immunity in a large number of cases.

¶ The micro-organisms most commonly found in patients suffering from "colds" are Pneumococcus, Pfeiffer's Bacillus, Micrococcus catarrhalis and Bacillus septus and these are included in the **Anti-Catarrh Vaccine** prepared in the Department for Therapeutic Inoculation, St. Mary's Hospital, London, W, especially for the prophylaxis of colds in adults.

A slightly modified formula is supplied under the title **Anti-Catarrh (Public Schools) Vaccine.**

¶ Vaccine treatment of respiratory infections often helps to abort an attack. **Cold Vaccine (Mixed)** is specially prepared for therapeutic use in connexion with common "colds" and bronchitis. It is suitable for routine use, as its composition has been chosen so as to avoid the necessity of a bacteriological examination.

¶ It is generally agreed that the serious and sometimes fatal complications of influenza—such as bronchitis and pneumonia—as well as many of the less severe symptoms, are caused by infection with Pfeiffer's Bacillus, Pneumococcus and Streptococcus. On this account the **Anti-Influenza Vaccine (Mixed)**, *St. Mary's Hospital Formula,* which contains these three organisms is of great value as a prophylactic of influenza.

Further particulars of these and other Vaccines prepared in the Department for Therapeutic Inoculation, St. Mary's Hospital, London, W, will be sent on request.

SOLE AGENTS:

PARKE, DAVIS & COMPANY

50 Beak St., London, W.1.

Inc. U.S.A., Liability Ltd. Laboratories: Hounslow, Middlesex.

Fig. 15. Advertisement for vaccines, from the September 1930 issue of the *Proceedings of the Royal Society of Medicine*. Note the promotion of a (prophylactic) anti-influenza vaccine, made from Pfeiffer's bacillus (*B. influenzae*) amongst other bacteria.

boils. Many of the vaccines manufactured in Wright's laboratory were of this therapeutic type. There were special vaccines for pyorrhoea, boils, pneumonia, bronchial colds, influenza, gonorrhoea, sore throats, intestinal troubles, tuberculosis and even cancer.[19] There were also 'Anti-catarrh vaccine' and 'Anti-catarrh (Public Schools) vaccine' – the difference between them (apart from their packaging and price) was said to be only in their strength.[20] Alexander Fleming himself developed a vaccine for acne, a 25 cc bottle of which retailed for £1 5s in 1914[21] – a reminder of just how profitable the vaccine business could be (see Figs. 15 and 16).

This development of a new vaccine for the treatment of acne is a good example for showing in detail the practical procedures involved in some of the daily activities of Wright's laboratory. Let us reconstruct what Fleming did, using primarily a paper which he published in the *Lancet* in 1909, supplemented by an account given at the Royal Society of Medicine, in which Fleming used his success in acne vaccine treatment to defend Wright's vaccine therapy programme.[22] The aim of his *Lancet* paper was to show that therapeutic vaccines were only effective if one used the correct vaccine. For Fleming, a correct vaccine was the one that contained the specific bacteria which cause that particular pathological condition. He drew this conclusion from his experience in treating acne with vaccines. The standard therapeutic vaccine used for treating acne contained killed staphylococci. Many doctors had been getting poor results in treating acne with this vaccine, and thus had become despondent about vaccines and expressed doubts about the efficacy of vaccine therapy in general. To combat dissidents and critics of vaccines, Fleming was now claiming that their poor results were due to the fact they had been using the wrong vaccine: acne, according to Fleming, had been shown to be caused by acne bacilli, rather than staphylococci, and the new treatment with vaccine containing killed acne bacilli produced startlingly effective results. Therefore, according to Fleming, vaccine therapy was effective, provided that one used the correct vaccine made from the correct bacterium. However, this could only be done by someone who had special knowledge of bacteriology, who could accurately identify the true infective agents and who could

[19] Macfarlane, *Fleming*, p. 66.

[20] W. C. Noble, *Coli: Great Healer of Men: The Biography of Dr Leonard Colebrook FRS* (London, 1974), p. 21.

[21] Hare, 'Scientific activities', p. 349.

[22] Alexander Fleming, 'On the etiology of acne vulgaris and its treatment by vaccines', *Lancet* (1909, 1), pp. 1035–8; Discussion on vaccine therapy, *Proceedings of the Royal Society of Medicine*, 3 (1910), General Reports Section, pp. 137–8.

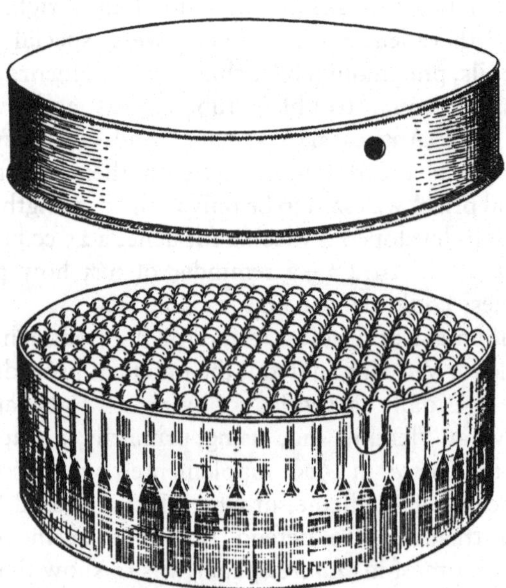

Fig. 16. Large-scale production of vaccines in Wright's laboratory: method of filling a batch of vaccine bulbs simultaneously. 'We have here a batch of vaccine bulbs packed closely together into a glass dish, which is provided with a valvular lateral opening, which can be opened and closed by turning round the cover. The vaccine bulbs are turned upside down, and their ends are, as will be seen, open... We turn the lid round, so as to open up the inlet, and introduce through this sufficient vaccine to provide for each bulb the quantum allotted to it... The filling is done by placing the dish under the bell of an air-pump and exhausting the air, and then re-admitting it.' (Wright, *Handbook of the Technique of the Teat and Capillary Glass Tube*, pp. 192–3.)

produce a specific vaccine made from these agents for his patients.[23] In other words, Wright's laboratory was the only laboratory in London where vaccine therapy was administered correctly and effectively. And patients who sought therapy should detour through Wright's laboratory – just as farmers had been persuaded to detour through Pasteur's laboratory to combat anthrax.[24]

How did Fleming undertake the construction of this new acne vaccine? He took regular swabs from the pustules of his patients. He examined the morphology of the bacteria under the microscope; and he attempted to classify them and correlate their presence with the

[23] Fleming, 'Etiology of acne vulgaris'.

[24] '"If you wish to solve your anthrax problem, come to my laboratory... If you don't... you will be eliminated."' Latour, 'Give me a laboratory', p. 147.

acne lesions.[25] In this instance, Fleming found a particular bacterium in his patients' pustules and he believed that this bacterium was the true cause of acne. He then experimented on how to grow it in an artificial medium. This was a laborious and painstaking process, since acne bacilli did not grow readily in routine bacteriological media under standard conditions. Furthermore, contaminant bacteria tended to outgrow the fastidious and delicate acne bacilli. In order to obtain a pure culture, Fleming first had to find a special culture medium, the proper temperature and special procedures to separate the contaminant bacteria.

He found that the skin had to be sterilised in a special way to separate contaminants: wiping it over with pure lysol and washing this off quickly with spirit. The acne pustules had to be freshly pricked. The content from the pustule had to be transferred onto a culture medium with a sterilised loop and had to be planted *in masse*, because 'if the pus be spread thinly over the surface of the medium, no growth of the bacillus will be obtained'. Furthermore, the incubation temperature was found to be crucial: the bacillus had to be incubated at 37 °C. At lower or higher temperatures, growth ceased. Finally, amongst all culture media, Fleming found that oleic acid glycerine agar produced the best yield, and he believed that was because its constituents resembled the fatty secretions of the sebaceous glands and mimicked the environment within an acne pustule.[26] After having acquired a pure culture, he farmed these bacilli to produce a sufficiently large quantity to make a vaccine. The harvested bacilli were then killed by heat and acid, and a standardised quantity of the microbes was introduced into a dose of vaccine. Fleming inoculated his patients with the new vaccines in a clinical trial and monitored their progress.

Fleming's work on acne was typical of the procedure for the production of bacterial vaccines in Wright's laboratory. However, the range of vaccines which the laboratory produced extended beyond bacterial ones. For instance, a famous set of vaccines, allergy vaccines, was created in the laboratory by John Freeman, who claimed that

[25] The criteria Fleming used to identify the bacterium were as follows: '1. It is constantly present in the pus as shown by examination of films. 2. It is frequently the only organism present in pus. 3. It can frequently be recovered from the pus in pure culture. 4. Inoculated into the skin of a susceptible individual it produces a pustular folliculitis and examination of the pus shows no other organism to be present. 5. Inoculated into animals it produces an abscess at the seat of inoculation ...'. Fleming, 'Etiology of acne vulgaris', p. 1037. These are modified versions of 'Koch's postulates', on which see Thomas D. Brock, *Robert Koch: A Life in Medicine and Bacteriology* (Madison, Wis., 1988), pp. 179–82.

[26] Fleming, 'Etiology of acne vulgaris', pp. 1035–6.

ii. *Advertisements.*

IMMUNISATION AGAINST HAY FEVER

THE DEPARTMENT FOR THERAPEUTIC INOCULATION, ST. MARY'S HOSPITAL, LONDON (Director : Sir Almroth E. Wright, M.D., F.R.S., &c.), prepares for supply to the Medical Profession, through the Agency of Messrs. PARKE, DAVIS & Co.,

"POLLACCINE"

(Pollen Vaccine for Hay Fever)

to be administered subcutaneously for the production of immunity to pollen toxin,

BOTH AS A PROPHYLACTIC AND CURATIVE OF HAY FEVER.

N.B.—"Pollaccine" is polyvalent for all the grains and grasses, and it is the pollen from the gramineæ which causes hay fever, in England, at any rate. In very severe cases, prophylactic treatment should be commenced in the early winter ; in milder ones, later in the winter, or even in spring, may suffice.

A HAY FEVER REACTION OUTFIT

is also supplied, which affords a means of determining (*a*) whether a patient is susceptible to pollen toxin ; (*b*) the degree of such susceptibility ; (*c*) the dosage of "Pollaccine" suited to any case.

Further particulars will be supplied on request by

PARKE, DAVIS & CO.,

50-54 Beak Street, Regent Street, London, W.I.

Fig. 17. Advertisement for hay fever vaccine, from the February 1925 issue of the *Proceedings of the Royal Society of Medicine*.

patients with allergy could be cured by immunisation with the very substance to which they were allergic. His insight was inspired by a lecture, given by a Dutch allergist, Storm van Leeuwen, in St Thomas's Hospital.[27] Van Leeuwen believed that asthma was precipitated by an allergy to moulds growing in the foundations and floorboards of houses. When Freeman returned to the laboratory he discussed with Wright his idea of immunising patients with mould vaccines. Wright was so impressed with the idea that he supported Freeman by employing a full-time mycologist (mould expert) in the laboratory: C. J. La Touche. Freeman's allergy patients were encouraged to bring in moulds from their homes; these would be farmed in the laboratory and extracts prepared from them would be made into vaccines for desensitisation, in the same manner that bacteria were farmed to produce vaccine. Apart from mould vaccine, Freeman also produced pollen vaccine for hay fever – a vaccine that was frequently advertised in contemporary medical journals (see Fig. 17).

The principles of prophylactic and therapeutic vaccination thus resulted in a wide range of activities. Bacteria farming, the study and understanding of bacteria, clinical therapy, large-scale synthesis, and advertising: all these activities were necessary for the development and commercial production of vaccines and for the extension of vaccine therapy to new areas. Nevertheless the vaccine programme had ramifications beyond these. As we will now see, a further set of activities were required to defend the principles of the vaccine programme whenever it came under attack.

Ramifications of the vaccine programme

Despite being the basis of a flourishing industry, Wright's vaccines were not universally acclaimed. There were dissidents and critics from both the old and the new quarters of the medical profession. An old-fashioned physician, Kingston Fowler, was prompted in 1910 to mount an onslaught against Wright's therapeutic vaccines, saying:

> Vaccines have been used for a long time in my wards at the Middlesex Hospital ... but if I were pressed to produce from my personal experience the evidence upon which my belief in their value is founded, I fear I should be unable to do so ... to-day patients may be roughly divided into those who are swallowing the Bulgarian bacillus, or rather who think they are, and those who are being injected with a vaccine – a fact highly flattering to Professor Metchnikoff and Sir Almroth Wright, but not marking a great advance in the scientific spirit of the profession ... I should like to take this opportunity of airing a belief to which I have often given utterance in teaching – viz.

[27] Hare, *Birth of Penicillin*, p. 83.

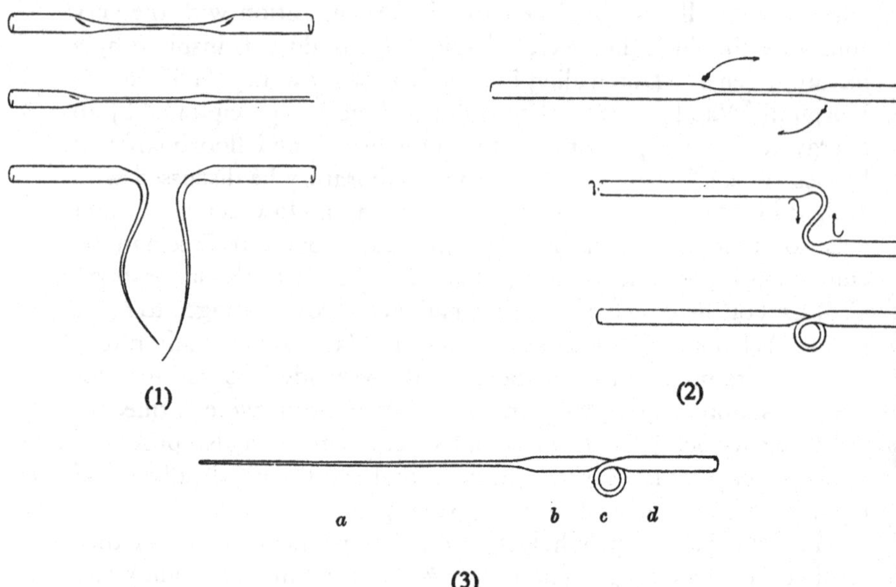

Fig. 18. Illustrations from Wright's *Handbook of the Technique of the Teat and Capillary Glass Tube*, showing techniques of glass-working. (1) shows three types of fault which may arise if the tube is not drawn out properly; (2) shows how to create a loop in a capillary stem; and (3) shows a typical product of this technique: a looped pipette suitable for measuring the bactericidal power of the blood. Here (a) is the capillary stem, where the fluids are measured and mixed; (b) is the chamber, which can be used as a reservoir for nutrient and as a cultivation chamber; (c) is the loop which acts as a trap for airborne microbes; and (d) is the handle, to which a rubber teat may be fitted.

that the difficulty in estimating the value of a new remedy is greatly exaggerated, and that when a drug has been in use for a definite purpose for several years, and opinion is still unsettled as to its value, it is usually because it has none... The history of medicine in... recent times, however, appears to prove that the tendency to exploit for selfish purposes each new discovery in therapeutics, and to recommend it as a panacea for almost every ailment of mankind, is ineradicable from the minds of the weaker brethren.[28]

It was imperative for the fortune of Wright's laboratory that such critics and dissidents be countered. For this reason, the work of the laboratory included not only the routine production of vaccines, the development of the technology of bacterial farming and the identification of bacteriological causes of known diseases for the production of new vaccines, but also a varied series of researches into immune

[28] Discussion on vaccine therapy, *Proceedings of the Royal Society of Medicine*, 3 (1910), General Reports Section, pp. 108–9.

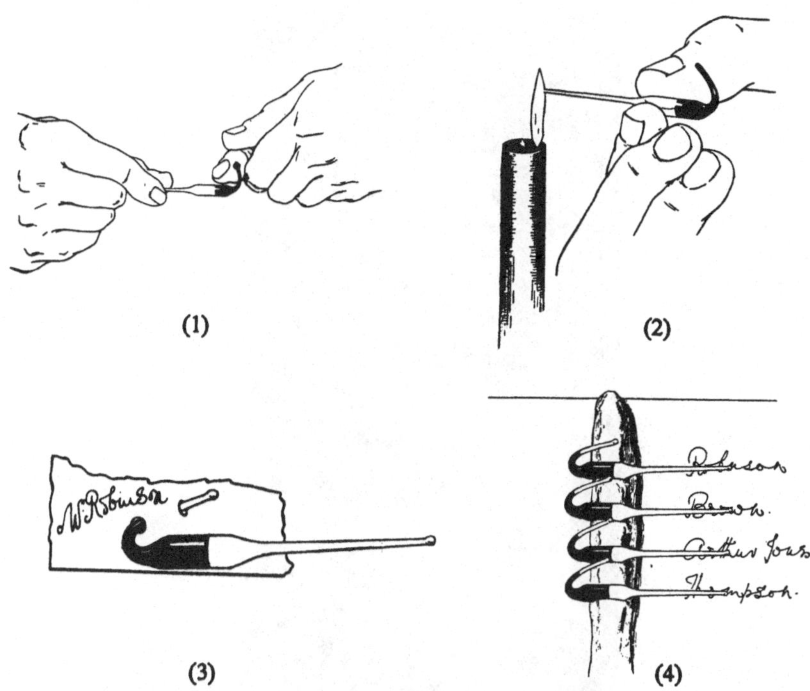

Fig. 19. Illustrations from Wright's *Handbook of the Technique of the Teat and Capillary Glass Tube* showing (1) the correct way to take a blood sample, (2) the correct way to seal a blood capsule, and (3) how to avoid confusion, by attaching a label to a blood capsule or (4) mounting the capsules in a roll of Plasticine.

physiology. Certain research projects were selected, emphasised and brought to full fruition with the construction of immuno-physiological facts which could answer critics and substantiate the claims to efficacy of particular vaccines or vaccine therapy as a whole.

To demonstrate how Wright constructed 'scientific facts' in order to promote his interests, we can look at his use of the physiological phenomenon of agglutination (i.e. clumping together) of typhoid bacilli as a blood test to demonstrate the efficacy of his famous typhoid vaccine. Around the turn of the century, Ehrlich had demonstrated that the body produced a substance to neutralise foreign protein in the blood – a substance later referred to as 'antibodies' or 'agglutinins'. Pfeiffer then showed that the body neutralised and inactivated the microbes of typhoid and cholera by producing agglutinins. Wright devised a special laboratory technique to make the agglutination phenomenon easily and reliably visible, and

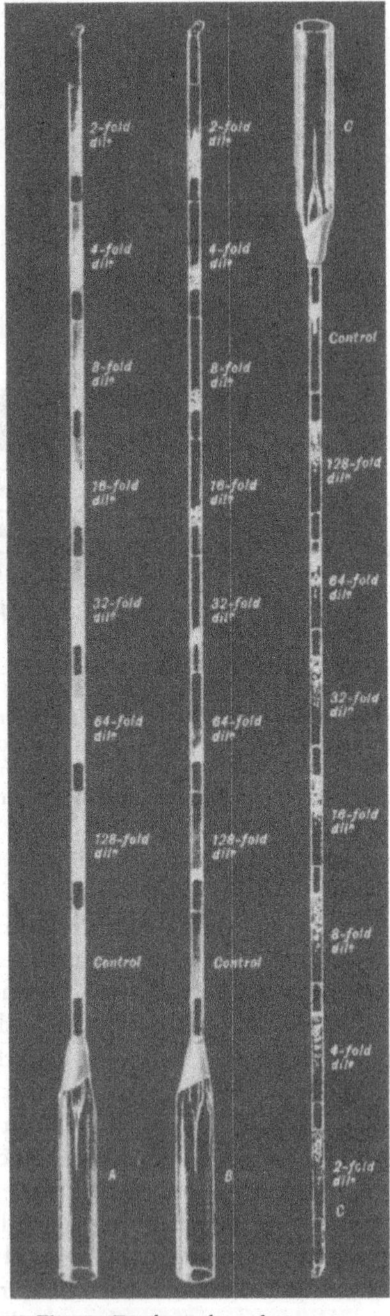

Fig 20. For legend see facing page.

to make it visible in other laboratories he described the procedure in detail in his *Handbook of the Technique of the Teat and Capillary Glass Tube*.[29] It was his pioneering use of capillary pipettes, fitted with rubber teats, which made it possible to test for agglutination with just a single drop of blood, and the early chapters of the *Handbook* explained precisely how to construct various kinds of pipette out of standard glass tubes. The meticulous detail and the many illustrations (see Figs. 18–21) were essential in order to make the test simple to carry out and the effect of agglutination easy to observe and to reproduce with minimal risk of failure – a 'black box' in Latour's terminology. This work on immuno-physiology and the publication of a book on laboratory techniques were not undertaken in the pure disinterested pursuit of knowledge. When Wright invented his anti-typhoid vaccine, it was the agglutination test which he used to show how his vaccine was effective: his anti-typhoid vaccine could convert an individual's blood from the deficient state (i.e. without the agglutinins specific to typhoid) to an immune state (i.e. with the presence of large quantities of agglutinins, thus showing the bactericidal power of the blood). This effect could be made visible with glass pipettes in all other laboratories. In other words, by seeking to make the perfected experimental procedure and apparatus accessible to as many people as possible, Wright was seeking to win allies and convince people of the efficacy of his typhoid vaccines – the vaccines which brought him his knighthood, his Fellowship of the Royal Society, his vaccine laboratory and factory in St Mary's, the patronage of Rupert Guinness, and his extensive profits during the war (see Fig. 22).

But when Wright wanted to extend this test to prove the efficacy of vaccine in other infections, such as those caused by streptococci and staphylococci, the agglutination test did not work: there was no

[29] A. E. Wright, *Handbook of the Technique of the Teat and Capillary Glass Tube: And its Applications in Medicine and Bacteriology* (London, 1912).

Fig. 20. The agglutination test. The figure shows 'throttled pipettes filled in each case with a series of mixtures consisting of one unit volume of a suspension of typhoid bacilli mixed with progressively increasing dilutions of serum derived from a typhoid patient... In *A* are shown the phenomena of agglutination as seen very shortly after the tube has been filled in. *B* shows the agglutination and sedimentation effect after an interval of 24 hours... *C* shows the effect of turning the tube upside down. In the control mixture there is here obtained a very fine rain of separate bacterial elements; in the test mixture a hail of agglutinated bacterial masses.' (Wright, *Handbook of the Technique of the Teat and Capillary Glass Tube*, frontispiece.)

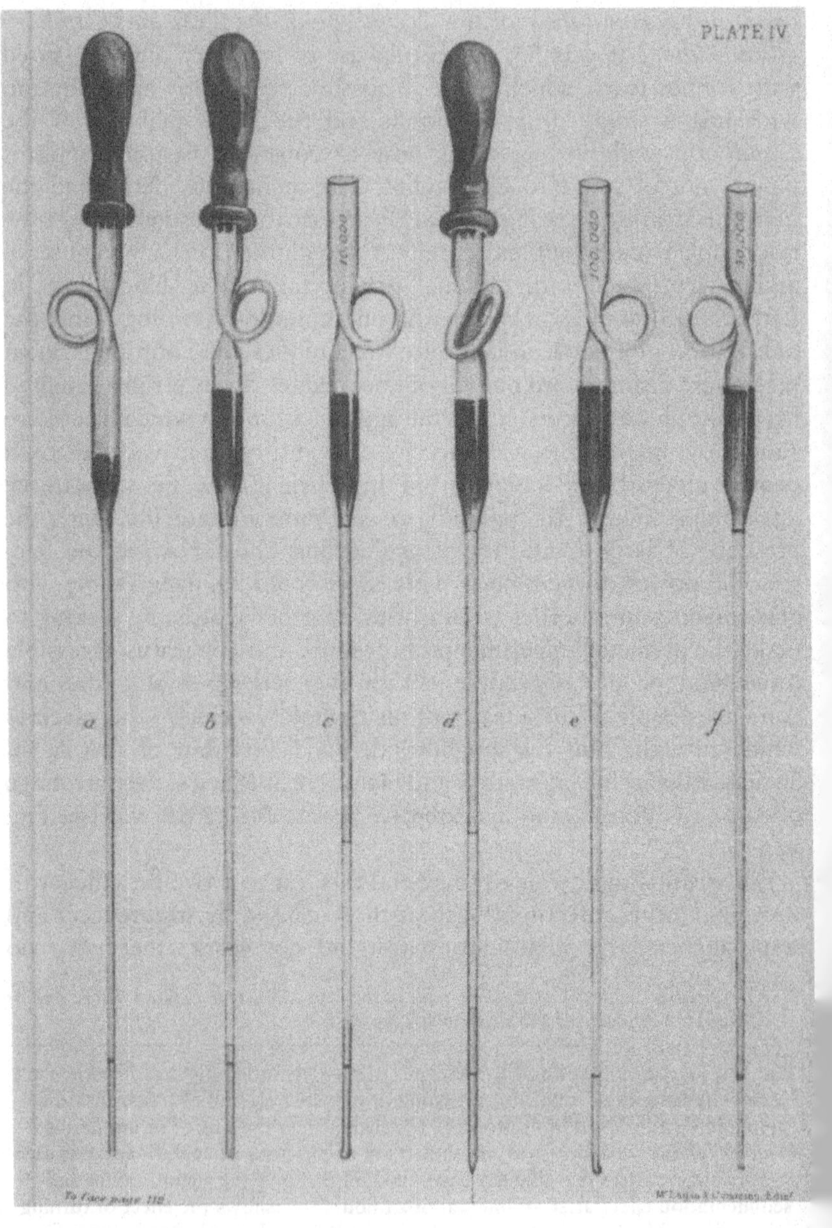

Fig. 21. For legend see facing page.

clumping effect on these bacteria after vaccination or in patients recovered from such infection. At that time, Metchnikoff at the Pasteur Institute observed that white blood cells killed bacteria by engulfing them (phagocytosis). Wright later demonstrated that their ability to do so was dependent on the presence of a substance which he called 'opsonin' in the patients' serum. Opsonin coated the surface of the bacteria and increased the ability of the white blood cells to engulf it; as the character based on Wright puts it in Bernard Shaw's play *The Doctor's Dilemma*, white blood cells only eat bacteria when they are buttered with opsonins.[30] Wright demonstrated that 'opsonisation' had this role in the killing of bacteria in a large number of infections. This 'opsonisation' theory had a certain function for Wright: it enabled him to devise a laboratory test for his other vaccines – those that could not be proven by the agglutination test. If such a test could be black-boxed, it could prove the efficacy of his other vaccines, just as the agglutination test had proven the efficacy of his typhoid vaccine in the past.

'Opsonic index' was an expression invented by Wright to demonstrate *in vitro* a change in the status of the patient's defence mechanism. It was a mathematical ratio, denoting the presence of

[30] Bernard Shaw, *The Doctor's Dilemma* (Harmondsworth, 1979), p. 98: 'Sir Patrick: Aye, phagocytes [white blood cells]: yes, yes, yes. Well, I heard this theory that the phagocytes eat up the disease germs years ago: long before you came into fashion. Besides they don't always eat them. Ridgeon: They do when you butter them with opsonin.' Wright coined the term from the Latin 'opsono' (I prepare for table, I render palatable), *Handbook of Technique*, pp. 122–3. On opsonins and vaccine therapy in general, see Peter Keating, 'Vaccine therapy and the problem of opsonins', *Journal of the History of Medicine*, 43 (1988), 275–96.

Fig. 21. Measuring the bactericidal power of the blood. (a) 'Looped pipette which is being filled in with litmus mannite broth.' (b) 'The nutrient fluid has been carried up into the cultivation chamber and one unit volume of serum and one unit volume of a dilution of the typhoid culture have been measured into the stem of the pipette.' (c) 'The serum and the dilution of the typhoid culture have been mixed and blown out, and have now been reaspirated into the stem, and the end of this has been sealed in the flame.' (d) 'After 24 hours in the incubator the test-mixture is being drawn up into the incubation chamber. To this end the capillary stem has been throttled, and the teat has been reimposed on the mouthpiece of the pipette in the collapsed condition.' In (e) and (f), 'the pipettes have been returned to the incubator for 24 hours'. In (e), 'the litmus mannite broth has remained clear and unchanged in colour', showing that in this particular dilution of the culture the bacilli have been completely killed off. In (f), with a lesser dilution, the bacilli have not all been killed off, as evidenced by a change in colour (more evident in the original colour illustration); typhoid bacilli produce acid when grown in litmus mannite broth, hence changing the colour of the litmus. (Wright, *Handbook of the Technique of the Teat and Capillary Glass Tube*, p. 112.)

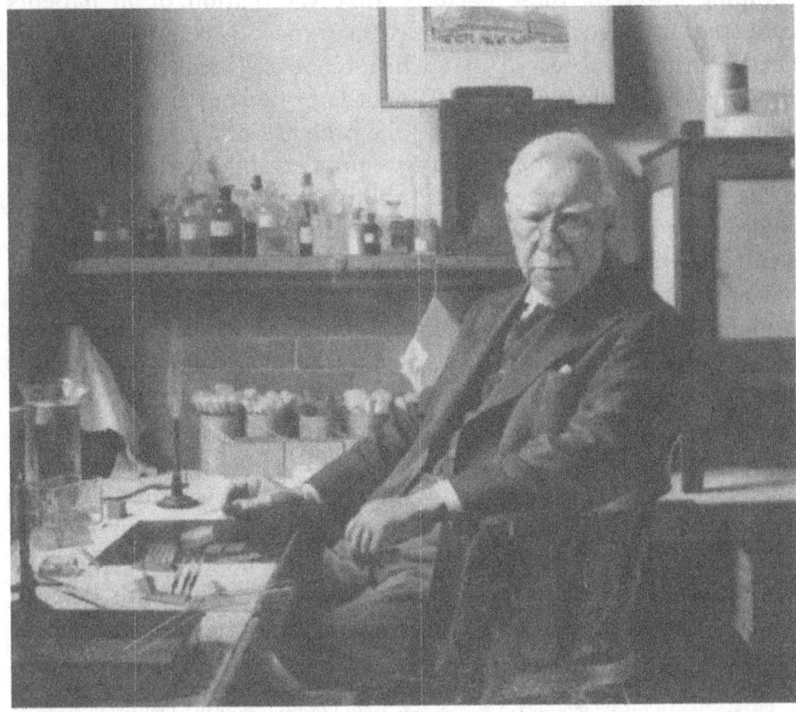

Fig. 22. Portrait of Sir Almroth Wright by Sir Gerald Kelly R.A., now in the Library of the Inoculation Unit, St Mary's Hospital. Notice how Wright's characteristic equipment functions as his emblem: he is depicted with a pipette in his right hand, with glass slides and blood capsules (mounted in Plasticine) in front of him. Compare this picture with the illustration of the apparatus for measurement of the opsonic index (Fig. 23). The picture on the wall shows his Inoculation Unit in its grand new location from 1933; see Fig. 14.

specific opsonins which enhanced the ability of white blood cells to kill specific bacteria. Wright claimed that a patient who suffered from a particular infection had an abnormally low opsonic index with respect to that particular bacterium: his white blood cells were less efficient in killing that bacterium. If a therapeutic vaccine was given to this patient, the immune system became stimulated to produce opsonin. Wright claimed that with the enhanced production of opsonin, as shown by an increased opsonic index, the patient could then fight his infection more effectively. Thus the opsonic index provided a way of demonstrating how well the administration of therapeutic vaccines promoted the body's self-defence mechanism.

The technique for measuring an 'opsonic index' was also described in Wright's *Handbook* (see Figs. 23 and 24), but it proved to be a more difficult black box to close than the 'agglutination test'. Another set of workers, represented by Kjer-Peterson and also by Shattock and Dudgeon, did not believe Wright's claims.[31] They thought that the apparent changes of opsonic indices were due to random variation, and that if statistical tests were applied to these results, the observed differences would fall into the standard deviations around the norm, making these differences totally insignificant. Therefore, opsonins did not exist and vaccine therapies were ineffective. There were great amounts of research work, experiments and publications from Wright's laboratory to counter-claim against the dissident camp. Even Fleming, who had then just joined Wright, published a joint paper with Noon in 1908 to defend the validity of vaccine therapy in general and opsonic indices in particular.[32] Around the same time, Fleming also defended the opsonic index in his own paper on acne. Acne was a convenient clinical condition to use because the lesions were always superficial – marks on the skin that could be easily and directly observed – so that the clinical progress of this condition could easily be assessed. In his paper, Fleming juxtaposed a graph of the change in his patients' opsonic index with anecdotal descriptions of his patients' progress. The text related how severe acne completely resolved after treatment with his new acne vaccine – a vaccine made from acne bacilli, the 'correct' causal pathogen. The graph showed how after vaccine therapy the opsonic index rose dramatically from its previous deficient state.

On the surface, the debate over opsonic indices was one of academic technicalities in immunology. However, taking it in the opsonist context of Wright's vaccine programme and his vaccine factory, it had a more important connotation: the opsonic index was the only 'scientific fact' that could prove in a laboratory the efficacy of many of his therapeutic vaccines, and thus this debate directly impinged upon the laboratory's vested interest in vaccines. If a patient's blood could be shown, in a laboratory, to be defective in opsonin before the vaccination, and it could be shown to become high in opsonins and hence super-effective in killing bacteria after vaccination, then the efficacy of the vaccine was established as a 'scientific fact'. If the efficacy of the vaccines was a 'fact', then the sale

[31] Colebrook, *Wright*, p. 58.

[32] L. Noon and Alexander Fleming, 'The accuracy of opsonic estimations', *Lancet* (1908, 1), pp. 1203–4. See also Alexander Fleming, 'Some observations on the opsonic index, with special reference to the accuracy of the method, and to some of the sources of error', *The Practitioner*, 80 (1908), pp. 607–34.

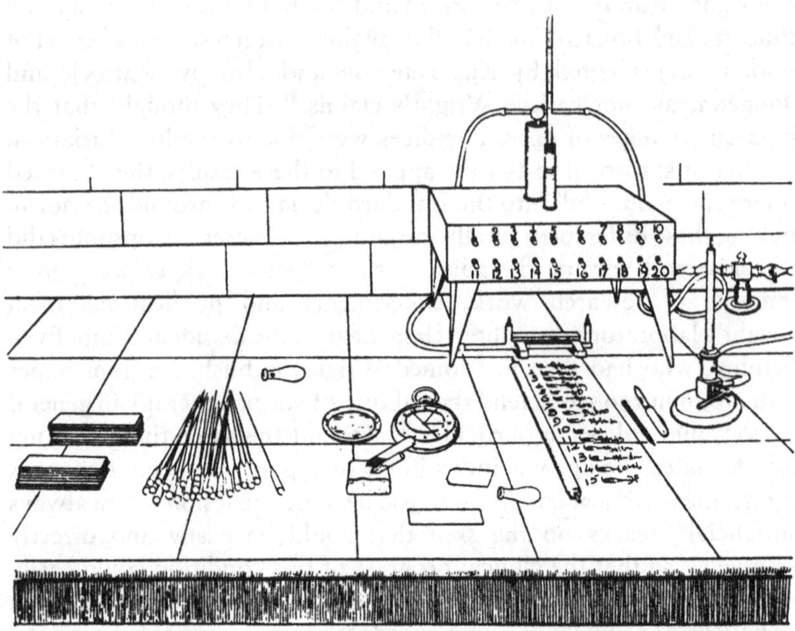

Fig. 23. Apparatus for measurement of the opsonic index. To the left are capillary pipettes and glass slides. At the rear is the 'opsoniser', or opsonic incubator, in front of which are the blood capsules (numbered) and a long roll of Plasticine for securing them in sequence once opened. A tube of washed leucocytes and a tube containing a bacterial suspension are mounted at an angle in another block of Plasticine.

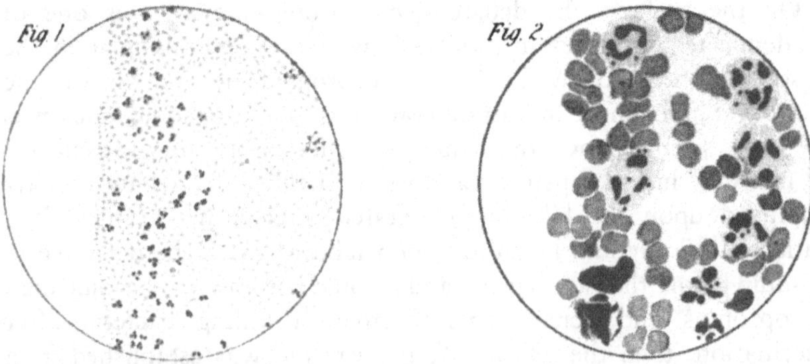

Fig. 24. Microscopic observations for measurement of the opsonic index. (1) 'The edge of an opsonic film (under a comparatively low power), showing the leucocytes gathered to the end.' (2) 'A portion of the edge of an opsonic film (under a high power), showing phagocytosis of the staphylococci.' The technique involved estimating the average number of bacteria ingested by each leucocyte. (Wright, *Handbook of the Technique of the Teat and the Capillary Glass Tube*, plate 5, following p. 152.)

of vaccine would be guaranteed, and the destiny of the laboratory secure. Much of the effort of the laboratory thus went into defending the efficacy of the opsonic index.

The vaccine programme and the attack on antiseptics

Other works published by Wright's team, although seemingly unrelated to vaccines, in fact served the same function of supporting vaccine therapy. During the First World War, Wright's team produced a large number of articles attacking the treatment of war wounds with antiseptics.[33] War wound infection was a very important condition during the First World War, as it was one of the biggest killers of many otherwise young and healthy soldiers. Opinions were then sharply divided between the military surgeons and Wright's research team in Boulogne. For the surgeons, the standard treatment for war wounds at that time was with local application of antiseptic solution, whereas the Wright team claimed that antiseptics impeded the immune response within war wounds, rendering infection rampant and causing fatal septicaemia.

The surgeons' practice was based on the belief that antiseptic solution killed harmful bacteria lodged in the wound and hence could

[33] Alexander Fleming, 'Some notes on the bacteriology of gas gangrene', *Lancet* (1915, 2), pp. 376–7; 'On the bacteriology of septic wounds', *Lancet* (1915, 2), pp. 638–43; 'The physiological and antiseptic action of flavine (with some observations on the testing of antiseptics)', *Lancet* (1917, 2), pp. 341–5; (with A. E. Wright and L. Colebrook) 'The conditions under which the sterilisation of wounds by physiological agency can be obtained', *Lancet* (1918, 1), pp. 831–8; 'The action of chemical and physiological antiseptics in a septic wound', *British Journal of Surgery*, 7 (1919–20), pp. 99–129; 'A comparison of the activities of antiseptics on bacteria and on leucocytes', *Proceedings of the Royal Society*, series B, 96 (1924), pp. 171–80. Almroth E. Wright, 'An address on wound infections: and on some new methods for the study of the various factors which come into consideration in their treatment', *British Medical Journal* (1915, 1), pp. 625–8, 665–8, 720–3 and 762–4; 'Memorandum on the employment of bandages for the irrigation of wound-surfaces with therapeutic solutions and the draining of wounds', *British Medical Journal* (1915, 2), pp. 564–7; 'A lecture on wound infections and their treatment', *British Medical Journal* (1915, 2), pp. 629–35, 670–6 and 717–21; 'Memorandum on the treatment of infected wounds by physiological methods (Drainage of infected tissues by hypertonic salt solution, and utilisation of the antibacterial powers of the blood fluids and white blood corpuscles)', *Lancet* (1916, 1), pp. 1203–7; 'The question as to how septic war wounds should be treated (being a reply to polemical criticism published by Sir Watson Cheyne in the *British Journal of Surgery*)', *Lancet* (1916, 2), pp. 503–13; (with H. H. Tanner and Ralph C. Matson) 'On a rose-irrigator for supplying a therapeutic fluid continuously and at a standard temperature to the whole surface of a wound', *Lancet* (1916, 2), pp. 821–4; 'A lecture on the treatment of war wounds, supplemented by additional matter relating to antiseptics and the method of Carrel', *Lancet* (1917, 1), pp. 939–49; 'New methods for the study of emigration and of the bactericidal effects exerted in the wound by leucocytes', *Lancet* (1918, 1), pp. 129–33; 'A lecture on the lessons of the war, and on some new prospects in the field of therapeutic immunisation', *Lancet* (1919, 1), pp. 489–501.

control wound infection. This rationale was founded upon Lister's antiseptic technique in surgical operations, developed in 1865 on the inspiration of Pasteur's germ theory, in which carbolic acid was used to sterilise the open surgical wound during operations. Lister's technique was shown to be effective in reducing the post-operative infection of 'hospital gangrene', the then most prevalent killer, and through his work the role of antiseptics in controlling septic wound infection became firmly established, and was later accepted as a standard treatment for war wounds during the First World War. To many of the surgeons of this era, Lister's authority was absolute and beyond dispute. And to challenge Lister was to challenge modern surgery *per se*.

Not surprisingly, when Wright's team criticised the use of antiseptics they were met with a great deal of hostility. They showed that antiseptics killed white blood cells as well as bacteria, thus diminishing the effectiveness of the body's immune defence and exacerbating wound infection, and they recommended that a saline solution should be used instead. This research may appear to be totally unrelated to vaccines, and other historians have interpreted it in this way.[34] But in fact Wright and Fleming made these findings and recommendations because they looked at war wounds from the viewpoint of the vaccine programme. Indeed Wright had gone to Boulogne specifically in order to develop a septic-wound vaccine.

At the outbreak of war in 1914, Sir Alfred Keogh suggested that Wright should give the service of his laboratory in St Mary's Hospital to produce anti-typhoid vaccines for the Forces. Wright had agreed to this. In addition, he had proposed that the War Office should also use his septic-wound vaccines.[35] Wright believed that this vaccine would enhance the body's defence against 'septic bacteria' and hence such vaccine could possibly be used both as a prophylactic and therapeutic vaccine for septic infections from war wounds. Keogh was uncertain of the efficacy of the septic vaccine and suggested that Wright set up a laboratory in France to research on wound treatment. Wright was made a colonel. He organised a team of assistants and they left for Boulogne to set up his laboratory near the front. Initially, they produced works on wound physiology, the bacteriology of wound

[34] For example, L. J. Ludovici, *Fleming: Discoverer of Penicillin* (London, 1952).

[35] Macfarlane, *Fleming*, p. 82; Noble, *Coli: Great Healer of Men*, p. 32.

infections and fever – subjects that bore a direct relation to septic vaccines. But the focus of their research later shifted to the detrimental effects of antiseptics on white blood cells in the wound cavity.[36]

As for the cause of this marked change, we can uncover it indirectly in a paper published by Wright after the war.[37] In this paper, Wright discussed the findings of his research. His research had been intended to demonstrate that immunisation with his septic vaccine was an effective treatment of war wounds. This paper reveals that he had conducted systematic researches in Boulogne to validate the use of septic vaccine. But unfortunately, vaccines were found to be ineffective in both prevention and control of wound infection. In other words, Wright's septic vaccine project had failed.

Wright's attack on the use of antiseptics arose from this. The failure of septic vaccines was, he claimed, due to the fact that white blood cells could not get into the wound cavity in sufficient number to engulf harmful bacteria. Therefore, the problem of wound treatment lay not only in sensitising white blood cells' ability to engulf certain bacteria by immunisation, but also in getting a large enough number of white blood cells there and maintaining them active in the wound cavity. His explanation drew support from various experiments and tests that demonstrated poor emigration of white blood cells into the wound cavity and also how the presence of antiseptic impeded the phagocytic function of the 'sensitised white blood cells' (sensitised, that is, by immunisation). Because of their involvement with vaccines, it was in the interest of Wright's team to monitor the activities of white blood cells in wound cavities, both before and after immunisation as well as before and after the application of antiseptic. If they found that the white blood cells' activity in the wound cavity was invariably reduced, it would of course be in their interest to identify causes other than immunisation as being responsible for this. For these reasons and because of their special interests, they devised special experiments to demonstrate the activity of white blood cells in wounds and also the effect of antiseptic on them. Moreover, once they had constructed these 'facts', it was also in their interest to propagate them; therefore they were published in medical journals and generated a very fierce dispute.

[36] Of the papers cited above, Fleming's early ones on war wounds were on the bacteriology of septic wounds and gas gangrene and also on skin grafting. Wright's early papers were on bandages and irrigators, and on the treatment of war wounds and its physiological basis. In mid-1917 Fleming started to publish papers that attacked the use of antiseptics. Wright started to attack antiseptics in mid-1916.

[37] Wright, 'On the lessons of the war'.

Thus the question of the efficacy of septic vaccine became overshadowed by the dispute over the antiseptic treatment. In retrospect, the original context of this project was removed; historians and biographers gave accounts of these counter-antiseptic researches without considering the original context of the development of Wright's septic vaccine. The antiseptic enterprise was thus misconstrued as the non-vaccine project that prepared Fleming later to look for a 'magic bullet' or a 'perfect antiseptic'.[38] However, as we have seen, it was the vaccine programme which underpinned the research of Wright's team on something as apparently unrelated to vaccines as antiseptics.

Seeing the activities of Wright's laboratory as the diverse ramifications of a vaccine programme allows us to understand in a more coherent framework the apparently unconnected individual research projects undertaken by different members of the team and in different phases of their careers in the laboratory. This framework allows our analysis to penetrate beneath the surface of the research activities in Wright's laboratory to unmask the implicit interest that also dictated the outcome of these projects and bound the apparently unrelated research projects together. In other words, this framework and its underlying implicit interest constituted 'the condition of possibility' for each individual project: what was perceived as possible, what was allowed, what was encouraged and what was prohibited (though it often operated on these in a tacit and implicit manner). The research in bacteriology, immunology and immune physiology undertaken by Wright's laboratory was directed by the vested interests in promoting vaccines – rather than purely for the sake of disinterested scientific knowledge and objective truth, as some authors have claimed.[39]

[38] See for example Maurois, *Fleming*, p. 108: 'he would dearly have liked to find the "magic bullet"'. Macfarlane, *Fleming*, p. 122: '[Penicillin] might be the long-sought "perfect antiseptic"'.

[39] For example, Colebrook, *Wright*. Noble, *Coli: Great Healer of Men*. Ludovici, *Fleming*. Alexander Fleming, 'The discovery of penicillin', *British Medical Bulletin*, 2 (1944), pp. 4–5.

II: ALEXANDER FLEMING AND THE CONSTRUCTION OF PENICILLIN

All the same, the spores didn't just stand up on the agar and say 'I produce an antibiotic, you know.'[40]
(Alexander Fleming)

Fleming's career in Wright's laboratory

Fleming joined Wright's laboratory in 1907, aged twenty-six, after graduating from St Mary's Hospital Medical School, and he was to stay there for the rest of his life.[41] At that time, the laboratory was still in its two-room museum stage. One year later, it moved into the Clarence Wing and expanded into the first research laboratory in Britain that was attached to an in-patient research ward.[42] On the one hand, there was the laboratory providing both a service of routine diagnostic testing and the research for the most advanced form of therapy; on the other, there was a ward of in-patients on whom these latest therapies were tested, and with progress and response monitored by the laboratory. Fleming started publishing as a co-author of three papers to defend Wright on the issues of therapeutic vaccines and of the opsonic index;[43] then he also undertook his own project to create a new vaccine for acne (the one that retailed at £1 5s in 1914!).[44] In 1919, twelve years after joining the laboratory, he was given the post of Assistant Director of the Inoculation Department. With this, Fleming not only inherited full charge of the department's commercial activities, together with a great deal of clerical and administrative work as the 'production manager' of the 'vaccine factory', but also came much closer into touch with the commercial market and the sales figures of the vaccines.[45] In 1927 he was appointed to the new

[40] Maurois, *Fleming*, p. 131.

[41] This account is based on the three biographies mentioned above, together with Claude E. Dolman, 'Alexander Fleming' in *Dictionary of Scientific Biography*, vol. v (New York, 1970); L. Colebrook, 'Alexander Fleming, 1881–1955', *Biographical Memoirs of Fellows of the Royal Society*, 2 (1956), p. 117; and Hare, 'New light' and 'Scientific activities': supplemented by the information extracted from two of Fleming's own accounts – Fleming, 'The discovery of penicillin', and a speech in British Library, Add. MS 56122.

[42] Colebrook, *Wright*, p. 177.

[43] A. E. Wright, S. R. Douglas, S. Freeman, J. H. Wells and Alexander Fleming, 'Studies in connexion with therapeutic immunization', *Lancet* (1907, 2), pp. 1217–36; Noon and Fleming, 'The accuracy of opsonic estimations'; Fleming, 'Some observations on the opsonic index'.

[44] Fleming, 'Etiology of acne vulgaris'; Discussion on vaccine therapy, pp. 108–9.

[45] Hare, 'Scientific activities', p. 354.

chair of bacteriology which Wilson had procured for the medical school from London University.

In his private life, Fleming now lived in a flat in fashionable Chelsea and owned a country house in Suffolk. He was also a member of Chelsea Art Club, where he often generously entertained friends and colleagues. His wife gave birth to a son in 1924 after several years of childless marriage, and Fleming planned to send him to Eton. But Fleming only received a small salary from the laboratory and from the university, and by now he did not have a large private practice – although he had made a considerable amount when he and Colebrook had used salvarsan to treat syphilis before the First World War.[46] Thus the profit made by the vaccine factory in the laboratory was an important source of Fleming's income.[47] In other words, Fleming had now both a professional and a personal commitment to maintain the sale of vaccines.

It was against this background that Fleming designed the experiments which led to his construction of two new substance-identities: 'lysozyme' and 'penicillin'. I will argue that the earlier work on lysozyme was crucial to Fleming's seeing anything of interest about the dish in which the *Penicillium* mould was growing (it provided a 'visual analogue' which he recognised), and that it also shaped his initial attempts to construct an identity for the substance produced by the mould. It is the construction of lysozyme, therefore, to which we must first turn.

The construction of lysozyme

The accounts of the discovery of lysozyme offered in the books by André Maurois and Gwyn Macfarlane have been derived from the retrospective accounts given by V. D. Allison, a junior colleague of Fleming. Maurois based his story on the manuscript recollections made by Allison for his book,[48] whereas Macfarlane quoted an extract from a public lecture given by Allison in 1973. This lecture was given some fifty-three years after the incident. In this lecture, Allison recalled:

[46] Wright was a personal friend of Ehrlich and obtained the first supply of salvarsan in Britain; he gave this new drug to Colebrook and Fleming to try out on syphilitic patients. With their own direct supply of this drug and their technical expertise, Fleming and Colebrook held a virtual monopoly of this form of treatment, attracting patients from all over London. Hare, 'Scientific activities' p. 349; Macfarlane, *Fleming*, pp. 71–2.

[47] Macfarlane, *Fleming*, p. 97.

[48] Maurois, *Fleming*, pp. 109–10.

> Discarding his cultures one evening, [Fleming] examined one for some time, showed it to me and said, 'This is interesting.' The plate was one on which he had cultured mucus from his nose some two weeks earlier, when suffering from a cold. The plate was covered with golden-yellow colonies of bacteria, obviously harmless contaminants... The remarkable feature of this plate was that in the vicinity of *the blob of nasal mucus* there were no bacteria; further away another zone in which the bacteria had grown but had become translucent...[49] [emphasis added].

Allison's account shows a remarkable similarity to the legend of the discovery of penicillin. The appearance of the agar plate described in this account is remarkably similar to the pattern on the agar plate on which penicillin was first noticed. Moreover, Allison's account is of a Eureka moment when a natural phenomenon of great significance was spotted by an unusually observant scientist and a remarkable substance discovered. According to Allison, the bacteria found on the plate were 'obviously' chance contaminants, and by implication the pattern on the plate was a naturally occurring phenomenon, i.e. not an experimental artifact, so that Fleming noticed this pattern by chance rather than specifically looking for it or specifically designing experiments to demonstrate it.

I challenge this assumption on the basis of two arguments. Firstly, in a paper published in the *British Journal of Experimental Pathology* in 1929, Fleming made reference to 'the usual way' of spreading 'the infected material, sputum, nasal mucus etc. on the plate'.[50] The photograph in this paper confirms that the infected material was evenly spread all over the entire surface of the plate and certainly not as a discrete blob in the centre of the plate. As this is the usual laboratory practice in bacteriology, and as Fleming himself described this as 'the usual way', we can be certain that when he cultured his own nasal mucus during the cold, this evenly spreading method was the one that he had initially used (and not a discrete blob). The plate which Allison saw was therefore not the original plate on which Fleming cultivated his nasal mucus and on which the bacteriolytic effect of his nasal mucus was first noticed; if it had been, the mucus would have been spread in 'the usual way' – evenly across the entire surface of the plate – and the bacteriolytic effect of mucus would not have been visible (because one would only see a smear of lysed

[49] Macfarlane, *Fleming*, p. 99.

[50] 'A definite quantity of the penicillin may be incorporated with the molten culture medium before the plates are made, but an easier and very satisfactory method is to spread the infected material, sputum, nasal mucus, etc., on the plate in the usual way and then over one half of the plate spread 2 to 6 drops... of the penicillin.' Alexander Fleming, 'On the antibacterial action of cultures of a Penicillium, with special reference to their use in the isolation of *B. influenzae*', *British Journal of Experimental Pathology*, 10 (1929), p. 233.

bacteria, and where the mucus was present and where it was absent would not be obvious).

Secondly, there are actually records of Fleming designing experiments that produced the appearance of the plate Allison remembered. In a paper on lysozyme in the *Proceedings of the Royal Society* in 1922, Fleming described an experiment in which he placed a drop of diluted nasal mucus in the centre of an agar plate, which had been thickly planted with *M. lysodeikticus* (a bacterium which Fleming found to be particularly sensitive to lysozyme). The result showed that where the blob of nasal mucus was placed, there was a complete inhibition of bacterial growth; and 'this inhibition extended to about 1 cm of radius around the central zone'.[51] This experiment was almost identical to the one recorded in Fleming's lab book for '21/11/21' which described adding 'AF' nasal mucus to a plate planted with a bacterium 'AF coccus', which became lysed and translucent after incubation. The pattern described was the same as the one which Allison was shown. But we must note that here the pattern was experimentally produced, not a spontaneously occurring natural phenomenon.

On the basis of these two observations, I maintain that Fleming did not 'discover' lysozyme through a chance contaminated plate. I suspect that Allison's recollection and his retrospective account were heavily tinged by the later legend of the discovery of penicillin and distorted by the foreshortening effect of retrospect that simplified and telescoped, across the gulf of fifty-three years, the complex research process into a single Eureka moment.

Instead, I will suggest there was a different sequence of events – a sequence I reconstruct from the historical documents and Fleming's manuscripts. The manuscripts records reveal that Fleming was engaged on the development of new vaccines around 1921.[52] At this time there were many articles about influenza in the medical journals: some reporting a new influenza epidemic, some on the bacterial aetiology of influenza, some on treatment and some on the deadly consequences of this condition. This interest is understandable since there were two influenza pandemics in 1918 and 1919 following the

[51] Alexander Fleming, 'On a remarkable bacteriolytic element found in tissues and secretions', *Proceedings of the Royal Society*, series B, 93 (1922), pp. 306–17.

[52] From March to May 1921, Fleming had been systematically culturing the stools from patients with diarrhoea and arthritis; and he correlated the bacteriological findings in their stools with their clinical symptoms, possibly with the view to developing a therapeutic vaccine for this clinical condition. '16.3.1921'–'11.5.1921' Fleming, British Library, Add. MS 56154.

First World War, killing 20 million people – more than the war itself.[53]

Despite pandemics, epidemics and the general advances made in bacteriology, the cause of this deadly disease was still uncertain in the early 1920s. In 1892, Pfeiffer had identified a bacterium which he called *B. influenzae*, suggesting that this bacterium was responsible for influenza. Later, research work during the two pandemics suggested that the aetiology was more complicated, as it was found that *B. influenzae* was not present in all cases; moreover, it was also found in other infections and in healthy asymptomatic individuals. This new finding renewed interest in the viral theory of the cause of influenza. This had been inferred from an experiment done by Kruse in 1914. Kruse claimed that the common cold (coryza) was due to a filter-passing virus, and he demonstrated that the disease could be transmitted to healthy individuals via drops of the clear diluted bacteria-free filtrate prepared from the nasal mucus of a patient suffering from a cold. Around 1921 the debate on the aetiology of influenza was between the supporters of the bacterial theory and the supporters of the viral theory; and amongst the bacterial theory supporters, there was a further division between Pfeiffer's supporters who believed that *B. influenzae* was the cause and those who believed that some other bacterium was responsible.[54]

During this time, Wright's laboratory had been consistently producing and marketing the 'Anti-Influenza Vaccine (mixed)' that consisted of 'Pfeiffer's Bacillus [i.e. *B. influenzae*], Pneumococcus and Streptococcus'.[55] If we consider Fleming in the context of Wright's laboratory, and Wright's laboratory in the context of the pandemic of life-threatening influenza and in the context of the debates centring around the aetiology of this condition, we can understand why Fleming would take an interest in developing a new 'flu' vaccine and also be investigating the aetiology of flu.

Sometime in 1921, Fleming developed symptoms like those of flu. With a view to investigating the bacterium responsible for this and also possibly developing a new vaccine if a new bacterium was

[53] Macfarlane, *Fleming*, p. 93; his source is Ministry of Health, *Report on the Pandemic of Influenza, 1918–19* (London, 1920).

[54] David Thomson and Robert Thomson, 'Investigations on the aetiology of influenza', *Lancet* (1927, 1), pp. 1125–6; Paul Fides and James McIntosh. 'The aetiology of influenza', *British Journal of Experimental Pathology*, 1 (1920), pp. 119–26; H. B. Maitland, Mary L. Cowan and H. K. Detweiler, 'The aetiology of epidemic influenza: experiments in search of a filter passing virus', *British Journal of Experimental Pathology*, 1 (1920), pp. 263–81.

[55] See advertisement illustrated in Fig. 15, from the *Proceedings of the Royal Society of Medicine* on the inside of the front cover of the issue for October 1929.

identified (we can recall how Fleming developed his new vaccine for acne), Fleming decided to systematically swab and culture his own nasal mucus.[56] And 'for the first three days of the infection there was no growth, with the exception of an occasional staphylococcus colony'. However, 'the culture made from the nasal mucus on the fourth day showed in 24 hours a large number of small colonies which, on examination, proved to be large gram-positive cocci'.[57] And this would suggest that this bacterium was the real causal agent for his flu/cold, though it was rather difficult and delicate to grow, hence its absence from the earlier plates. As Fleming took sufficient care to secure a supply of this strange bacterium, he evidently did not simply dismiss it as a chance contaminant from the laboratory atmosphere that was unworthy of serious attention. Initially, Fleming called this bacterium 'AF coccus' (evidently 'AF' stands for Alexander Fleming, suggesting a bacterium derived from his own nose, as there is evidence in his notebook that he used these initials to refer to himself, and initials in general refer to people rather than laboratory animals).[58] This 'AF' bacterium was later renamed *Micrococcus lysodeikticus*. Now, since the condition which Fleming suffered from was retrospectively diagnosed as coryza, the common cold (the symptoms of which are almost indistinguishable from those of flu in the early stages), we can be reasonably sure that it was a mild condition and that he was beginning to recover from this condition after four or five days or at most a week. And at this point, it would have been reasonable for Fleming to conclude that he had developed an immunity against this condition.

Around this time there was fierce debate about the mechanism by which the body acquired immunity against an infection. A new theory was proposed in 1917 by d'Herelle who suggested that a living ultramicroscopic filter-passing virus was responsible for causing lysis (breaking-down) of the infective bacteria and giving the body

56 Fleming's account in 'On a remarkable bacteriolytic element' just briefly mentioned that the mucus came from 'a patient suffering from acute coryza [common cold]' (p. 306); but reading this account together with other descriptions (those by Allison and the evidence from Fleming's notebook – British Library, Add. MS 56154 – in which he repeatedly used his own initials 'AF' to denote the nasal mucus and this bacterium alleged to be derived from this patient), the 'patient suffering from acute coryza' can be concluded to be Fleming himself. See note 58 on Fleming's use of initials.

57 Fleming, 'On a remarkable bacteriolytic element', p. 306.

58 A loose page in British Library, Add. MS 56154 records an experiment in which Fleming tested his staphylococcal vaccines in rabbits. The rabbits were named according to their external characteristics 'Red/Ear', 'Black', 'Wild', 'Brown' etc. His early notebooks such as 56139 (3.12.1907–08) used 'AF' to denote himself.

immunity against a particular bacterium.[59] He called this virus 'bacteriophage', meaning 'bacteria-eater', signifying a virus that feeds on living bacteria as a parasite and lyses them. This theory was first proposed to explain what became known as 'the d'Herelle phenomenon'. Having taken an emulsion of a stool from a dysentery patient and filtered it, d'Herelle noticed that the clear bacteria-free fluid obtained was capable of dissolving *B. dysenteriae* Shiga – the bacterium that causes dysentery. He correlated the presence of this bacteriophagic element in his patients' stools with their recovery from dysentery. He also noticed that only living bacteria underwent lysis. Hence he used the living virus theory to explain this phenomenon, suggesting that bacteriophage had an important role in explaining how a host acquired immunity during an infection; and also implying that bacteriophage had a potential therapeutic value that could be exploited in the treatment of infectious disease.

Fleming suspected that bacteriophage might have developed in his nasal secretion, in the same way that opsonins and agglutinins developed in blood, and so be responsible for the immunity and his recovery from the cold. To test this hypothesis, Fleming repeated d'Herelle's experiment, though not literally. Instead of using a stool emulsion from a patient recently recovered from dysentery and adding this to the dysentery bacterium, Fleming (having just recovered from a cold) used his own nasal mucus and added it to his 'AF coccus' – the unidentifiable bacterium that had been found in his previous nasal mucus culture during his cold. This claim that Fleming was investigating the bacteriolytic effect of bacteriophage in his own nasal mucus is supported by an entry for an experiment on '21/11/21' in his lab notebook numbered 56154 in the British Library. This entry is headed 'Bacteriophage'. In it, Fleming planted six streaks of three different strains of bacteria (i.e. two streaks of each strain) on an agar plate and placed drops of his own diluted nasal mucus across them. The three kinds of bacteria used were: pneumococcus, staphylcoccus and the mysterious strain which he had called 'AF coccus'. In this experiment, he incubated these bacteria with the diluted nasal mucus for 18 hours and 48 hours; and he looked for any changes at these intervals. Fleming sketched down the appearance of the plate (see Fig. 25). He recorded:

'Staphyloid coccus [AF coccus] completely inhibited where drop of supernatant or sediment of nasal mucus.

[59] Anonymous editorial, 'The phenomenon of d'Herelle', *Lancet* (1921, 2), p. 1173.

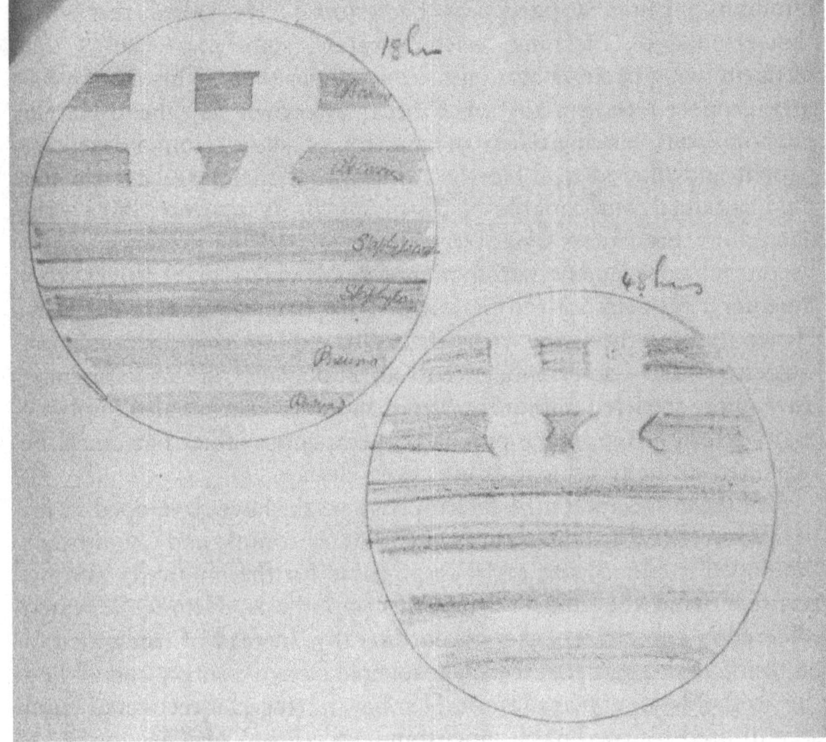

Fig. 25. Sketch from Fleming's laboratory notebook, showing the result of his 'bacteriophage' experiment, later construed as the discovery of lysozyme.

No growth at all in these areas and growth ceases abruptly. (no falling off). Staphylococcus and Pneumococcus – No inhibition.'[60]

This was the first recorded experiment in which the bacteriolytic effect of nasal mucus was experimentally demonstrated. Immediately after this entry, we find the record of the experiment in which a blob of nasal mucus was placed on a plate thickly planted with this 'AF coccus' (probably the one that Allison saw).

We should note that these were special experiments designed, contrived and perfected in order to demonstrate the bacteriolytic effect of nasal mucus, which is not itself naturally visible. The experiment described in the *Proceedings of the Royal Society* (or the plate Allison saw) was deliberately contrived to show up the bacteriolytic effect: the agar plate was thickly planted with the sensitive bacterium *M. lysodeikticus* (AF coccus), with the aim of

[60] Fleming, British Library, Add. MS 56154, vol. XLIX (16.3.1921 to 2.2.1922).

enhancing the contrast between the lysed region and the dense growth of the unaffected region; and again it was a discrete and centrally placed blob of nasal mucus which served to make the effect more visible. In the experiment marked 'Bacteriophage', the discrete thick bands of bacteria and discrete blobs of centrally placed nasal mucus served the same function. If the sensitive bacteria had been thinly and randomly spread on the agar plate and the nasal mucus smeared evenly or sprayed randomly, such bacteriolytic effects would not have been visible. Therefore, only by the design of the experiment was Fleming able to demonstrate (make visible) the bacteriolytic effect of bacteriophage; and from what the heading suggests, he was most likely to have been investigating its presence in his own nasal mucus after his recovery from his cold as a part of the immuno-physiological project within Wright's vaccine programme.

Having established the bacteriolytic effect of his recovered-from-cold nasal mucus, Fleming's next step was to find out whether this effect was specific to this strange bacterium. To test this, he designed other experiments. In the same lab book (British Library, Add. MS 56154), apart from the experiment described above, he recorded another experiment in which he compared the effects of nasal mucus on 'AF coccus' and a wider range of bacteria: 'coli [a bowel bacterium], pneumo [pneumococcus], staph [staphylococcus], strepto [streptococcus]'. Later, he tested whether this bacteriolytic property was specific to himself just recovered from the cold, and he started using nasal mucus from his colleagues. To his surprise theirs too had the same bacteriolytic property. As tears drain into the nasal cavity before they are swallowed, Fleming postulated that the bacteriolytic substance might have come from the tears. This led him to test tears and the result was positive. He then tested saliva, sweat and other body tissues and secretions, and found that they all had this bacteriolytic property.

At this point, the bacteriophage model was no longer tenable. There were two sets of crucial experiments that severed the link between 'bacteriophage' and Fleming's 'bacteriolytic agent in body secretions'. The first showed that this agent lysed both dead and living bacteria and that its lytic action was sustained within a wide temperature range (4 °C–65 °C); d'Herelle on the other hand had defined his bacteriophage as a living virus which fed parasitically upon living but not dead bacteria, and the range of temperature within which it would act was narrower. The other set of crucial experiments showed that this supposed bacteriophage denatured at

70 °C and that it was precipitated by alcohol, picric acid and other chemicals that precipitated protein, from which Fleming concluded that it was in fact a protein and an enzyme, not a virus.[61] From this point onwards, Fleming's 'bacteriophage' had to be turned into something else. In this process, a new substance had to be created and constructed in these secretions. Fleming constructed this substance first by creating a new name, 'lysozyme'. At this point in its history, 'lysozyme' signified nothing more than an enzyme which lysed an unusual and unidentifiable bacterium (AF coccus); the rest of its properties and its new identity were still to be constructed and grafted onto this substance, provided the new properties and identity constructed were congruous with the previously established properties.

However, the existence of this substance had first to be made self-evidently natural, observable by a seemingly natural process rather than one created by human ingenuity and artifice. To do this, the test or indicator (the AF coccus) used to show up this substance had to be made, in Gooding's parlance, 'transparent', i.e. 'unobtrusive though not necessarily invisible';[62] the test had to be made unobtrusive and transparent for lysozyme to show up directly in front of the eyes. In Latourian parlance, this test had to be made into a 'closed black box'. To close the black box, 'AF coccus' was now renamed by Wright *Micrococcus lysodeikticus* (lysis indicator); its contingent origin and its relationship with the flu vaccine and bacteriophage were omitted in all publications about 'lysozyme'. In Fleming's papers, *M. lysodeikticus* simply became 'a convenient indicator for work in connection with [lysozyme's] distribution and properties'.[63] In reality, the existence of lysozyme was dependent on its indicator, and the privileged status of 'AF coccus' as *M. lysodeikticus*, the lysozyme indicator, was, in turn, dependent on the bacteriolytic effect of the lysozyme phenomenon. Yet for Fleming to construct 'lysozyme' as 'a fact', he had to start by making *M. lysodeikticus* into a closed black box by employing the rhetorical devices of the scientific literature. Once the indicator was a closed black box, 'lysozyme' could be split

[61] Alexander Fleming and V. D. Allison, 'Observations on a bacteriolytic substance ("lysozyme") found in secretions and tissues', *British Journal of Experimental Pathology* 3 (1922), pp. 252–60. Macfarlane, *Fleming*, p. 102.

[62] 'An experiment is transparent when the apparatus and procedures appear to contribute nothing to what the experiment shows. Like the preparations and manipulations of a magician, they are unobtrusive, though not necessarily invisible...' Gooding, 'Faraday as an experimentalist', p. 107.

[63] Fleming and Allison, 'Observations on a bacteriolytic substance', p. 252.

off as a scientific fact with a natural existence independent of the laboratory, the scientist, the contrived experiments, and its laboratory indicator. Lysozyme was then retrospectively claimed to have existed at the time of the Eureka moment of its discovery, while in fact Fleming had been looking for 'bacteriophage' when he was doing research to develop a 'flu vaccine' during the flu epidemics.

At this point in time, 'lysozyme' could have gone in many different directions, such as becoming an antiseptic, a laboratory test, an immuno-physiological fact, a selective culture medium...or the project could have been abandoned or aborted. Amongst all these options, Fleming succeeded in turning lysozyme into an immuno-physiological fact because he succeeded in constructing a natural function upon this substance, and thus confirming its status as a lytic-enzyme, i.e., as a naturally occurring body enzyme with a natural bodily function. This 'fact' was made visible by experiments that demonstrated the sensitivity of a wide range of bacteria to lysozyme. By systematically tabulating the virulence of the bacteria against their sensitivity to lysozyme, Fleming showed that the bacteria sensitive to lysozyme were non-virulent ones, whereas the bacteria resistant to lysozyme were virulent. By inference, he concluded that lysozyme was part of the natural defence of the body and the virulence of a bacterium was to be determined by its sensitivity to lysozyme rather than any other intrinsic virulent characteristics.

This particular identity of 'lysozyme' was in line with Wright's vaccine programme. Its status as a scientific immuno-physiological fact contributed to and strengthened the defence which Wright mounted against the attacks on vaccine therapy. Wright subsequently cited this immuno-physiological fact as part of the integral body defence mechanism, showing the complexity and the sophistication of this mechanism, in his defence of the efficacy of vaccines and also in his attacks on antiseptics and chemotherapy.[64] However, Fleming's attempts to turn the identity of 'lysozyme' once again into something else – antiseptic – were not received with the same enthusiasm, and efforts to construct its antiseptic properties were abandoned. Consequently 'lysozyme' emerged from Wright's laboratory as an immuno-physiological fact, while its original identity as a bacteriophage, its origin in the research context of developing a flu vaccine, and the aberrant pathways it moved through, were all removed or erased.

[64] Almroth E. Wright, 'A discourse on Ehrlich's "chemotherapy": and on certain general principles which require to be brought into application in all treatment of bacterial disease', *Lancet* (1927, 2), pp. 1327–34, esp. at p. 1331.

Lysozyme was not discovered: it was slowly constructed in Fleming's laboratory, undergoing metamorphosis, assuming different identities, with many different possible properties to be grafted onto it; and the identity into which it was finally settled, with a congruous set of properties packaged together and incongruous anomalous elements removed, was an identity in line with the interests of Wright's vaccine programme.

The construction of penicillin

Sometime in September 1928, Fleming encountered a strange mould amongst the scattered dots of golden-yellow colonies of *Staphylococcus aureus* on an agar plate. He was engaged at the time in a series of intense researches on the staphylococci – an important group of bacteria that cause common skin infections, like boils, carbuncles and abscesses, and are also responsible for serious and often fatal general infections, like those from war wounds. Fleming had special knowledge of these bacteria because of his work on war wounds during the First World War, when Wright, as we recall, set up his laboratory in Boulogne to work on his septic vaccines. Since then, Fleming's work on war wounds had become well known, and by the late 1920s he had established himself as an authority on staphylococci. Around 1927, he was invited to write a section on staphylococci in a book published by the Medical Research Council, called *A System of Bacteriology*. In order to accomplish this assignment, Fleming started on a good deal of reading and experiments on staphylococci. During his research, Fleming came across a paper which correlated the virulence of these bacteria with the variations in colours of their colonies.[65] This article suggested that when culture plates after incubation were left at room temperature, the bacterial colonies might change their colour and such changes were claimed to be indicative of the characteristics of the strain and also its virulence. Fleming decided to repeat this experiment himself and he enlisted the help of a junior colleague, D. M. Pryce, to do this. Half way through this project, in February 1928, Pryce changed jobs and left the laboratory.[66] Around 3 September 1928, he returned to the laboratory to visit Fleming and to enquire about the progress of the project. Fleming casually picked up

[65] Joseph W. Bigger, C. R. Boland and R. A. Q. O'Meara, 'Variant colonies of *Staphylococcus aureus*', *Journal of Pathology and Bacteriology*, 30 (1927), pp. 260–9; Hare, *The Birth of Penicillin*, p. 63; Macfarlane, *Fleming*, p. 118; Fleming, 'The discovery of penicillin', p. 4.

[66] Macfarlane, *Fleming*, p. 119; Hare, *The Birth of Penicillin*, p. 63.

a few already discarded culture plates and showed them to Pryce. As Fleming was making this cursory second inspection, he was struck by the unusual appearance of a plate. He remarked: 'That's funny', and pointed out to Pryce how the colonies of staphylococci disappeared around the large blob of mould. After this, he showed this plate to a number of people in the laboratory; but neither Pryce nor anyone else in the laboratory paid much attention or attached any great significance to this plate – or at least not until some twelve or thirteen years later.

What Fleming had seen was a visual analogue of one of his early experiments on lysozyme (or more correctly on bacteriophage) where he had thickly planted the plate with the golden-yellow *M. lysodeikticus* and had placed a drop of nasal mucus in the centre of the plate (Fig. 25). The 1928 plate showed an almost identical pattern, with a circular central blob and a surrounding transparent zone of lysed bacterial colonies; even the colour of the bacterial colonies was the same – golden-yellow! The only difference between them, to an informed observer like Fleming, was that lysozyme could not inhibit the growth of *Staphylococcus aureus* whereas the mould had inhibited its growth. And to someone like Fleming who had been trained to read specific meanings in these patterns, this pattern would signify that the mould produced an unusual variant of lysozyme which was more powerful than any other form of lysozyme he had previously encountered: it was capable of inhibiting a *virulent* bacterium! No wonder this mould and this finding were very exciting for Fleming – not because he spotted a potential antibiotic, but because he recognised an extraordinary variant of lysozyme: a substance which he had constructed, which he had been working on for seven years and which he knew more about than anyone else in the world.

The evidence in his lab book shows that Fleming then proceeded to repeat most of the experiments which he had conducted on lysozyme. He started by testing the bacteriolytic activity of the mould against a wide range of bacteria. Next he added the filtrate of the mould broth to a thick opaque suspension of staphylococcal culture, and saw that after incubation for two hours at 45 °C, the opaque suspension turned almost clear. However, when he tested the mould broth filtrate against the sensitivity of *M. lysodeikticus* – the established indicator of lysozyme – it was found to be only mildly sensitive. Its anomalous nature was further confirmed; just as crucial experiments had differentiated 'lysozyme' from 'bacteriophage', so crucial experiments were differentiating 'the mould broth filtrate' from 'lysozyme'.

One of them was to test whether the nature of this lytic agent was that of a protein. Proteins are denatured at 70 °C: lysozyme lost all its bacteriolytic activity when heated to this temperature; in repeating this experiment, Fleming found that his 'mould broth filtrate' was heat-resistant. Moreover, it dissolved in alcohol, in which lysozyme (being a protein) would have precipitated.

The previous experiments now had to be reinterpreted in a different light: this 'mould broth filtrate' was not a variant of lysozyme. A new identity now had to be given to this substance. The first step was to give it a new name. The resident mycologist in the laboratory, C. J. La Touche, had identified the mould as being *Penicillium rubrum* ('red paint brush'), and so Fleming decided to call the substance 'penicillin'. This penicillin was not penicillin-the-antibiotic which we are familiar with now; it was much more humble. As Fleming wrote: 'for convenience and to avoid the repetition of the rather cumbersome phrase "Mould broth filtrate," the name "penicillin" will be used'.[67] In other words, 'penicillin' in February 1929 implied nothing more than 'mould broth filtrate' and the rest of its properties (including those we know now) were constructed later in the laboratory.

Let us now consider what Fleming was about to do with 'penicillin'. The identity and properties of penicillin were not immediately obvious nor directly visible. Laboratory apparatus and scientific experiments had to be devised to demonstrate them. Though apparatus and procedures often appear to contribute nothing to what an experiment shows, yet experimenters are well aware that experiments rarely work first time or as expected: the technical and observational processes that constitute an experiment are reworked until they can readily reproduce the desired results.[68] Furthermore, scientific experiments are not simply a transparent instrument through which Nature reveals herself. They are created specifically to manifest and demonstrate specific phenomena and properties of a substance. Of all the properties of 'penicillin' that could possibly be discovered, Fleming designed only certain experiments to uncover some. And what he uncovered was inevitably determined by the design of the experiments which, in turn, was a result of the questions he was asking. And the latter, in turn, were the outcome of the interplay of a complex and diverse set of factors, such as his experiences, his knowledge, expertise, current medical debates and so on. But there was an important over-arching factor that dominated this activity: it was the

[67] Fleming, 'On the antibacterial action of cultures of a penicillium', p. 227.
[68] See Gooding, 'Faraday as an experimentalist'.

general interests of the laboratory where Fleming worked, as Fleming only saw properties of 'penicillin' that were considered to be relevant and useful within the framework of this laboratory.

We can recover the questions which Fleming was addressing from the experiments reported in his first paper on 'penicillin', titled 'On the antibacterial action of cultures of a *Penicillium*, with special reference to their use in the isolation of *B. influenzae*'. One of the experiments described was the test of the inhibitory power of penicillin on a range of bacteria. The bacteria found to be resistant to penicillin were *B. influenzae*, acne bacilli, whooping cough bacteria (*Bordetella pertussis*), some bowel bacteria (enterococci) and a few others. From all these resistant organisms, Fleming picked out *B. influenzae* and devised a further experiment with it. *B. influenzae* was very slow-growing on solid media like an agar plate. Its colonies were often so small and transparent that not only were they difficult to see, but they could also easily be overgrown and masked by more luxuriant species such as those commonly found in the nose, throat and sputum. Consequently, this made it very difficult to isolate this bacterium in a laboratory either for making a diagnosis or for farming it for vaccine production purposes. In the next experiment, Fleming planted a mixture of *B. influenzae* together with some penicillin-sensitive organisms that were commonly found in the throat and nose. He then treated the lower half of the agar plate with penicillin. After incubation, the untreated upper half showed a mixture of growth with very large colonies of common throat and nose bacteria that almost completely masked the presence of *B. influenzae*; while in the lower half of the plate treated with penicillin there was only a pure growth of *B. influenzae* (Fig. 26). Here Fleming commented:

> It sometimes happens that in the human body a pathogenic microbe may be difficult to isolate because it occurs in association with others which grow more profusely and which mask it. If in such a case the first microbe is insensitive to penicillin [like *B. influenzae*] and the obscuring microbes [like common nose and throat bacteria] are sensitive, then by the use of this substance these latter can be inhibited while the former are allowed to develop normally.[69]

The message was that penicillin makes it infinitely easier to isolate *B. influenzae* 'when they have not been seen in films of sputum and when it has not been possible to detect them in the plates not treated with penicillin'.

To make sure his readers got the message, he illustrated this statement with another experiment, a clinical trial conducted with Dr

[69] Fleming, 'On the antibacterial action of cultures of a penicillium', p. 233.

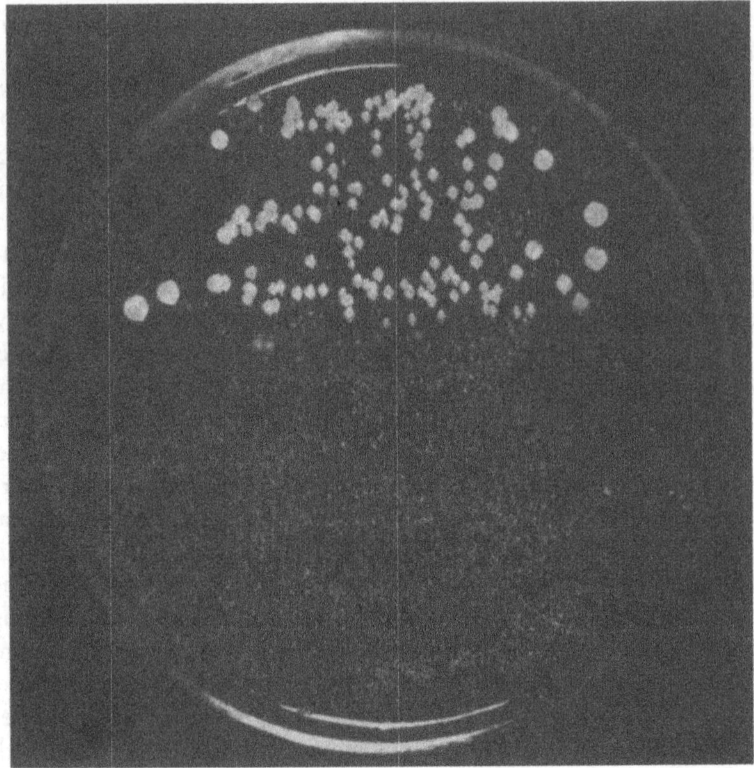

Fig. 26. Fleming's demonstration of the usefulness of penicillin for the culturing of *B. influenzae*. This plate was *evenly* planted with *B. influenzae*, but its growth is only visible in the bottom half, where staphylococcal growth was inhibited by the application of penicillin as a sort of 'weedkiller'.

McLean on twenty-five nurses warded for 'influenza'. Swabs from these nurses' noses were cultured on Fleming's special plates (in which the lower half was treated with penicillin and the upper half was left untreated). The result was that, in the lower half treated with penicillin, twenty-two out of twenty-five showed profuse growth of *B. influenzae*; while, in the upper half, only eight out of twenty-five showed the growth of this bacterium. The message was loud and clear: not only was penicillin useful in demonstrating the presence of *B. influenzae*, but there were a lot of *B. influenzae* cases undiagnosed in 'influenza' patients. The implication of this was profound: *B. influenzae* could well be the true cause of 'influenza' after all! If this was the case, the anti-influenza vaccines produced in Wright's laboratory could well be useful against this deadly disease that had caused epidemics killing millions of people.

This paper was published in May 1929 – the first paper ever published on the epoch-making penicillin. The special status of this paper in our age can be reflected by the price – one to two thousand pounds – that the original now fetches on the collectors' market,[70] and also by the fact that some libraries keep this volume of the *British Journal of Experimental Pathology* off the open shelf.[71] All historians who have worked on the discovery of penicillin make reference to this paper. But many find it illogical and incomprehensible that Fleming should have been concerned with isolating *B. influenzae* in a laboratory when he had in his hand such a powerful antibiotic that could revolutionise modern medicine. This paper has often been quoted by historians with reference only to the short sections at the end of it in which Fleming hinted at the potential use of penicillin as an antiseptic in therapy. Most of the historical research so far has dismissed or overlooked the importance of the main bulk of this paper – isolating *B. influenzae* from 'influenza' patients.[72] This part only makes sense when we see it in the context of the current concerns and disputes of the medical debate around 1929 and the place of Wright's laboratory in this.

In the *Lancet* and *British Medical Journal* between 1927 and 1929, we find the record of two epidemics of 'influenza': in the winters of 1926 and 1928. The epidemics were mirrored by an increase in the number of publications on influenza. These articles were about the high mortality, the aetiology, the complications, the prophylaxis and the treatment of the disease. The mortality in these epidemics was not as high as the pandemic of 1918 and 1919; nevertheless in 1928 there were in excess of 12,000 deaths reported and attributed to 'influenza' in England and Wales alone.[73]

In these epidemics, the role of vaccines was debated. Some dismissed them as simply ineffective both therapeutically and prophylactically and recommended simple measures such as isolation and quarantine instead.[74] Others, like the Royal College of Physicians in Edinburgh,

[70] Macfarlane, *Fleming*, p. 131.

[71] For example, the library of the London School of Hygiene and Tropical Medicine.

[72] Even Macfarlane, who notes Fleming's insistence on the use of penicillin as a bacteriological 'weedkiller', sees this as a strange paradox. Macfarlane, *Fleming*, pp. 127 and 137.

[73] Parliamentary Intelligence: 'Mortality from influenza', *Lancet* (1929, 1), p. 903.

[74] Alfred A. Masser, 'Prophylaxis of influenza', *Lancet* (1929, 1), p. 414; Anonymous editorial, 'The etiology and prophylaxis of influenza', *British Medical Journal* (1929, 1), pp. 1007–8; E. R. Lyth, 'Prophylaxis of influenza', *British Medical Journal* (1929, 1), p. 584.

after conducting a trial on vaccine prophylaxis, found that there were fewer complications in patients who had been immunised.[75] As for the treatment of this condition, no one seemed to know much. But one thing that appeared to be certain was that therapeutic vaccines had been abandoned in immunotherapy. In their place, some recommended anti-streptococcic serum to be administered intravenously in patients who had developed severe fever. The majority of articles suggested that the simple measure of taking aspirin and bedrest was the best form of treatment. In very severely ill patients, chemotherapy was recommended, including the use of two new drugs: Neo-Salvarsan and Mercurochrome.[76] Interestingly, around this period several papers that came out of Wright's laboratory attacked the use of Neo-Salvarsan, Mercurochrome and chemotherapy in general.[77] Even Wright, who had not published for quite a while, joined in the battle and opened fire on Ehrlich's salvarsan – the paradigm of a successful chemotherapy agent which Ehrlich used to call 'the magic bullet'.[78]

Furthermore, there was a renewed debate on the aetiology of the disease. Several more possible causal pathogens had been reported and each attracted its own followers, generating a very heated debate. The virus theory was gaining more support, though *B. influenzae* still attracted a number of conservative followers; a new organism called *B. pneumosintes* was reported by Olitsky in the Rockefeller Institute; and a pneumococcus-like streptococcus was discovered by Thomson and Thomson in London.[79] However, on the whole, *B. influenzae* was falling out of favour. And one of the main reasons for disfavouring *B. influenzae* was its *absence* from bacterial cultures made from the nose and throat swabs of 'influenza' victims.[80]

That was the situation when Fleming encountered penicillin and constructed its properties. In other words, it was in the context of these deadly influenza epidemics, Wright's laboratory and its vaccine

[75] Anonymous report, 'Influenza vaccine: an Edinburgh experiment', *Lancet* (1929, 1), p. 793.

[76] A. H. Douthwaite, 'Treatment of influenza: the prevailing epidemic in London', *Lancet* (1929, 1), p. 359.

[77] Leonard Colebrook, 'NeoSalvarsan in the treatment of puerperal septicaemia', *British Medical Journal* (1925, 2), p. 1246; L. Colebrook and R. Hare, 'On the bacteriocidal action of mercurochrome', *British Journal of Experimental Pathology*, 8 (1927), p. 109.

[78] Wright, 'A discourse on Ehrlich's "chemotherapy"'.

[79] G. S. Wilson, 'An attempt to isolate *Bacterium pneumosintes* from patients suffering from influenza', *Lancet* (1927, 1), pp. 1123–4; Anonymous editorial, 'A new cause of influenza', *Lancet* (1929, 2), p. 1321; Thomson and Thomson, 'Investigations on the aetiology of influenza', David Thomson and Robert Thomson, 'A bacteriological investigation of the present influenza epidemic', *Lancet* (1929, 1), pp. 388–90; Lyth, 'Prophylaxis of influenza'.

[80] Maitland *et al.*, 'The aetiology of epidemic influenza', p. 263.

factory, Fleming's role as the production manager in it, the general doubts expressed about the role of vaccines in controlling this condition, the general anti-chemotherapy campaign launched by the laboratory and the £105,000 investment which the laboratory had made in its new Institute building that required substantial funds to maintain, that Fleming had succeeded in turning penicillin into a diagnostic reagent and bacterial farming reagent – all of which worked in perfect accord with his personal, professional and institutional interests.

Or put this another way: if *B. influenzae* had eventually been recognised as the true cause of this life-threatening infection – 'influenza'; if vaccine therapy and prophylaxis had been made to be really effective in controlling diseases; and if these had been seen as the consequences of Fleming's paper in 1929 advocating the use of penicillin as the means of isolating *B. influenzae*; then the identity of penicillin, the properties of penicillin and the discovery story of penicillin would have been completely different. The identity of pencillin would have been that of a diagnostic reagent and a bacterial farming 'weedkiller',[81] not that of an antibiotic; its antibiotic/chemotherapeutic property would probably not be known, or if known, would not be emphasised (just as its reagent and farming properties are not widely known now). And Fleming would have been congratulated by modern historians for having discovered a flu diagnostic reagent and an effective 'weedkiller' for use in making vaccines. And above all, the Eureka moment when Fleming looked at the plate in 1928 would have become the discovery of a special culture medium that had subsequently delivered mankind from the perils of 'influenza'; it would not have been the discovery of an antibiotic.

But the wheel of fortune happened to turn the other way. *B. influenzae*, despite all the plausible evidence, was decided to be responsible only for the secondary infection in 'influenza'. Vaccine therapy, despite its sound theoretical basis, was found to be ineffective in general. As a consequence, attention turned to focus on chemo-

[81] Fleming, 'On the antibacterial action of cultures of a penicillium'; Alexander Fleming, 'A simple method of using penicillin, tellurite, and gentian violet for differential culture', *British Medical Journal*, (1942, 1), pp. 547–8; Fleming, 'The discovery of penicillin'; Macfarlane, *Fleming*, p. 127. In a draft for a speech delivered in 1944, Fleming wrote: 'We immediately used penicillin in the laboratory for the purpose of isolating insensitive bacteria such as the influenza or whooping cough bacilli. The penicillin inhibited the common bacteria from the throat and sputum (streptococci, pneumococci and diphtheroid bacilli) and allowed the influenza or whooping cough bacilli to grow freely.' Fleming, British Library, Add. MS 56122, f. 53. In the alternative version, f. 69, the phrase 'We immediately used' is altered to 'We have continuously used'.

therapy. As it happened, an effective agent – sulphonamide – was found in 1935. Both vaccine therapy and immunotherapy have since then been superseded by new chemotherapeutic agents. In the new tide of chemotherapy, penicillin was turned into an antibiotic in the laboratory of Florey and Chain at Oxford. In this process, penicillin-the-antibiotic became split off from the laboratory, the experiments and the contingent historical circumstances in which its chemotherapeutic properties were constructed. Then, in retrospect, penicillin-the-antibiotic was projected back to the moment when Fleming looked at his agar plate: this moment has since been mythologised as the monumental Eureka moment when penicillin – the epoch-making antibiotic – was discovered.

No wonder the original construction of penicillin has been difficult to understand, since it has been hidden from us by the walls of not just one black box but two. Opening the box first of Florey and Chain's penicillin and then that of Fleming's, we can see the significance of the business role of Wright's laboratory, not as a bias or distorting factor in the logical pursuit of truth, or as an economic base which somehow generates a theoretical intellectual superstructure, but rather as part of the ordinary process by which facts are constructed. We have seen how the vaccine programme defined the group of people who needed to be convinced of the laboratory's claims (those people who opposed vaccine therapy); how it identified some of the technical and intellectual resources which the laboratory needed to develop (the agglutination test, the opsonic index, *M. lysodeikticus*); and how it shaped the identity constructed for the new substances which the laboratory produced (lysozyme, penicillin). Though the circumstances of penicillin's construction are now doubly distanced from us, it is still possible to see how the business interest and the vaccine programme of Wright's laboratory gave penicillin its original existence, and its original identity.

Reflexions

9

The costly ghastly kitchen

BRUNO LATOUR

One must be brought up in laboratories and live in them, to appreciate the full importance of all the details of procedure in investigation, which are so often neglected or despised by the false men of science calling themselves generalizers. Yet we shall reach really fruitful and luminous generalizations about vital phenomena only in so far as we ourselves experiment and, in hospitals, amphitheatres, or laboratories, stir the fetid and throbbing ground of life... If a comparison were required to express my idea of the science of life, I should say that it is a superb and dazzlingly lighted hall which may be reached only by passing through a long and ghastly kitchen.[1]

(Claude Bernard)

I take it that our aim is to explain the link between the laboratory and medicine: we want to understand how it is that laboratories make themselves indispensable to medicine at the end of the nineteenth century.

My remarks are divided into closing remarks and opening remarks. The closing remarks are about the things I would like to see closed and entombed: certain classical sociological notions. The first one is the notion of 'profession'; one cannot get much mileage out of it, because all kinds of people are being professionalised during the nineteenth century, from bank-tellers to doctors. So this is not specific. The second notion I would like to see entombed is that of 'institutions', because again everything in the nineteenth century is being institutionalised. As we can see from Richard Kremer's and Paul Weindling's chapters, even the buildings are remarkably unspecific (as Foucault showed).[2] From fire-stations to schools everything looks approxi-

This is an edited version of the closing talk delivered at the conference from which this volume took its origin.

[1] Claude Bernard, *An Introduction to the Study of Experimental Medicine*, trans. Henry Copley Greene (New York, 1949; first published, 1927; original French edition, 1865), p. 15.

[2] Michel Foucault, *Discipline and Punish: The Birth of the Prison*, trans. Alan Sheridan (London, 1977; original French edition 1975).

mately the same, with the same differentiation of function, the same sort of invention of new partitions, new accounting rules, new panoptica. So to say that the laboratory gets funding in medicine because of the institutionalisation of physiology, is merely to repeat that physiology developed in the nineteenth century. Every single discipline is doing the same in the nineteenth century: getting a profession, institutions and buildings. So it is a nineteenth-century feature; it is not specific.

We could give the same kind of unspecific explanation using 'the rising social status' of physicians. It is very difficult to get any mileage out of the notion of 'rising': the physicians have been rising all the time. And as I showed in one very specific case, with the same rising social status you have to explain how it is that physicians are so sceptical about vaccine in 1880 and so enthusiastic about serum in 1890.[3] The same profession, the same 'rising status', the same groups are sceptical about the first and suddenly shift their enthusiasm to the second, which means that the *content* in some ways is more important than the 'rising social status'.

There is the same limitation with 'laboratory revolution' as an explanatory notion, because it is clear that medicine is revolutionised constantly. Every new school of medical thought in France, since the eighteenth century, is constantly positioning itself as being revolutionary. So 'revolution' as an explanatory category is certainly a non-issue.

The notion of 'laboratory revolution' is very difficult to characterise. An alternative way of analysing it might be to say that the art of doing medicine is constantly *becoming more complicated*. This at least is empirically tractable. There are more and more actors and more and more mediators to take into account in the business of curing. First there is clinical medicine, and then anatomo-pathology, and then physiology, and then bacteriology; the number of mediators interposing between an actor and his goal, between a doctor and his patient, instead of getting fewer is multiplied. So we can observe a series of mediators being added, but it is very doubtful if we can see a 'laboratory revolution' in any clear-cut way. Perhaps even the notion of a 'laboratory' defined by its hardware and special room does not seem to have really meant much, since you might have a lab and not use it. It is not even easy to see what are the minimum elements necessary to count as a laboratory. We can go from the end

[3] Bruno Latour, *The Pasteurization of France*, trans. Alan Sheridan and John Law (Cambridge, Mass., 1988; original French edition 1984).

of the eighteenth century to the physics labs of the end of the nineteenth century, and we can find multiple definitions of what a laboratory is. But is this what we want to do: do we want to find the minimum essence of the laboratory? I do not think that that is very worthwhile. It seems to me much more interesting to look at the *positioning* of the laboratory – the movement of the laboratory – where the laboratory goes. Do the people go to the lab, or does the lab go to the people, and in what sort of ways; and what sort of practices are spread in between? This seems to me to be more interesting. So, without the network of practices in which it is engaged, the mere existence of a laboratory is not in itself a particularly interesting sign.

These are my closing remarks. Now for the opening remarks. The first opening remark is the question: 'why the lab, instead of nothing?' Why can't doctors be left to mind their own business, without interrupting their path and being shifted to the lab? Why is the laboratory tied to medicine at all? What are the movements laboratory proponents are making in order to capture all sorts of interests? Despite what we have heard and read about antivivisectionists and so on, it seems that from the 1850s to the end of the century the number of opponents to the detour through the lab was relatively small. And it is still more surprising that there was so little material opposition, if you consider that there is a double reduction involved in the laboratory. First, it is a special closed place that claims to be relevant to the practice of people who are *outside*; and second, *inside* the laboratory it is a place where small pieces of bodies are standing for the whole patient. There is a double metonymy at work here, a double translation, as we say in our jargon. And it is very surprising that more people do not say: this is a blind alley; nothing happens in the laboratory; it's splitting hairs; it is completely irrelevant to the practice of medicine; there is no relation between a patient and a Petri dish. Can we observe and document more of that sort of discourse against the double reduction of laboratory practice? It is especially surprising to me because of the problem of the time-lag: how come laboratories were believed to be essential, years or even decades before doing anything of value for medicine? When was the detour through the laboratory starting to pay off for the physicians? The question itself may be absurd if considered in terms of 'usefulness', but it is still an important question if considered in terms of self-fulfilling prophecy.

The problem of the diffusion of laboratory innovation can be solved quite easily if we say that the laboratory as an essential part of physiology and medicine is ultimately a self-fulfilling prophecy. If enough people – physiologists, state officials, doctors, hygienists – make in common the prophecy that the laboratory is relevant, it will become so, especially through the medium of standardisation. For if you start to add obligatory tests, and then start to train students in the practices of the laboratory, and impose routine checks in the hospital ward, then twenty years later you can get an obligatory passage point for the laboratory without ever having to argue about relevance or 'real usefulness' (which means nothing anyway). So I think a large part of what we describe as the 'extension' of laboratories has to be studied in terms of standardisation processes. A nice comparative case would be not physics but psychology. For example, IQ tests, which might well not be reliable in themselves, are nevertheless indispensable and have been made indispensable, with hundreds of students being trained in making them, and they have even come to be reflected in education systems, especially in Britain. So again the notion of 'real usefulness' can be dispensed with, but not the question of why laboratories are attracting and dragging behind them any sort of interest at all. For it seems to me that we should constantly remind ourselves of the question: why has the laboratory been *made* to be essential? How has its relevance been imposed? And since we do not find the expected number of opponents in the later period, it means either that after 1850 it is no longer the case that laboratories have to be made relevant – which would mean that everything interesting had happened before, and that it was in the first half of the century that the self-pleading for special places was made – or that the whole question of 'usefulness' depends on the secondary mechanism of 'attribution'. When a bridge holds, engineers say, it is due to the strength of mathematics; but when it breaks down, it is very rare that mathematics are held responsible. This mechanism of 'attribution' is secondary compared to the primary mechanism of alliance-building.

The second opening remark is the distinction between the laboratory as cultural training ground, and the laboratory, as I would say, as a retooling site. The story of the laboratory which had a lens-less microscope, which was displayed in a cabinet but was not to be used, is a nice emblem for the first, the cultural training ground, aspect. Is the laboratory used to lengthen studies and make a training appear serious so that, while nothing really happens in it, it is somehow good for training students, it furnishes the mind? In that case it does not occupy any strategic position at all; it does not retool the business of doing medicine – which would be the second aspect.

And here I cannot resist throwing in the comparison between factory and laboratory. It is striking that the whole century is also creating these specialised places called factories, which include specific places to make new machines. Laboratories are becoming special places to make specific goods – in this case, facts – for a new emerging market, the scientific market. In this view, the laboratory does not exist just to train students, but it is producing the means to deeply modify the practice of medicine. This quasi-Marxist argument might allow us to rethink the notion of 'instrument': by comparing it with machines. Because laboratories – and here we have a way of getting back to the content of the laboratory – are places where extreme milieux are produced. The physiology laboratory is not as striking as the furnace of chemistry, of course, or the big instruments of physics, but it is a very good place for torturing animals, for making chemicals react, for inducing bacteria to grow, for putting actors to the question. It is an extreme place, the laboratory, and you cannot make the facts if you do not have the machines, any more than you can make iron without the big furnaces and the big hammers. This argument that you need a specific place to produce facts is not alluding to a superstructure influenced by an infrastructure. This place is both at the same time: making specific facts for a market which is being created at the same time. It seems to me that laboratories are doing the same sort of thing for science as factories are doing for capitalism, if I may be allowed this completely outmoded opening remark. In any case, it is an argument much more tied to practice, and to the making of phenomena in the nineteenth century, than to presentation and values.

The third opening remark is the one million dollar question: can we link together the issue of 'discipline', the issue of the minimum elements that are carved out in a laboratory and the issue of the 'method of pain'? Can we bring the question of pain, the tortured, extreme condition undergone by the animal, which is so typical of physiology, to bear on the question of the relevant unit of investigation, and link the two to the question, 'what is a discipline?'? So the one million dollar question is: what does it mean to scientificise medicine at all? In a sense of course, it seems that it is an unanswerable question if we talk about *method*, and I think that everyone would agree that if you put together du Bois-Reymond, Claude Bernard and Pasteur, they would not disagree very much about scientific method – what it is, why it involves a laboratory. The difference between them would be trivial compared to the enormous difference of *what they do* to the elementary units they carve out in the laboratory; the difference of method, the epistemological question of method, is small compared to the enormous difference of what they ask the non-humans they are disciplining to do. So we do not want to answer the question 'what does it mean to scientificise medicine?' directly; but we might want to answer the question about these three different ways of turning medicine in the physician's cabinet into a laboratory science. The lab does not exist just for cultural or symbolic reasons; it is not like learning Greek or Latin. It has to have some sort of strategic importance – not only because it is a ghastly kitchen, as Claude Bernard said, but because it is *costly* kitchen. It is a costly ghastly kitchen. I am not bringing back a 'usefulness' argument again here. People equipped with a laboratory are able to do things which the others cannot, just as the factory owners equipped with an iron furnace, or a Bessemer process furnace, were able to do things the others could not do. It is not 'usefulness' that is in question; it is strategy. And again, it is not the problem of the *extension* of laboratory practices which is important. That is simply explained by a sort of positive feedback mechanism: you cannot compete with others who have been thus equipped with laboratories. But it is the *specificity* which we have to explain.

It seems to me that much of what we call physiology is actually classical microscopic studies; very little of it is actually the active pulsating animal broken into small parts, which we associate with Claude Bernard's work. We keep seeing physiology as defined by this tortured, reduced, pulsating animal. And I have been very struck by the argument that it is metonymically the same as a whole. It is interesting, as Mary Hesse has shown,[4] that scientists are so obsessed by metonymy. The part means the whole. The extracted mechanism means the complete animal. The liver means the functioning liver. What is specific to physiology is this: that even though it is cut into pieces it is still an *active* organism, as in Claude Bernard's experiments. So it is possible to make a small unit still relevant to medicine: still active, and still representing the whole. And this is the complete converse of anatomy; because in anatomy you are dealing with small building blocks, but they are not supposed to be active. So it is an invention which is to anatomy what the steam engine is to windmills. Once you have made your preparations, cut up your experimental animal, maintained it in existence for a long time – and part of

[4] See for example, Michael A. Arbib and Mary B. Hesse, *The Construction of Reality* (Cambridge, 1986), chapter 8, and p. 212.

Stewart Richards's chapter which is very interesting talks about the length of time these animals have to be kept alive – then these preparations are *representative of the whole*, and are therefore still relevant to medicine. And what can you do with this that you cannot do with the anatomo-pathology argument? It seems to me that if we could answer that, we would have the answer why it is that physiology is doing things no other discipline can do, without falling into an argument about 'usefulness'. The laboratory physiologists are bringing into medical dispute a new definition of what a unit is: it is not a patient, it is not a tissue, it is an active organ. The active organ allows a solution to the paradox of being at the same time a reductionist and a non-reductionist. The independent organ retains some of its characteristics – it is holistic and vitalist – but nevertheless is fully tractable – it is anti-holistic and anti-vitalist. Isolated parts are still functional and thus are good models to represent medical practice. So it seems to me that the content here – what people do with the disciplined cut-out part of the body, the central element – if we could find that, if we could characterise that, we could understand why the physiologists are so strong. And then the question of how they convinced the state officials, and how they convinced their colleagues, would become understandable and so make clear the relative lack of opposition I mentioned earlier.

When discussing the lab, we tend to talk seriously about disciplines and unseriously about politics, and I want now to talk seriously about both. The notion of 'discipline' is very interesting in this context if we can see what is disciplined simultaneously: bodies, tortured animals, colleagues. Colleagues, in a sense, are no less tortured by the torture inflicted on the animals. I mean: you torture your colleagues, especially anatomists, quite nicely out of the game, because you have tortured quite nicely the little beast down there in the laboratory. So the disciplining of *buddies* and the disciplining of *bodies* is linked. And very important, it seems to me, is the disciplining of *students*. The laboratory is a very nice way of keeping track of 400 students.[5] *Instruments* are no less important as means to discipline, simplify, reify, mobilise, all bodies of knowledge. So it seems to me that if we could take the notion of discipline out of the sociological realm, where discipline is a sort of human-to-human link, and bring it to bear on strategic ways of disciplining-animals-to-discipline-colleagues-to-

[5] See Merriley Borell, 'Instruments and an independent physiology: the Harvard Physiological Laboratory, 1871–1906' in Gerald L. Geison (ed.), *Physiology in the American Context, 1850–1940* (Bethesda, 1987), pp. 293–321.

discipline-students-to-discipline-instruments, then the strategic path of the laboratory will appear. Do the thought experiment. If you take the laboratory *away*, then you have undisciplined students, who start throwing things around; you have colleagues who don't care about what you are doing; you have all these nice little animals doing all sorts of things, jumping about and so on; and you have the state officials deeply *un*interested. As for the physicians, they are able to mind their own business without having to be detoured through the laboratory. We can get quite a lot more mileage out of Foucault's notion of discipline, it seems to me, than out of the notion of discipline as in the Ben-David tradition, where you basically isolate a profession, and then have trouble linking it to the context, to the politics.

If we wish to qualify in what way politics and content interact we have to be more precise. There is a big difference here between the beginning and the end of the nineteenth century. A number of historians have studied the link at the beginning of the century between building-blocks in medicine and building-blocks in society.[6] And there are lots of ways in which you can easily see the relation between what the elementary units in anatomy are, and what the elementary units in politics are. But I have always been struck by the fact that the available political interpretations are much less specific and clear as you move on in the century. Is there any way in which physiology is made important because it redefines the elementary unit which is representative of the whole – the organ – as a *functional* unit? If so, then this is indirectly political, in the sense that it redefines politics: because it has to do with the designation of 'representative', of what is the smallest unit you need in order to get the whole. This is not directly politics as at the beginning of the century, where people were arguing in the same breath about recomposing society and recomposing the body. It is more complicated than that, because they are not dealing with building-blocks, they are dealing with strategic actors doing things: for instance, the microbes, the glycogenic function of the liver. It is very clear in the case of bacteriology, as I showed in my study of Pasteur, because the bacteriologists were recomposing a society made of billions of active entities. But it seems to me just as striking for physiology, because the physiologists are recomposing the patient from dozens of different organs which are nevertheless *active* organs, and selecting them out as representative of

[6] See for instance, John V. Pickstone, 'Bureaucracy, liberalism and the body in post-Revolutionary France: Bichat's physiology and the Paris School of Medicine', *History of Science*, 19 (1981), pp. 115–42.

the whole. The end of the nineteenth century is very interesting for physiology and for politics, where this time you define not building-blocks, but an *active* entity, which can still be made tractable and disciplined in the laboratory. Politics is not out there in society. Politics is down there in the laboratory where a new definition of what is a part and what is a whole is forged in front of one's colleagues, around the suffering of a dog.

To link the closing remarks and the opening remarks: it seems to me that we cannot use notions like 'institution' and 'profession' and so on, because they do not tell us much about the content. Now when we get back to the content, it does not have to look like the 'reality' of the old realist school. It seems to me that we have become hesitant of talking about the *things*, because that would be falling back into the internalist argument and that bygone vision of reality. But I would like to describe the realists as 'absentee landlords'. They believe the real things are their property, and social historians are left with the social – social status, institutions, professions and so on. But they are absentee landlords none the less: they do not do anything with the content, they just sit there, far from it, and they simply say 'this is our property: you can't even touch it'. But when you hear the content, the things, getting back into the discussion again they are extraordinarily different from the 'reality' of the realist absentee landlords. So there is no need for us to be impressed by the landlords and abstain from talking of the content in new ways. I do not think social historians should pay too much attention to sociology, or at least be limited to it. We should have no hesitation in talking about the *things*, because the things are not the property of the absentee landlords. The things are these bizarre actors that the authors have been describing here in many of the chapters. We should invade the latifundia of the realists and cultivate something else on their fallow land. 'New internalism', an internalism in which nothing is left outside, might be a way of describing these multiple ties between politics and laboratory practices.

10

The laboratory revolution in medicine as rhetorical and aesthetic accomplishment

NICHOLAS JARDINE

Divers sont les savoirs qui baignent dans l'élément de la science
(Claire Salomon-Bayet)

In the 1840s the only laboratory of which the average European or American medical man would be likely to have a direct acquaintance was that of the pharmacist. By 1900 a host of types of laboratories – physiological laboratories, pharmaceutical and pharmacological laboratories, forensic laboratories, public health laboratories, microbiological laboratories – was securely entrenched in the institutions of medicine. Laboratories had become indispensable for medical qualification and for authentication of a wide range of diagnoses and prognoses. Above all, laboratories had become, in Latour's phrase, 'obligatory passage points' for researchers wishing to be credited with medical discoveries: as Pasteur observed, 'laboratories et découverts sont des termes corrélatifs'.

The following historiographical reflexions and suggestions, inspired by the treatments in this volume of the 'laboratory revolution' in medicine, focus on two questions. What kind of achievement was the laboratory revolution, and in what terms may we most profitably seek to account for it? And how did it transform the content of medicine – both content as embodied in the ranges of questions real for medics, and content as manifested in their lived experience?

For an earlier historiography the questions I have raised about the laboratory revolution in medicine were unproblematic. The installation of laboratories in the institutions of medicine was seen as the means whereby medicine became scientific. Those who executed that installation were seen as having recognised a truth, the truth that it is

Acknowledgements: I am indebted to Andrew Cunningham, Perry Williams, Jim Secord, Andy Warwick, Sue Morgan and Sonia Uyterhoeven for much kind guidance through unfamiliar territory.

the experimental methods of the laboratory that are the most powerful instruments of scientific progress in applied sciences such as medicine. Laboratory education and the pursuit of laboratory-based research turned medics into scientists and it turned medicine into a scientific discipline capable of sustained progress both in the questions it addressed and in the answers it delivered.

Such a historiography is in disarray and few of the contributions to this volume show even a latent sympathy with it. There are, of course, many reasons for this disfavour. One is the current aversion of historians to presentist narratives of the accumulation of knowledge. Another is the growing distrust of the naive realist view that laboratory experimentation competently conducted puts us in direct touch with nature as she really is. But it is worth noting some more local reasons for distrust of the traditional story of the laboratory revolution, reasons that should convince even the most dedicated historical presentists and the naivest philosophical realists.

The beginning of the period with which we are concerned was marked by a plethora of programmes for making medicine 'scientific'. Warner (chapter 3 above) alludes to one of them – the American programme for a scientific medicine based on a French-style medical empiricism antipathetic to laboratory practices. Lenoir (chapter 1 above) touches on another, the natural historical programme of Johann Lukas Schönlein and his associates and pupils, a programme that recognised only an ancillary role for laboratory practices in medicine. In 1840 Ferdinand Jahn, an aberrant member of the natural historical school, listed as follows the competing schools promising to provide scientific foundations for medicine:

Metaphysicians, Idealists, Iatromechanics, Iatrochemists, Experimental Physiologists, Natural Philosophers, Mystics, Magnetizers, Exorcisers, Galenists, modern Paracelsian Homunculi, Stahlianists, Humoral-pathologists, Gastricists, Infarct-men, Broussaisists, Contrastimulists, Natural Historians, Physiatricists, Ideal-Pathologists, German-Christian Theosophists, Schoenleinian Epigones, Pseudo-Schoenleinians, Homoeobiotics, Homoeopathists, Isopathists, Homoeopathic Allopathists, Psorists and Scorists, Hydropathists, Electricity-men, Physiologists after Hamberger, Heinrothians, Sachsians, Kieserians, Hegelians, Morisonians, Phrenologists, Iatrostatisticians.[1]

Of all these only one, experimental physiology, definitely entailed a central role for laboratories in medicine. Given the plurality of

[1] Ferdinand Jahn, *Sydenham. Ein Beitrag zur wissenschaftliche Medizin* (Eisenach, 1840), p. 2; cited in W. Pagel, 'The speculative basis of modern pathology', *Bulletin of the History of Medicine*, 18 (1945), pp. 1–43, at p. 3. On the natural historical school see J. Bleker, *Die naturhistorische Schule 1825–1845. Ein Beitrag zur Geschichte der klinischen Medizin in Deutschland* (Stuttgart, 1981).

programmes of the 1840s for the scientific reform of medicine, and the lack of consensus on the actual or potential relevance to medicine of the fruits of laboratory research, we are bound to ask how it happened that in the following decades laboratories came to be regarded as the crucial instruments of medical reform. A historiography which treats recognition of the potential benefits to medicine of laboratory practices as an adequate explanation of the laboratory revolution is evidently at fault.

A similar objection may be voiced against the view of the traditional historiography on the impact of the laboratory revolution on the content of medicine. Though laboratories substantially affected the self-images of many medical men, even in the later phases of the laboratory revolution few came to regard themselves as scientists. Indeed, it is my impression that even today few medics do so. Nor can we ascribe to the laboratory revolution any generally perceived substantial advancement of medicine. Even by 1900, a date at which the laboratory revolution was effectively accomplished, the roster of acknowledged practical pay-offs attributed to laboratory researches remained sparse in diagnostics and prognostics and yet sparser in therapeutics, as clinicians opposed to laboratory education and laboratory practices in medicine continued to protest well into the present century.[2] And it is sparser still if we insist on viewing the matter from a present-day standpoint rather than from the standpoint of medics around 1900.

In sum, whatever its philosophical merits or demerits, the traditional historiography is in deep historical trouble over the laboratory revolution in medicine. Neither the general recognition of the potential value of laboratories to medicine which it presents as a cause of the revolution nor the scientific status and achievements of medics which it presents as the consequence of the revolution seem to have happened on cue.

[2] On clinicians' resistance to laboratory training and practices see, for example, C. J. Lawrence, 'Incommunicable knowledge: science, technology and the clinical art in Britain, 1850–1914', *Journal of Contemporary History*, 20 (1985), pp. 503–20; G. L. Geison, 'Divided we stand: physiologists and clinicians in the American context', in M. J. Vogel and C. E. Rosenberg (eds), *The Therapeutic Revolution: Essays in the Social History of American Medicine* (Philadelphia, 1979).

...to find out in each case the existing means of persuasion
(Aristotle)

The contributions to this volume suggest an interpretation of the laboratory revolution in medicine as a rhetorical and aesthetic accomplishment.

I am here using 'rhetorical' and 'aesthetic' in extended senses. Rhetoric I take, in line both with the broadest of its classical usages and with the prevalent usage of many sociologists of the sciences, to be concerned with all discursive forms of persuasion. Aesthetics I take to be concerned with all the ways in which men may be affected and moved by their perceptions. Aesthetic subjects may be perceptibles of any kind – natural or artificial, human or non-human, transitory or permanent, familiar or strange, things or representations. Aesthetic response includes, of course, contemplative reception of works of fine art – of the beautiful, sublime and authentic. Importantly for our purposes, it includes the engaged reception of live performances, spectacles and demonstrations. Equally importantly, it includes what Walter Benjamin memorably called 'distracted reception': response to and appropriation of popular art, familiar scenery, the architecture in which we live and work, the machines and instruments with which we are in day-to-day interaction.[3]

A rhetorical and aesthetic interpretation of the entrenchment of laboratories in the institutions of medicine would incorporate elements from three currently fashionable historiographies: the historiography of texts and discourses, the historiography of networks and the historiography of social interests. From the first it would borrow a minute concern with the rhetorical conventions and strategies at play in the writings of those who promoted the cause of a laboratory-based medicine, and in particular with the strategies whereby such texts project, define and control their readerships.[4] From the historiography of networks it would borrow a concern with the processes of delegation whereby the skills of persons become 'black-boxed' into instruments and whereby the actions of persons are facilitated and controlled by instruments; and it would follow

[3] Walter Benjamin, 'The work of art in the age of mechanical reproduction', in *Illuminations*, ed. H. Arendt, trans. H. Zohn (London, 1970; original German edition, 1936), pp. 219–53.

[4] Serious textualist historiography appears not yet to have hit the history of medicine. Fine specimens of this genre in the history of chemistry are O. Hannaway, *The Chemists and the Word: The Didactic Origins of Chemistry* (Baltimore, Md, 1975) and W. C. Anderson, *Between the Library and the Laboratory: The Language of Chemistry in Eighteenth Century France* (Baltimore, Md, 1984).

network theory in attending closely to the processes of 'translation' through which proposals for innovation and reform are selectively interpreted and modified in the interests of those who sponsor and enact them.[5] From the historiography of social interests, the historiography whose impact is most in evidence in the present volume, the approach would borrow a minute concern with the actual interests – professional, factional and political – of those who promoted, sponsored, resisted and enacted the laboratory revolution.[6]

There are, however, important respects in which the historiography I am advocating would break with existing emphases in textualist, network-theoretic and interest-theoretic historiographies. It would have no truck, for example, with 'pan-textualism', the treatment of authors and readers and of natural and social entities as 'projections' from the autonomous realm of texts. In particular, it would view with deep suspicion the textualist tendency to conflate the interests and motivations that are projected in texts with the real interests and motivations that explain the production of texts and their persuasive efficacy. It would resist the network theorists' principle of symmetry between the activities of persons and things, insisting on a sharp distinction between the roles in the transformation of disciplines of the deliberate actions of persons and of the efficacies and powers of things. And it would resist also the tendency of interest theorists to treat interests as historical 'givens', overlooking the extent to which the promotion and enactment of innovations and reforms may form and consolidate, deform and dissolve social interests. (Lenoir's contribution to this volume, in emphasising the extent to which programmes for the scientific reform of German medicine combined appeal to existing interests with projection of new social and political orders, provides a valuable corrective to this tendency.)

There is a further and more fundamental point of divergence between interest theory and the proposed historiography. For our approach would call in question a fundamental tenet of interest theory. Interest theorists assume that it is primarily through appeals to their interests that people are moved to commitment and action, an assumption which is often reinforced by a treatment of declarations of rational and moral grounds for commitment and action as *post*

[5] B. Latour, *The Pasteurization of France*, trans. A. Sheridan and John Law (Cambridge, Mass., 1988; original French edition, 1984) pioneers the network-theoretic approach to the history of medicine.

[6] An exemplary application of interest theory to the history of medicine is A. Desmond, *The Politics of Evolution: Morphology, Medicine and Reform in Radical London* (Chicago, 1989).

factum legitimations that conceal the true grounding of such commitments and actions in social interests. On the proposed approach, appeal to interests would lose its exclusive prerogative as a mover of men. Appeal to social interests would take its place as a rhetorical strategy alongside appeals to reason and appeals to morals and ideals. (I should emphasise, in passing, that I do not mean to imply that appeals to reason and morals are 'merely' rhetorical in any pejorative sense: as noted above, rhetoric is here taken to cover all discursive means of persuasion.) Moreover, the proposed historiography would seek to do justice to the fact that the effectiveness of such appeals depends not merely on the strength with which those addressed are committed to the relevant interests, rationalities and morals, but also on the media through which those appeals are made. Thus the success of appeals through texts will depend upon the affective powers of narrative, layout, illustrations, etc.; and the success of appeals through addresses and live demonstrations will depend on the affective powers of oratorical gesture and intonation, of the staging and performance of experiments, etc. In short, the proposed historiography would take seriously the roles of aesthetic appeals as stimuli to commitment and action.

As shown by the contributions to this volume of Kremer and Lenoir, copious material for the study of the rhetorical accomplishment of the laboratory revolution in medicine is provided by the specific proposals, counterproposals and negotiations concerned with the setting up and funding of physiology laboratories and the reform of medical education to incorporate laboratory training.[7] Another obvious, but as yet little explored, resource for the study of the rhetoric and aesthetics of promotion of laboratory-based medicine in this era of sermonising scientists is provided by the public addresses of such virtuoso orators as T. H. Huxley, Rudolf Virchow and Emil du Bois-Reymond, along with the responses their addresses provoked in the periodical and newspaper literature.[8]

Two more indirect vehicles of persuasion deserve close attention. Certain scientific instruments, the microscope, the clinical thermometer, the stethoscope, the sphygmograph, the electrocardiograph,

[7] See also A. M. Tuchman, 'From the lecture to the laboratory: the institutionalization of scientific medicine at the University of Heidelberg' in W. Coleman and F. L. Holmes (eds), *The Investigative Enterprise: Experimental Physiology in Nineteenth-Century Medicine* (Berkeley, Calif., 1988), pp. 65–99; T. Lenoir, 'Science for the clinic: science policy and the formation of Carl Ludwig's institute in Leipzig', in *ibid.*, pp. 139–78.

[8] Of particular interest in this connection is M. Subbiah, 'Popularizing Science: Thomas Henry Huxley's Style', unpublished Ph.D. thesis (Oklahoma State University, 1987).

became successively established in the period 1840 to 1910 along with the white coat as symbols of 'scientific' medical practice. But it is misleading, not least on chronological grounds, to regard this as a consequence of the laboratory revolution in medicine. Rather, such instruments are to be seen as tokens of medical practitioners' commitment to a precise, quantitative, cause-seeking medicine, and as emblems of the enhanced professional status and authority of the 'scientific' medic: in Shortt's words, they were the 'Trojan horses' of the laboratory revolution.[9] In this connection great interest attaches to the ways in which instrument makers and marketers and textbook protagonists of instruments targeted their wares on the medical fraternity. This targeting clearly involved appeal to professional interests as well as appeal on grounds of medical utility and efficacy. And these rhetorical appeals are clearly mediated through aesthetic appeal. No one glancing at advertisements for microscopes of the period, the French ones elegant and decorous, the German ones chunky, metallic and functional, could doubt that we have here symbols of professional status and authority and icons of scientific precision.[10] And when we turn to the instruments of vivisection, their description and their demonstration, we see in play elements of the aesthetics of the theatre and the initiation rite.

The use of history to promote, legitimate and consolidate the introduction of experimental methods into medicine is, I believe, of outstanding importance in the formation of a medicine disciplined by the laboratory.[11] The following tentative remarks are based on my reading of the historical treatments of physiology and allied disciplines to be found in Claude Bernard's *Introduction à l'étude de la médecine expérimentale* of 1865 and *Rapport sur les progrès et la marche de la physiologie générale en France* of 1867, Sir Michael Foster's *Lectures on the History of Physiology during the Sixteenth, Seventeenth and Eighteenth Centuries* of 1901, and in the lectures and addresses of Rudolf Virchow, T. H. Huxley and Emil du Bois-Reymond.[12]

[9] S. E. D. Shortt, 'Physicians, science and status: issues in the professionalization of Anglo-American medicine in the nineteenth century', *Medical History*, 27 (1983), pp. 51–68.

[10] This observation is based on a comparison of the nineteenth-century microscope catalogues of Maison Nachet et Fils, Paris, and Carl Zeiss, Jena.

[11] Complementary to the following account is the treatment by Bleker, *Die naturhistorische Schule*, ch. 6, of the deployment of the history of medicine to defend and contest the claims of the natural historical school to provide a scientific foundation for medicine. Another fine study of the polemical uses of history in medicine is J. Martin, 'Explaining John Freind's *History of Physick*', *Studies in History and Philosophy of Science*, 19 (1988), pp. 399–418.

[12] I have used *Disease, Life, and Man: Selected Essays by Rudolph Virchow*, trans. with intro. by L. J. Rather (Stanford, Calif., 1959); *T. H. Huxley, Science and Education*, intro. by C.

A first impression of these works is of an extraordinary diversity of aims and strategies. Foster presents experimental physiology as a subject with a long history, much of it English. From the time of Vesalius and Harvey there have been those who 'work their way by careful observations and patient experiment or trial out of exactly determined anatomical facts, up to the real meaning of the facts'; and it is with von Haller that we see the emergence of 'modern physiology'. For du Bois-Reymond, on the other hand, the history of experimental physiology is short and German. The founder was the immortal Johannes Müller, and the subject was brought to maturity by his pupils, including du Bois-Reymond himself. For Bernard the history of the subject is, needless to say, almost entirely French. It rests on a tripod of 'sciences physio-chimiques' (represented by Laplace and Lavoisier), 'sciences anatomiques' and 'expérimentation sur l'organisme vivant' (represented by Bichat). It is itself largely the product of the labours of his teacher Magendie and of Bernard himself. For Virchow scientific medicine is born with his own inauguration of a cellular pathology in the 1840s. However, the nationalist fervour of Bernard and du Bois-Reymond is lacking; Virchow is, for example, liberal in his tributes to the non-German founders of morbid anatomy and general pathology – notably Morgagni for his 'comprehensive presentation of pathological data' and John Hunter 'who introduced the experimental method into pathology'.

The polemical targets of these authors are likewise very different. For the religious Nonconformist Foster one prime target is dogmatism, especially as represented by the 'bloodhounds of the Catholic Church'; another is the approach to physiology based on the gross anatomy of the human body as opposed to that based on the comparative anatomy and histology of the whole animal kingdom. For Bernard the prime targets are experimentally ill-founded hypotheses and 'vitalism' according to which the spontaneity of life can evade the laws of physics and chemistry; subsidiary targets include excessive reliance on medical statistics and on the insight and tact of experienced physicians. For du Bois-Reymond the prime target is the mysticism and speculation of the *Naturphilosophie* that beset the physiology of his youth, leading men to address questions beyond the bounds of mortal cognisance. Virchow is more ecumenical, much concerned to promote a balance between scientific principles and

Winnick (New York, 1964); Emil du Bois-Reymond, *Reden*, ed. Estelle du Bois-Reymond, 2 vols. (Leipzig, 1912).

clinical experience, opposed both to what he sees as the reductive materialism of du Bois-Reymond and his allies and to all speculative system-building.

The selection of material in these histories clearly represents the disciplinary specialities of their authors: histophysiology in Foster's case, chemical physiology in Bernard's, biophysical physiology in du Bois-Reymond's, physiological pathology in Virchow's. The differences in orientation come out also in the disciplines they present as scientific exemplars for physiology. For Bernard the model discipline is analytical chemistry, for du Bois-Reymond experimental physics, for Virchow cellular pathology, for Huxley the new science of biology, for Foster, at least by implication, comparative anatomy and histology.

Finally, there are substantial differences between the methods that these authors use history to promote. To be sure, all repeatedly convey their commitment to 'the experimental method'. However, Bernard's concern with the hunting-down of the proximate causes of vital phenomena through vivisectional analysis finds little echo in the others' writings. Bernard's experimental method corrects the errors to which vulgar common sense gives rise; Huxley's experimental method, by contrast, is 'organised common sense'. Du Bois-Reymond's pleas for a physiology founded on exact quantitative determinations of the physical parameters of living processes mark off his experimental method sharply from the others. Huxley and Foster differ from the others in their insistence that experimental physiology be conducted on a basis of comparative anatomy. And there is a wide spectrum in the attitudes of these authors to analogical argument in the conduct of experimental physiology – ranging from du Bois-Reymond's and Bernard's flat rejection to Virchow's enthusiastic endorsement.

Underlying these divergences, however, we may detect a range of common tactics in these authors' uses of history to promote a laboratory-based medicine. Most obviously, all promote 'the experimental method' by appeal to the exemplary discoveries it has yielded and the disastrous errors that have arisen at the hands of those who failed to employ it. All of them, even the iconoclastic free-thinking Huxley, appeal in connection with the experimental method to disciplinary father- and founder-figures, figures who are often ruthlessly recreated and modernised in the author's own image.[13] (A

[13] On nineteenth-century construction of disciplinary father-figures in medicine see L. S. Jacyna, 'Images of John Hunter in the nineteenth century', *History of Science*, 21 (1983), pp.

striking example is provided by du Bois-Reymond's life of Johannes Müller, a cautionary tale of Romantic speculative enthusiasm succeeded by wholesome experimental penance, a story which has evident resonances with du Bois-Reymond's own mature disillusionment with his youthful enthusiasm for holistic physiology and radical politics.)

There are striking parallels too in the ways in which these histories negotiate certain obstacles and dilemmas in the promotion of laboratory-based medicine. For example, there is an obvious tension between the official image of the new natural science as a disinterested pursuit of knowledge and any portrayal of science as a means of furthering the practical goals of medicine. In these histories we find repeated emphasis on the moral and intellectual qualities inculcated by education in and practice of the experimental method; but direct promotion of experimental physiology by appeal to its clinical and therapeutic pay-off are rare. We have here a modicum of confirmation of the claim that introduction of laboratory training into the pre-clinical curriculum was conceived in the period primarily as a means to the advancement of the professional autonomy and authority of medics rather than as a direct means to the practical improvement of medicine.[14]

Common strategies are evident also in the ways in which these authors use history to negotiate a basic dilemma in polemical tactics. How are opponents of laboratory-based medicine, including the many protagonists of rival programmes for the scientific reform of medicine, to be countered without dropping the mask of 'scientific' impartiality or conveying the dangerous impression that they represent positions worthy of serious consideration? One recurrent strategy is relegation of the opinions of live opponents to the past, either charitably, as representative of an earlier stage in the development of physiology (Bernard's strategy in countering his vitalist opponents), or uncharitably, as diseases or excesses which once

85–108, and C. J. Lawrence, 'Cullen, Brown and the poverty of essentialism' in W. F. Bynum and R. Porter (eds), *Brunonianism in Britain and Europe, Medical History*, suppl. 8 (London, 1988), pp. 1–21.

14 See, for example, Shortt, 'Physicians, science and status'; J. H. Warner, 'The idea of science in English medicine: the decline of "Science" and the rhetoric of reform', in R. French and A. Wear (eds), *British Medicine in an Age of Reform* (London, 1991), pp. 136–64; S. V. F. Butler, 'White coated doctors: the transformation of medical training in the mid-nineteenth century', paper delivered at the conference 'Medicine and the Laboratory', Cambridge, September 1988; S. W. Uyterhoeven, 'The anti-vivisection movement and physiology in late Victorian England: the reception of Burdon-Sanderson's *Handbook for the Physiological Laboratory*', unpublished M. Phil. thesis (Cambridge, 1990), ch. 1.

afflicted physiology (du Bois-Reymond's preferred tactic). More subtly, guilt is often conveyed by association. In du Bois-Reymond's vitriolic denunciation of Goethe's dabblings in natural philosophy, Goethe's failings are set out in such a way as to be applicable to all opponents of his own physical-reductionist approach and Goethe's doctrines are so characterised as to cast aspersions on the entire morphological-genetic approach to the study of natural phenomena. When Huxley makes of Priestley a symbol of the contributions to science of radical Dissenters we are invited to share his own Dissenting attitude to Establishment control of higher education. And when Foster denounces the 'bloodhounds of the Catholic Church', the reader may well call to mind the established clerical fellows of the Cambridge colleges who had tried to thwart his establishment of experimental physiology in the Cambridge curriculum.

A further dilemma in historical promotion of laboratory medicine arises from the conflict between two effective rhetorical strategies, that of 'normalisation' whereby laboratory-based medicine is presented as a natural development in a long tradition of sound scientific medical practice, and that of 'dramatisation' whereby it is presented as a revolutionary break with the unscientific past of medicine opening up exciting new possibilities for a scientific medicine.[15] The balance of normalisation and dramatisation ranges widely, from Foster's relatively undramatic normalised history via Virchow, Bernard and Huxley to du Bois-Reymond's aggressively dramatised history. But there is a common strategy in achievement of the balance, that of presenting the history of medicine, physiology and pathology as a battle between error, superstition and mysticism, on the one hand, and a reasonable deployment of the faculties on the other. For in these well-worn terms the introduction of laboratory experimentation into medicine can be presented as at once the continuation of the tradition of sound inquiry based on reason and the senses *and* as the revolution that promises the extirpation of medical mystique and error.

[15] On 'normalising' histories see T. S. Kuhn, *The Structure of Scientific Revolutions* (Chicago, 1962), ch. 11. On dramatic and epochal histories of the sciences from the Romantic period see D. von Engelhardt, *Historisches Bewusstsein in der Naturwissenschaft von der Aufklärung bis zum Positivismus* (Munich, 1979), sect. 3. (For all his denunciations of Romantic *Naturphilosophie* and historicism, du Bois-Reymond's historical reflections on the sciences use many of the tropes of Romantic historiography.)

One day all that will be of as much value, and no more, as the amount of belief existing today in the masculinity or femininity of the sun
(Nietzsche)

What changes in the content of medicine did the laboratory revolution bring about? Historians of science and medicine these days are wary of pleas for a renewed concern with content, fearing that they conceal hankerings after the noble simplicities of old-fashioned internalist and intellectualist chronicles of discovery and the succession of theories. However, the changes of content that I have in mind do not have to do with discoveries and doctrines. Two other and more fundamental sorts of change of content cry out for investigation. First there are changes in what I shall call 'the scene of medical inquiry' – the ranges of questions that were validated and invalidated, rendered 'real' and 'unreal' for medics by the laboratory revolution. Secondly, there are changes in the lived experience of medicine brought about by the laboratory revolution, changes in what it was like to be involved in medicine – as teacher, clinician, general practitioner, pharmacologist, microbiologist, orderly, nurse, patient, experimental animal, etc.

What is it for a question to be locally real, to belong to the scene of inquiry of a community of practitioners of a discipline? Elsewhere I have proposed a detailed account of scenes of inquiry and of the ways in which the historian may come to understand past scenes of inquiry.[16] On that account the scene of inquiry of a community consists of those questions with which they can see in principle how to get to grips. Local scenes of inquiry depend both on the communal beliefs which constitute presuppositions of questions and, more fundamentally, on the communal practices of inquiry through which attempts may be made to resolve questions. Change in local scenes of inquiry comes about through change in presuppositions and through change in practices of inquiry. Thus, to take a simple example, questions about the number, nature and modes of operation of vital forces became locally real when certain communities of medics and natural historians came to believe in the existence of vital forces and came to practice forms of inquiry which enabled them to see how, in principle, they might acquire evidence relevant to the resolution of questions about vital forces. Those questions ceased to be real for inquirers when they ceased to believe in the existence of vital forces or ceased to regard questions about them as potentially resoluble by their methods of inquiry.

[16] N. Jardine, *The Scenes of Inquiry: On the Reality of Questions in the Sciences* (Oxford, 1991).

Rather than setting out my own example of the way in which the laboratory revolution made new questions real for medics I shall lazily lift my example from Cunningham's fascinating and provocative contribution to this volume. Cunningham claims that historians cannot coherently attribute beliefs about or experience of the disease we know as 'plague' prior to 1894, the year in which the specific micro-organism responsible for plague was identified by experimental operations based on Koch's rules for the demonstration of specific pathogens. Translating into our terms, this is the claim that all questions about plague, in *our* sense of the term, were unreal before 1894.

This claim is, on my account, too strong. However, my account licenses a related but more circumspect claim. There is a vast range of questions real for present-day medics about the aetiology and epidemiology of plague which presuppose the assignment of plague to the class of diseases uniquely caused by specific pathogenic micro-organisms. None of these questions was locally real prior to the local acceptance of this presupposition. They were locally realised only when communities of inquirers were formed who accepted this presupposition and developed practices of inquiry that enabled them to see how, at least in principle, they might get to grips with them.

On my reading of the evidence this weaker claim entails a gradual and piecemeal realisation of questions about the ways pathogens cause and spread diseases including plague in the second half of the nineteenth century. Despite its moderation my claim justifies Cunningham's main historical and historiographical conclusions. The practices which led to the realisation of such aetiological and epidemiological questions were, as he insists, all laboratory practices: without the development of specialised laboratory equipment and specific laboratory routines, no one could have seen how in principle to get to grips with any of them.[17] And the kind of historiography of medicine to which he objects is effectively outlawed. On my account, as on his, it is incoherent to project into the pre-laboratory period concern with the causation and spread of diseases by pathogens in the case of plague and other diseases, let alone to discern successive anticipations of our aetiological and epidemiological doctrines.

[17] The formation of laboratory-based methods competent to resolve questions about the pathogenic aetiology of diseases is explored in detail in a series of articles by K. Codell Carter: 'The Koch–Pasteur dispute on establishing the cause of anthrax', *Bulletin of the History of Medicine*, 62 (1988), pp. 42–57; 'Edwin Klebs' criteria for disease causality', *Medizinhistorisches Journal*, 22 (1987), pp. 80–9; 'Koch's postulates in relation to the work of Jacob Henle and Edwin Klebs', *Medical History*, 29 (1985), pp. 353–74.

On my account it is local practices of inquiry that we must investigate if we are to understand the ways in which the laboratory revolution shifted the scenes of medical inquiry.

To start with we should note that there may be only modest mileage to be had from consideration of the declared general epistemologies of the principal spokesmen for a laboratory-based medicine. The very generality of the methodological pronouncements of Claude Bernard, T. H. Huxley, Emil du Bois-Reymond and others make it hard to see how communal commitment to their various versions of 'the experimental method' could be used to account for the local realisation of specific new questions in medicine. At best, it may be that the successful promotion of such empiricist commitments can be used to account for the dissolution of questions once real. Thus Claude Bernard and Emil du Bois-Reymond explicitly argue that questions about the essence and origins of life are improper for men of science because all such questions lie entirely beyond the reach of experimental inquiry. (English readers are often startled when they find Bernard dismissing Charles Darwin's speculations on these grounds along with the speculations of such *Naturphilosophen* as Oken and Carus.) Moreover, as a now extensive body of recent sociological work has shown, there are often major discrepancies between publicly expressed methodology and the actual practices of inquiry, presentation and adjudication. It is methods in use rather than methods officially espoused (*logica utens* rather than *logica docens* in scholastic terminology) that are the prime determinants of perceptions of the relevance of evidence to questions and hence of their local reality.

If we are to understand the changes in scenes of medical inquiry brought about by the laboratory revolution we must consider specific methods and practices local to particular disciplines, institutions and factions. In particular, we need to consider how new methods and practices were introduced into and maintained in medical institutions.

As Weindling's contribution indicates, we may learn much about the details of daily routines of work and about the social and cognitive division of labour from the architecture and layout of medical institutions.[18] Thus we can gain valuable insights into the varied roles of the laboratory in medicine – as preparation rooms for demon-

[18] On the inference of didactic and experimental ideals, goals and practices from laboratory architecture and layout see the masterly studies by Sophie Forgan: 'Context, image and function: a preliminary inquiry into the architecture of scientific societies', *British Journal for the History of Science*, 19 (1986), pp. 89–113; 'The architecture of science and the idea of a university', *Studies in History and Philosophy of Science*, 20 (1989), pp. 405–34.

strations, as locations of hands-on learning, as places of restricted access and professional initiation. In this connection special interest attaches to the question of the precedents and models for the various types of medical laboratories. How far can the new medical laboratory practices be seen as extensions and transformations of practices already established in medicine: the practices of the anatomy theatre and its preparation room, the practices of hygienists, of pharmacists, etc? How far are they to be seen as imported from or modelled on the practices of other disciplines: on the laboratory practices of the Mechanics' Institutes and learned scientific societies that proliferated from the 1820s; on the practices of the German physiology institutes of the 1840s, '50s and '60s (themselves variously modelled on observatories, analytical chemistry laboratories and even on the disciplines of the classical philology seminar); on the physics laboratories of the 1860s and 70s (themselves often modelled on the practices of the factory bench)?[19]

Pride of place amongst the determinants of the new questions realised by the laboratory revolution must go to the new instruments and preparations thereby introduced into medical training and research. Precisely how were the new instruments used? How were they calibrated and standardised? How were they modified in the interests of greater reliability, durability, portability and mass-producibility? How were they adapted to new types of user and new types of application? How far was their use articulated in user manuals and textbooks; how far did competence in their use depend upon acquisition of tacit know-how? How was such expertise distributed within the medical profession, between practitioners and technicians, between laboratories of different types in different institutions and nations? Such issues are crucial for the understanding and explanation of the new scenes of medical inquiry.[20]

Tormented animals and other living preparations, Claude Bernard's 'throbbing and fetid ground of life': here the link with new

[19] On the models for German physiology institutes see Tuchman, 'From the lecture to the laboratory' and Lenoir, 'Science for the clinic'; on industrial models for physics laboratories see M. Norton Wise and Crosbie Smith, 'Measurement, work and industry in Lord Kelvin's Britain', *Historical Studies in the Physical Sciences*, 17 (1987), pp. 147–73.

[20] Relevant studies sensitive to these issues include: T. Lenoir, 'Models and instruments in the development of electrophysiology, 1845–1912', *Historical Studies in the Physical Sciences*, 17 (1987), pp. 1–54; R. G. Frank, Jr, 'The telltale heart: physiological instruments, graphic methods, and clinical hopes 1854–1914' in Coleman and Holmes (eds), *The Investigative Enterprise*; M. Borell, 'Instruments and an independent physiology: the Harvard Physiological Laboratory, 1871–1906' in G. L. Geison (ed.), *Physiology in the American Context* (Bethesda, Md, 1987), pp. 293–321.

scenes of medical inquiry is peculiarly direct. Their role is a double one: as 'objects' of demonstration they preside over the initiation of medical students into the goals, methods and agendas of experimental physiology; as 'subjects' of experimentation they define particular subject matters and fields of research. Thus in manuals and textbooks of experimental physiology we find that the range of questions addressed is closely tied to limited repertoires of standard frog, cat and dog preparations: at the elementary level the nerve–muscle preparation of the frog gastrocnemius, the various perfused heart preparations, etc.; at the more advanced level such ghastly wonders as Magendie's spinal preparation of the frog and the Sherrington decapitated dog. To study the way in which such preparations extended the scenes of medical inquiry it would be necessary to undertake some grim researches. Precisely how were living animals and living flesh rendered 'docile', immobilised, injected, dissected, stabilised, so as to constitute instruments for the exploration of particular replicable physiological effects? And how precisely were the responses of the docile animals and organs monitored, amplified, plotted, mapped and logged so as to provide convincing and publishable findings?

The laboratory manuals of the period are often, by present-day standards, extraordinarily explicit on questions of purchase, installation and operation of instruments and preparations. Indeed, the instructions on such topics as how to prepare a potato slice as a culture medium (Fig. 27) are often reminiscent of the hilarious accounts of such skills as walking upstairs in Julio Cortàzar's 'The instruction manual'.[21] But laboriously though the manuals seek to convey to medics the new skills, there is much in the way of procedural detail and conditions for competent performance that they do not, or cannot, convey. Further insight into local laboratory practices is doubtless to be gained from laboratory notebooks, students' lecture and demonstration notes, from the reports of visitors seeking instruction in foreign laboratories, etc.[22] But if we are to gain the maximum appreciation of the details of the skills and routines of laboratory medicine there is clearly no substitute for attempts to reconstruct and replicate the experiments ourselves.[23] (God, or failing Him the licensing regulations, forbid that historians of medicine should reconstruct and replicate in full the horrors of the nineteenth-century experimental physiology laboratory!)

What of the other type of change in the content of medicine brought

[21] J. Cortàzar, *Cronopios and Famas*, trans. P. Blackburn (London, 1978), pp. 1–26.

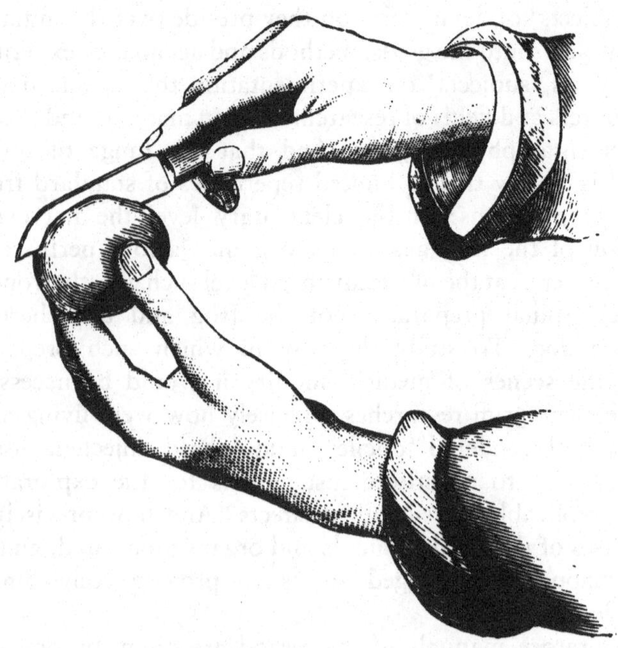

Fig. 27. How to cut a potato in half, as described in an 1887 manual of bacteriology. The potato is to be used as a culture medium, and the trick is to avoid contamination of the cut surfaces.

about by the laboratory revolution: change in the lived experience of those involved in medicine? My suggestion here is that the priorities of the historical research needed to understand and explain changes in scenes of medical inquiry scarcely differ from those needed for an appreciation of the changes in lived medical experience. Local and specific practices and routines, the architecture and layout of the institutions of medicine, temperamental instruments, tormented animals and pulsating preparations – knowledge of all this is crucial for any appreciation of changes in the lived experience of medicine.

But here a caveat is in order. Historical research alone cannot

[22] For evidence of the rich rewards of study of laboratory notebooks see, for example, F. L. Holmes, *Lavoisier and the Chemistry of Life: An Exploration of Scientific Creativity* (Madison, Wis., 1985), and D. Gooding, *Experiment and the Making of Meaning* (Dordrecht, 1990).

[23] David Gooding has repeatedly and effectively emphasised this point: see, for example, 'History in the laboratory: can we really tell what went on?' in F. A. J. L. James (ed.), *The Development of the Laboratory* (London, 1989), pp. 63–82.

enable the historian to appreciate and convey past lived experience. For such appreciation requires not only knowledge but also imaginative projection and response. Knowledge of past local environments and practices is a precondition for such appreciation. But success in achieving and inducing in others imaginative projection into the experience of past medicine depends on the ways in which past local environments are described and represented, past local practices reconstructed and re-enacted, past lives narrated and dramatised.[24]

Every thing is what it is and not another thing
(Bishop Butler)

I have argued for the fruitfulness of an interpretation of the laboratory revolution in medicine which stands in sharp opposition not only to the traditional presentist historiography of doctrines, discoveries and scientific progress but also to certain current textualist and sociological contenders for the place vacated by the traditional historiography. In part the contrast is one of goals. The proposed historiography has as its goal the understanding of change in the contents of disciplines, both the content that is constituted by the ranges of questions real for their practitioners and the content that is constituted by their lived experience: in sum, an understanding of changes in the worlds of past disciplines. Both understanding of past concepts and doctrines, on the one hand, and of past textual and social conventions, on the other, figure in such a historiography as means rather than ends. But there is a contrast that is, I think, yet more fundamental, a contrast in the conception of the sources of changes in disciplines.

On the historiographical proposals sketched here two sorts of incitement to human action play central roles – rhetorical incitement and aesthetic incitement. Rhetorical incitement as here conceived includes the entire range of persuasive strategies, appeal to ideals of rationality and morality, appeal to authority, appeal to social and factional interests. Rhetorical incitement is doubly social, social in the

[24] Methodological issues concerning the recovery of past lived experience have been little addressed in recent Anglo-American historiography of the sciences. It is, however, a central concern of French *histoire des mentalités*. The effectiveness of *mentaliste* techniques in recovering and conveying past lived experience in the sciences is revealed in two works influenced by the *mentaliste* approach: R. Darnton, *Mesmerism and the End of the Enlightenment in France* (Cambridge, Mass., 1969); K. Pomian, *Collectionneurs, amateurs et curieux. Paris, Vénise: XVIe–XVIIIe siècle* (Paris, 1987).

sense that it presupposes and works through social conventions of presentation and argument and social in the sense that it is targeted on the social goals, attitudes and assumptions of its recipients. But more is involved in rhetorical appeal and response than the blind play of conventions of persuasion and social interests. Successful rhetorical incitement involves actions, the actions of the persons who deploy persuasive strategies, who interpret and criticise them, who respond to or contest them.

Aesthetic incitement as here conceived includes the whole range of ways in which perceptible things – gestures, words, representations, instruments, preparations, displays and demonstrations – move persons through their appeal to the senses, the imagination and the emotions. There is now a quite substantial literature on the aesthetics of representations in the sciences: exemplary works include Rudwick's study of the roles of conventions and techniques of mapping in the formation of geology as a discipline and Lenoir's exploration of the links between the rise of realism in painting and optics and the involvement of scientists in the politics of practical interests of Bismarck's *Kaiserreich*.[25] In connection with the laboratory revolution in medicine a study of the traces, plots and graphs generated from the new instruments of experimental physiology would yield ample dividends. Equally if not, in the present instance, more important as an incitement to commitment, action and discipline is the as-yet unexplored aesthetics of the specific materials of the laboratory practices of medicine. We need an aesthetics of the 'real and active' things to which Latour has so eloquently directed our attention, an aesthetics of things in all their mundane particularity and contingency: prestigious new research institutes along with anatomy preparation rooms hastily converted to laboratories; beautifully designed and precisely calibrated microscopes along with ramshackle and unpredictable sphygmographs; gently twitching frogs along with struggling tormented dogs. Aesthetic incitement is again doubly social, social in the sense that it presupposes and works through social conventions for the staging and demonstration of things, their illustration and representation, and social in the sense that the modes of aesthetic response are, for the most part, socially instilled dispositions. But here again more is involved than the blind

[25] M. Rudwick, 'The emergence of a visual language for geological science, 1760–1840', *History of Science*, 14 (1976), pp. 149–95; T. Lenoir, 'The politics of vision: optics, painting and ideology in Germany, 1845–1880', forthcoming. See also the collection of articles edited by B. Latour and B. de Noblet, *Les 'Vues' de l'esprit*, special issue of *Culture Technique*, 14 (1985); Jardine, *Scenes of Inquiry*, ch. 10.

play of social conventions and dispositions. Aesthetic appeal and response depend upon the powers and appearances of the things themselves.

I have already protested at the ways in which currently fashionable historiographies treat persons as unreflective dupes of social and textual conventions. Things too receive raw deals: downgraded to social constructs by interest theorists; inflated by network theorists into members of society credited with goals and strategies; interpreted as projections from the 'intertextual universe' by post-modernists. These strange construals of things rest on genuine insights. Interest theorists are right in their view of the phenomena of science as representing not direct perceptions of the world but consensuses achieved and maintained by complex social interactions; and their *cui bono est*? is often effective in uncovering the hidden motivations of such negotiations. Network theorists are right to insist on the powers of things to embody human knowledge and skill, to incite and control the actions of persons. And, conversely, they are right to insist that persons, singly and socially, are not only intelligences, wills and bearers of interests but also material bodies interacting with other material bodies. Textualists are right to insist that all writing, even that which purports to convey unadorned the things and events of the real world, may be read as commentary, formed and informed by countless earlier texts. They are right too in emphasising the paramount importance of conventions of representation in the formation of the 'idealised' obedient and predictable things that figure in the annals of completed science. The historiography proposed here would exploit these insights – without maltreating things.

If there is a single philosophical moral to be drawn from my reflexions on the roles of rhetorical and aesthetic incitement in the laboratory revolution in medicine it is that a common-sense ontology suffices for historical understanding. This transformation of medicine, like other transformations of disciplines, is to be accounted for in terms of the predilections, plans and deeds of persons and of the powers and efficacies of things.

11

Gendered reflexions on the laboratory in medicine

HILARY ROSE

Janus's fourth dictum:
When things are true they hold. When things hold they start becoming true.
(Latour)[1]

Reflexions on actual and imaginary meetings

While the feminist critique of science over these past fifteen years has been richly abundant, it is still possible for most papers at a mainstream meeting in the historical and social studies of science – even an agreeable meeting such as the Cambridge conference where this book began – to cast the dimension of gender as unproblematic. Its discussion is left to the quiet aside, and the exchange in the safety of the women's room; or perhaps it generates a moment of anger when a suffragist becomes a 'suffragette', and yet again women indicate that sexist categories are not to be tolerated. The overall air of civility is such that it is as if the only thing that is wrong is the gender balance of the meetings; the content is fine, and women and men are working together sensitively and appreciatively.

Yet the situation can be read differently. Despite the pleasantness of the discussion, the hegemony of the old ungendered (i.e. masculinist) knowledge that we are listening to, and indeed learning from – for that's the complexity – is at the same moment under siege. Whether or not the debate between the critical knowledge produced by feminists and that of masculinism is formally enjoined at any specific meeting, there is both 'out there' – and for some of us sharply in our own heads – a struggle between accounts. For significant numbers of women and

Acknowledgements: My thanks to the Editors, Andrew Cunningham and Perry Williams, for their supportive and critical editing.

[1] Bruno Latour, *Science in Action: How to Follow Scientists and Engineers Through Society* (Milton Keynes, 1987), p. 12.

their allies whose lives and understanding have been touched by the women's movement and its theorising, Janus' fourth dictum holds, but perhaps not quite in the sense intended by Latour. For it too has its context(s).

Reflecting on this set of papers discussing the laboratory in medicine, the silences – with some deviant murmurings – suggest that gender does not, in Bruno Latour's sense, 'hold', so obviously cannot be 'true'. Yet in other contexts where scholarly work has explored the silences, gender does indeed hold and the analysis of patriarchical relations within science, both as a knowledge-producing system and as knowledge itself is indeed 'becoming true'.[2] In consequence, to reflect on these papers is for feminists to experience a sense of mild schizophrenia – of not quite being able to connect to the texts on offer. Fortunately, at the Cambridge meeting, as well as the texts there were also conversations and pictures – even a movie – and it was in these that the silences became less complete.

Thus our hosts, taking the view that all work and no play make very dull children (and conferees), encouraged us to enter the world of science fiction through showing the film *Things to Come*. This exceedingly masculinist vision of H. G. Wells (just why did the brilliant feminist Rebecca West put up with him and his phallic air-dictatorship?) projects a technologically innovative and socially conservative future. This gives me the excuse to make my argument by drawing on a rather different utopian tradition, whose political project makes a decisive break, not just from Wells – as if he were some figure from the past of whom we can all be safely critical – but from the all-pervasive socially conservative tradition of mainstream/malestream science fiction. Instead, let's imagine a meeting on the history of the laboratory in medicine in a feminist science-fictional

[2] The feminist/social-studies-of-science critique of science has now an extensive literature. Key texts would include the special issue 'Women, science and society', *Signs: Journal of Women in Culture and Society*, 4 (1978), pp. 1–216; Evelyn Fox Keller, *Reflections on Gender and Science* (New Haven, 1985); Sandra Harding, *The Science Question in Feminism* (Milton Keynes, 1986). Overviews of the literature are provided by Hilary Rose, 'Beyond masculinist realities', in Ruth Bleier (ed.), *Feminist Approaches to Science* (Oxford, 1986), pp. 57–76; Londa Schiebinger, 'The history and philosophy of women in science: a review essay', in Sandra Harding and Jean F. O'Barr (eds), *Sex and Scientific Inquiry* (Chicago, 1987), pp. 7–34. The mainstream literature refuses any acknowledgement of gender relations, and indeed one of the most interesting journals, *Social Studies of Science*, tolerates a degree of sexism in language which few other journals in the social or biological sciences would accept. Criticisms of this androcentricity may be found in Sara Delamont, 'Three blind spots? A comment on the sociology of science by a puzzled outsider', *Social Studies of Science*, 17 (1987), pp. 163–70; Evelyn Fox Keller's 1987 address to the Four S and Hilary Rose's 1988 address to the new Women's Studies section within the Four S and EAST.

utopia. It seems reasonable to claim that papers, conversation and images would be rather different. No doubt there would be an extensive literary and political debate concerning which feminist utopia would make the ideal location for the symposium; none the less, in view of the acclaim which has for good reason greeted their SF novels, surely Joanna Russ's Whileaway and Marge Piercy's Mattapoisett would be the two most favoured locations. Both Russ's *The Female Man* (1975) and Piercy's *Woman on the Edge of Time* (1979) take the view that there is nothing inevitable about the development of science and technology, or indeed in our relations to either science and technology or even to nature itself. Their feminist SF creates safe places, dream laboratories where we may safely experiment with different and other ways of living and thinking. From the safe freedom of the fictional utopia, both the past and the actual present may all the more effectively be examined under a critical microscope.

Despite their common features, the utopias of Russ and Piercy represent very different solutions to the feminist project of overcoming patriarchy, with different answers as to how and under what circumstances it is possible to move towards a society – and knowledges – no longer divided/deformed by gender. Whileaway (literally while the men are away) offers an alternative society which perhaps takes place now – for the linearity of time seems to have lost its grip – and is both separatist and replete with the fractured identities of post-modernism. Mattapoisett, also ambiguously located in time, has found another solution, envisioning a post-gendered society where difference is blurred both at the physiological and social levels. In this realist novel a utopian image is offered of a lactating bearded person feeding a baby, and the personal pronoun has of course become 'per'; so even realism at the hands of feminism is playful. Thus not only would the utopian conference be rather different from that of today's mainstream history of science, but that held in Whileaway and that in Mattapoisett would also be rather different (not least in composition) from one another.

In both, however, the claims of nineteenth-century physiology to be an experimental and exact method of producing knowledge, offering to medicine the chance to become truly scientific, and science's self-conception of its civilising influence on doctors, would be inconceivable. The intellectual framework would demand taking gender into account in constituting experimental science, and also experimental science into account in constituting gender. From their post-gendered/separatist vantage-points the papers might begin with some exploration of the overarching preoccupation of the nineteenth century, with 'Woman' cast both as the 'Other' and as 'Nature', a story in which women are conceived of as outside history, as objects but not subjects of history.

It would not be passed over in silence that Claude Bernard described 'nature as a woman who must be forced to unveil herself when attacked by the experimenter, who must be put to the question and subdued'.[3] In this phrase, Bernard reveals himself as a direct masculinist descendant of Bacon, and this would not be seen as accidental. Instead, in Mattapoisett or Whileaway, papers might explore what part this ideological commitment to violence against both 'Nature' and 'Woman' played in ensuring the greater claims to scientificity of physiology over and above those of an observational, and non-violent, discipline such as zoology.[4] While the British advocates of laboratory training had spoken of its benefits for medical training and the US advocates spoke more grandly of 'training the mind' in the scientific method, our utopian conference would pick up on the critical questions in these papers concerning the implication for medicine of physiology's highly reductionist conception of 'the' scientific method. Why was it more scientific to look within the organism for the origin of disease, and what did it mean for the organisation of medicine and the care of patients – not least women? The question asked by the nineteenth-century feminist and antivivisectionist Frances Power Cobbe would be very seriously addressed: 'How could one expect medical students brutalised by their exposure to vivisection to metamorphose overnight into respectable, courteous and caring doctors?'[5] Deconstructing science's civilising claim would be a prime analytical task.

Our conference might examine why it was that science, not least physiology, in the late twentieth century, was for the greater part still

[3] Claude Bernard, *An Introduction to the Study of Experimental Medicine*, trans. Henry Copley Greene (New York, 1957), pp. 22–3; as quoted in Coral Lansbury, *The Old Brown Dog: Women, Workers, and Vivisection in Edwardian England* (Madison, Wis., 1985), pp. 162–3.

[4] Bernard claimed that 'adopting the practice of vivisection, physiologists had caused their discipline to make the all-important transition to the level of experimental status'; by contrast, zoology was merely observational. Elliott suggests that vivisection 'did not arise out of medicine and the search for the explanation of disease, although Magendie and Bernard in particular always used this as a justification for their work. On the contrary, vivisection had its origins deep within science.' Paul Elliott, 'Vivisection and the emergence of experimental physiology in nineteenth-century France', in Nicolaas A. Rupke (ed.), *Vivisection in Historical Perspective* (London, 1987), pp. 48–77, at p. 75.

[5] Mary Ann Elston, 'Women and anti-vivisection in Victorian England, 1870–1900', in Rupke (ed.), *Vivisection in Historical Perspective*, p. 277.

produced by – or, more precisely, inscribed by – white middle-class men. And what was the significance of production by this rather peculiar subgroup within the population for the content of science? The papers would cast light on the resounding silence from the mainstream social studies of science concerning the contribution of both women scientists (from Hypatia to Rosalind Franklin) and working-class men and women technicians to the production of knowledge.[6] Historians have brought out the class and gender character of the witnesses to scientific experiment in the nineteenth century, and indicated how mere assistants could not validate science; yet there has been no corresponding analysis of laboratory life today, as to why working-class men and women (especially women technicians in biological laboratories) might in the late twentieth century only work as invisible producers. Despite a possibly less hierarchical construction of the contemporary laboratory, technicians may still not, in all too many, inscribe their names on the sacred texts.

Other papers would explore why the mainstream of social studies of science, even though it managed to escape internalism, none the less became stuck halfway in its move towards reflexivity. Why was it that, despite the new perspectives on nature associated with the new social movements, the accounts of the mainstream social studies remained for so long unraced and ungendered, and handled even the seemingly well-honed concept of class cautiously, if at all?[7] Thus even where the social studies of science embrace post-modernism, and endorse the constructionist account of truth claims, they exclude many of the 'differences' that post-modernism, whatever else it might be criticised for, is potentially able to include.

More positively, looking at the changes which helped overcome this patriarchal conservatism, papers might explore the systematic funding

[6] Even when empirical material on lab technicians is reported and seems to invite a gendered analysis, the opportunity is passed up. Thus in Latour and Woolgar's ethnography of a laboratory an exchange is reported between a scientist (male) and a technician (female). She thinks her contribution was crucial to the production of knowledge, he does not. We are not told, but it would seem likely that his, not her, name was therefore inscribed on the text (*Laboratory Life: The Social Construction of Scientific Facts* (London, 1979), p. 219). For the masculinist gaze of the mainstream social studies of science the issue of the power relation embedded in the language of the exchange is dissolved in the technical appearance of the discourse. Not for nothing did the feminist philosopher Mary O'Brien make the joke that 'mainstream' equals 'malestream'.

[7] This begins to change, at least in the alternative streams. In addition to the feminist literature in the social studies of science, which increasingly addresses issues of 'race', the taken-for-granted whiteness of men's accounts begins to be made problematic. See Martin Bernal, *Black Athena: The Afroasiatic Roots of Classical Civilisation* (London, 1987); and Ivan van Sertima, *Blacks in Science: Ancient and Modern* (New Brunswick, 1985).

of gendered research in the United States, as in the Rockefeller Fellowships in theoretical work, the Mellon grants or the Streisand chair, and remap the influence of key trusts and foundations on the restructuring of knowledge in the twentieth century. This US situation would be compared with the British experience, where there has been a general policy of financial starvation of theoretical or empirical feminist research, except in a few policy-approved areas – notably health and, above all, 'motherhood' and employment. The rather few empirical social studies of science carried out in Britain by feminists have been doctoral theses, where feminists have often rather successfully run off with the proferred freedom.[8] Funded post-doctoral work is a species scarcely permitted to come into existence. The examination of this peculiarly British masculinist research policy would indicate why well-meaning men, such as our hosts, would – and did – find it hard to secure empirical historical papers from feminists. Today women working in the history of science are working in a profoundly gendered knowledge system and it is more comfortable to discuss one's feminist scholarship elsewhere.

Such papers would examine the detailed practices through which masculinist truth-protectors, or constructionists (for both realists and constructionists keep firm hold on the knowledge production process), maintained the marginality of feminist scholarship, hoping perhaps that eventually the movement and its scholars would fade away.[9] What was the hope? That if the revolution was staved off, then normal (i.e. men's) science could get to work again? In consequence the most exciting section of this entirely utopian conference would be those historical papers analysing and debating the extraordinary processes – entirely unforeseen in the 1980s – whereby masculinist hegemony had suddenly yielded during the 1990s and how science and science studies had become post-gendered in the twenty-first century.

[8] See Wendy Farrant, 'Who's for amniocentesis? the politics of prenatal screening' in Hilary Homans (ed.), *The Sexual Politics of Reproduction* (Aldershot, 1985); and Kim Thomas, *Gender and Subject in Higher Education* (Milton Keynes, 1990).

[9] A paradigmatic example of the powerfully exclusivist nature of the debate between men is contained in Hilary Lawson and Lisa Appignanesi (eds), *Dismantling Truth: Reality in the Post-Modern World* (London, 1989). Here the social constructionists and the realists are lined up very sharply – and elegantly – against one another. It goes without saying that neither side takes any notice of the feminist theoretical debate of epistemology. This refusal enables the contributors to continue the classically masculinist and dichotomous stance of 'either/or'. In marked contrast, feminism's theoretical distaste for dichotomous reasoning, and its deepening commitment to inclusivity, means that its stance is one of 'both/and'.

A lab of our own?

But before I become carried away by our utopian conference, the facts are (and how interesting it is to use the word 'facts' in this sentence) that such conferences are not totally science-fictional events but exist today in reasonably coherent prefigurative forms. Many women academics, and indeed a number of men, have by this point in the twentieth century had the experience of taking part in feminist conferences and in consequence may have both a political and an epistemological appreciation of the different discourses of a taken-for-granted masculinism and a conscious feminism. What happens to those different discourses, how they weave around, accommodate and oppose one another, is another story. But the point I want to make is that even where a set of papers is largely located within gender-blind goalposts and the discussion is more or less tidy, some of us know the posts have been moved – and maybe into another dimension.

Thus whereas Bruno Latour once wrote 'Give me a laboratory and I' (singlehandedly?) 'will raise the world', feminists have collectively raised a great diversity of labs and are indeed here and now raising the world. From Virginia Woolf's claim for 'a room of one's own' in the early twentieth century, the new feminism has argued for, and collectively built, not just a lab but an academy of our own in the late twentieth. Indeed the existence of the feminist academy – in the form of the growth of women's studies – begins to trouble patriarchy. A Dutch sociologist, Professor Schuyt, at a recent international conference on the theme of the crisis of knowledge, 'Does the university still lead the way?', suggested that these 'group oriented neo-disciplines challenged the unity of the scientific method and community and the universalization of knowledge'.[10] He is of course right. Women's studies as a group-oriented knowledge does indeed challenge these claims. What Schuyt does not see is how far the existing sciences also might be fairly called group-oriented neo-disciplines – or, to put it more bluntly, men's studies. Viewed from within the perspectives of feminism, the continued and increasingly abundant production of feminist research, strengthened by its linkages with the women's movement, has led to a situation in which, for growing numbers of women, 'things' which hold and are true for many men increasingly don't hold for women, and we have more than doubts about their truthfulness.

[10] Reported in the *Times Higher Educational Supplement*, 30 September 1989, p. 9.

Maintaining ungendered history

Of course history, along with the social studies of science, is not 'science' but 'about' science; but this seems scarcely sufficient to exempt the production of historical knowledge from a Latourian analysis. In such a schema, a recalcitrant who doubts the 'fact' that the laboratory in medicine has nothing to do with gender relations, who suspects that masculinism reigns and is all the more powerful for reigning invisibly, has to be shown the scale of the technical and social forces against which her doubts are being pitted. Thus, as Latour reminds/warns us, having doubts about scientific truths is not a cost-free business. Drawing on a very revealing military metaphor, he writes 'technoscience is war'. Hence allies of the 'truth' are to be mobilised and its enemies isolated, and the price of doubting is exclusion. 'In general the technical appearance of the scientific literature is nothing but its social character, its display of armed phalanxes making it pointless to resist.' Scarcely surprisingly, he sees doubters as having no possibility of overturning the dominant truth-holders.[11] As the proto-sociologist Mandy Rice-Davies observed, robustly drawing on an interest theory of knowledge: 'Well he would, wouldn't he?'[12]

But while recalcitrants ponder what it is about medicine, laboratories, and men that made/make them all so reflective of and constitutive of masculinist hegemony, so that the masculinism is rendered (almost) invisible, hidden by the technical appearance of the discourse, it seems that tools increasingly sharpened by current analytical strategies could, if taken seriously, help dig the grave of masculinism. Above all, if reflexivity is taken seriously then all sorts of excluded 'facts' start entering. Of course if reflexivity is taken sillily, and the discipline does seem to be 'well endowed with silly men' (to only slightly mischievously rewrite Steven Shapin's brilliantly witty and distinctly sexist review of *Science in Action*),[13] they can observe every nuance in the division of labour, carry out discourse analysis, analyse power, scrupulously study content – and still produce gender-blind/masculinist knowledge.

[11] Latour, *Science in Action*, p. 62.

[12] Mandy Rice-Davies, a prostitute and a central figure in the Profumo affair, made this retort in the light of a public man's denial that he knew her.

[13] The original androcentric quotation was, 'This is one of the funniest books in a discipline which is well-endowed with funny-men'. Steven Shapin, 'Following scientists around', *Social Studies of Science*, 18 (1988), pp. 533–50.

Texts and talk

Interestingly, at the Cambridge meeting, the first moment when the possibility arose that something other than the exclusively technical was taking place came with Stewart Richards's introduction to his paper. Speaking as a participating 'I', both as an experimental physiologist and historian, Stewart recalled first the physiology centenary exhibition and his revulsion at the stench, and then the personal as well as intellectual problem of sorting out the nature of that revulsion. He observed that research which used the 'method of pain' needed to be seen to be detached and objective, and so served to make the object of study detached and objective. I found myself thinking that, distinct from the use or non-use of anaesthetics in the experimental laboratory, it seemed that the quality of our exchanges had up to that moment anaesthetised our discussion of the 'method of pain'. Parallel to an apologia for physiology, the defence of laying bare the nerve, there was a corresponding – and reflexive – courage in laying bare the moral and aesthetic response. Thus it was the spoken presentation of the paper which took reflexivity seriously, which made it possible to make connections between the mainstream and the feminist histories.

Did Mr Jekyll become Dr Hyde?

It was a rather beautiful Freudian slip which for me triggered the connection. Thus we were invited to consider what transmogrification came over John Burdon-Sanderson, the family man and physiologist, as he entered the University College laboratory door. 'Did', we were asked, 'Mr Jekyll become Dr Hyde?'

In answering that question, Frances Power Cobbe, a central figure in the twin struggles against vivisection and wife-beating, would have had few doubts. For Cobbe the brutal scientist and the brutal husband were one and the same person. Indeed Burdon-Sanderson's unhappy wife left her own message as to her views by leaving her money to an animal refuge. Not by chance, mainstream accounts of the anti-vivisection movement, such as that of Westacott,[14] ignore Cobbe's involvement in the campaign against violence to wives even while they acknowledge her feminism, thus denying what was for her a theoretically and politically linked struggle. The problem for Cobbe,

[14] E. Westacott, *A Century of Vivisection and Anti-vivisection* (Ashingdon, 1947).

and indeed for a long strand of feminist analysis extending to the contemporary theorists Andrea Dworkin and Mary Daly,[15] is precisely the nature of men. Her article 'Wife torture in England', published in the influential *Contemporary Review* in 1878,[16] exposed men's cruelty and sensuality, and has become a founding text for contemporary feminists engaged in the battered women's movement. It has been the feminist historian Mary Ann Elston who has remade the link, drawing attention to Cobbe's speculation, during the height of the Jack the Ripper panic, as to whether the Ripper was a physiologist 'delirious with cruelty'.[17]

At the same time, Cobbe's moral reasoning about the proper relationship between animals and people is very different from the perspectives of the contemporary animal rights movement, in which many feminists are actively involved. She and many of her fellow activists saw animals not as subjects with rights but as objects claiming our moral concern. In Cobbe's autobiography, she quoted with approval the eighteenth-century Quaker John Woolman:

> I believe, where the love of God is verily perfected and the true spirit of government watchfully attended, a tenderness to all creatures made subject to us will be expressed, and a care felt in us that we do not lessen that sweetness of life in the animal creation which the Great Creator intends for them under our government.[18]

Cobbe understood very well that to oppose the mechanistic construction of animals by the Bernards and the Magendies which legitimised using animals' bodies as if they were machines and therefore without feelings, it was crucial to produce an account of animal consciousness. Cobbe used the *Quarterly Review* to publish an article, 'The consciousness of dogs'. Her autobiography reports with some pleasure that Darwin thought well of this piece. Indeed at this point Cobbe thought well of Darwin, seeing him as 'a man who would not allow a fly to bite a pony's neck'.[19] While Darwin himself was revolted by experimental methods and indeed found surgery on children, without anaesthetic, quite intolerable (a significant part of

[15] Dworkin and Daly as cultural or radical feminists have simply given up on the possibility that men can be changed. Their ultimate theoretical appeal is to the biological basis of men's violent nature. Paradoxically, instead of inspiring an ideology of subordination as with contemporary sociobiology, it inspires an enraged and woman-centred politics – claimed to be both different from and better than that of men – or even non-radical feminists.

[16] *Contemporary Review*, 32 (1878), pp. 55–87.

[17] Elston, 'Women and anti-vivisection', p. 281.

[18] Westacott, *A Century of Vivisection and Anti-vivisection*, p. 24; Frances Power Cobbe, *Life of Frances Power Cobbe: as Told by Herself*, posthumous edn (London, 1904), p. 619.

[19] *Quarterly Review*, 133 (1872), pp. 419–51; Cobbe, *Life of Frances Power Cobbe*, pp. 489 and 491.

the reason why he abandoned medicine), Cobbe did not recognise that – to use Stewart Richards's distinction – although he was aesthetically repelled, morally he could and did defend physiology.

The machine metaphor was not unique to either the French or the British. It was of course echoed by Pavlov when he spoke of the methodological need for 'the partial destruction or complete extirpation of parts of the cortex', seeing it as the 'roughest form of mechanical interference'.[20] The suggestion has been made that the destruction of traditional sources of authority in the French Revolution meant that the professional intelligentsia had greater ideological power in France than in Britain, so that the antivivisection movement in Britain was able and needed to draw on aristocratic power, and indeed hinted at Royal support (shades of the Royal Family's interest in homeopathic medicine, to say nothing of Prince Charles's more recent green moments). However, the core of the debate turned on the conception of animal nature as incapable of being conscious of pain. The account by George Hoggan, who had observed Bernard's laboratory, of the great scientist as first experimenting on animals and then handing over the used animals to his assistants to carry out their less important experiments, suggests that Bernard had no conception of animals suffering pain. Francis Sibson, Consulting Physician to St Mary's Hospital, in his evidence to the 1875 Royal Commission on animal experimentation, spoke in similar vein of Magendie: 'I do not think that the idea entered his mind that he had a suffering being under him.'[21]

While it is not my purpose to trace the history of the antivivisection movement in Britain and its influence on state regulation of research, the state's involvement in animal welfare in the laboratory has a century-plus record in a way that is rather less marked in other countries. The British antivivisectionists were able either to create or build on a belief that animals could feel pain in a way that the French, for example, were not. Perhaps the considerable presence of women in the British movement with this sense of defending oneself along with the animals gave a particularly sharp and effective edge to the struggle in Britain. Mary Ann Elston makes the point that the ethicist Peter Singer, arguably the leading theorist of the contemporary animal liberation movement, fails to analyse this 'complex symbolic as-

[20] Passage from Pavlov, quoted by George Bernard Shaw, *On Vivisection* (Chicago, 1950). Shaw also tells H. G. Wells's pointed joke, 'If I had only one lifebelt, and GBS and Pavlov were drowning, I would save Pavlov.'

[21] Westacott, *A Century of Vivisection and Anti-vivisection*, pp. 31 and 27.

sociation between women, sentiment and nature'.[22] She is charitable to Singer. A harsher reading of his commitment to animal liberation would see it as rather transient, as by the time he had become involved in the ethical discussion of *in vitro* fertilisation it had pretty much faded out. In a book published with a leading obstetrician concerning the new reproductive technologies, he is entirely able to ignore the mice and frogs whose laboratory usage had made possible the human work and indeed he reveals himself as a straightforward androcentric and uncritical enthusiast for modern medical technology.[23]

However it should not be assumed that all nineteenth-century intellectual women or feminists shared Cobbe's opposition to physiology. George Eliot for example, who had already celebrated in *Middlemarch* the potentiality of the new scientific medicine with the story of Mr Lydgate's hopeful beginnings and the abandonment of his ideals to keep a frivolous wife, established a physiology scholarship in memory of George Henry Lewes. The debate was echoed within medicine. Elizabeth Blackwell, as a pioneering woman doctor, was opposed to vivisection and gynaecological examinations where women were strapped and bound, as both brutalising and degrading. Her sister clinician, Elizabeth Garrett Anderson, by contrast took the view that women should study physiology. None the less, the metaphor of rape is strongly present within the antivivisection literature written by women from the 1880s onwards, characterising the laboratory within medicine, and also medical practice on women.

Elston suggests that this debate between feminists was about a naturalised conception of the difference between men and women, not least at the moral level. For Cobbe, this difference was thus part of the divided spheres in which women were properly and naturally the guardians of morality. This naturalised conception of the moral superiority of women persists and, as I have indicated, is still influential within the radical feminist strand of contemporary feminism. But for Cobbe it meant that every woman who studied physiology was a double loss. Cobbe identified cruelty as *the* moral evil – by definition the cruelty of men, as women had naturally finer feelings. Consequently her campaigning work against vivisection was integral to her opposition to men's cruelty and sensuality, whether within the house as Mr Hyde or in the laboratory as Dr Jekyll. As Elston observes, for Cobbe the knowing cruelty of the scientist was

[22] Elston, 'Women and Anti-Vivisection', p. 260.

[23] P. Singer and D. Wells, *The Reproductive Revolution: New Ways of Making Babies* (Oxford, 1984).

more evil than that of the men who engaged in blood sports (to which she was opposed) or ate meat (she was not a vegetarian). The scientific doctor was truly more cruel and vile than the plain man.

'Laboratories and whorehouses are places in which you do what you like – which has its amusing sides.' (Conference participant)

Before I leave the discussion of Stewart Richards's paper, which precipitated all these connections and, as I have suggested, included cultural politics as well as aesthetic and moral responses in their negative representations of women and nature, I want to show how taking reflexivity seriously draws out emotional and sexual material which the rules of both science and the conference game render invisible. Thus Stewart, in talking about personal feelings, seemed to feel himself to be heretical and in consequence found it necessary to reassure us that he was morally still committed to physiology. By contrast, such disclosure is routine to feminist research and meetings, where personal feelings are integral to analysis to achieve what is sometimes spoken of by feminists as 'passionate objectivity'. The point of talking about this is not to expose one person's feelings but to explore the kind of emotions which are taken for granted and therefore invisibilised and also what may be released by talking about other sorts of feeling.

First, although there is a general ideological statement that the doing of science/history is dispassionate, this is simply empirically untrue: some kinds of emotion are routinely displayed and talked about. The point is that these are so normalised within science that the dominant discourse no longer recognises them as emotions. Thus aggression and anger can be routinely reported as part of doing laboratory science, and such emotions may be similarly displayed by participants at a meeting. It is true that the participants will often deplore this privately, wondering 'what has got into X today?' But the disapproval seems not to be sufficient to marginalise the displayer. No Latourian phalanxes seem to bear down. Are we to conclude that some kinds of emotion are not really heretical, but are excusable and invisible as emotions in the production of science, and just mildly *passé* in the best circles?

However, speaking of more tender feelings *is* heretical; it is only these which are described as 'being emotional', these that become dangerous; heaven knows what may be released. Indeed it was – at the Cambridge meeting. Discussing the motive power of research, a participant made the observation quoted above about laboratories and whorehouses. Now while the sayer was intensely embarrassed and apologised – so I don't want to drone on about the infamy of the remark – I do want to reflect on it, as it makes another set of connections around sexuality and the laboratory in medicine which only feminist historians have explored.

Nor is the remark exceptional in the discussion of science. Any reader of Feyerabend[24] must see that his philosophical prescription of 'anything goes' is profoundly linked to his lewd sexist conception of a new theory as a charming courtesan whose sole purpose is his delectation. These connections exist outside the goalposts of the mainstream meeting, and it is only when the rules start being breached that the goalposts start moving and the rules of disclosure become uncertain. Then New academic men speak in an unguarded way, sounding uncommonly like the Old ones. What feminists find disturbing is that Feyerabend is seen by so many as a liberatory figure within the philosophy of science when his metaphor is so much part of the old and sexist story of science. The chief difference is that where, from Bacon to the nineteenth-century physiologists, nature as woman was seen as passive, to be violently possessed by a male science, now she is supposed to be the voluptuous whore, to whom, and in whose workplace, 'you can do anything you like'.

It goes without saying that the 'you' who 'can do anything you like' is profoundly gendered. No one could for a moment consider that women were being invited to do anything we like. We, along with the animals, are the 'Other', both in the laboratory and in the whorehouse. As for the 'amusing sides', the invocation is of these privileged spaces where men may play out their sadistic fantasies on the Other, and it is this which gives the opportunity for men's pleasure and amusement. Coral Lansbury's examination of the symbolic nineteenth century reveals the links between the practice of strapping women for gynaecological examination (so opposed by Elizabeth Blackwell) and the frequent representation of women as well-groomed horses.[25] Consider Lady Dedlock in Dickens's *Bleak House* (that most savage but euphemistic account of relations between the sexes in Victorian England), the brutal practice of bearing reins exposed by Anna Sewell's *Black Beauty*, which young girls wept over then and

[24] Paul Feyerabend, *Against Method: Outline of an Anarchistic Theory of Knowledge* (London, 1978); and *Science in a Free Society* (London, 1982).

[25] Lansbury, *The Old Brown Dog*, p. 99.

now (did boys?), and the pornographic representation of women, as in *Fanny Hill*, as young mares to be flogged into submission, and their masochistic sexual pleasure.

As my example of Feyerabend sought to indicate, I do not think that our participant's lapse was totally exceptional. (The exceptional part was the genuine distress of its utterer.) The intensely gendered and often violent sexual metaphors through which science works are unfortunately alive and well. Evelyn Fox Keller, for example, has looked at the language of Nobel prizewinners' speeches of acceptance in which they speak of their relationship to science and nature. The representations of old theoretical models as faithful old wives and new ones as delightful young mistresses speak of sexuality as well as gender.[26]

Murmurings and alternative knowledges

But to return to the papers presented at Cambridge: there were murmurings as well as silences and they should be attended to, for they tell us a little about gender, physiology and the new social history of science. For example, Paul Weindling noted the presence of Eastern European women doctors at the Pasteur Institute and saw this as an example of its 'cosmopolitanism'. While it is clear that the institute was more inclusive than Berlin, it might be interesting to explore whether national inclusivity often carries with it gender inclusivity. Certainly the hospitable atmosphere of Gowland Hopkins's Cambridge laboratory in the interwar period offered a home both for Jewish scientists escaping Nazi-occupied Europe and for a number of immensely gifted women, including Dorothy Wrinch and Hopkins's eventual successor Margery Stephenson. In other papers women, not least as students, were seen as threatening. Bill Bynum quoted a letter from Michael Foster to Edward Schäfer in which he urges him to give up lecturing. For Foster, lecturing to women, along with lecturing in general, threatens masculinity, which should not be sacrificed but find its fullest expression in research. 'I see you are lecturing to women... don't do too much lecturing – *it destroys a man*... give all your energy to research'.[27]

But it was perhaps Timothy Lenoir's paper which, in its ambition to go beyond the usual argument that support for laboratory training

[26] Keller, *Reflections on Gender and Science.*

[27] Letter from Foster to Schäfer, undated, Contemporary Medical Archives Centre at the Wellcome Institute for the History of Medicine, London, PP/ESS/B6/11. The Editors are grateful to Sonia Uyterhoeven for locating this letter.

was a long-term investment in the future, promised but ultimately frustrated a gendered analysis. Lenoir claimed to look in a very concrete way at the implications of the new practices and ways of seeing things for a society in cultural and political crisis. He wrote: 'While accepting the importance of the politics of material interest as a strong motivating ideology, I have attempted to go beyond ideology to its concrete manifestations in the motivations, interests and actions, in short the life-world of particular groups.' Just so. But what would have made his analysis rather more concrete would have been to explore how these 'particular groups' of scientifically trained physicians also came to be gendered in the process of becoming an influential elite. Lenoir continually offered gendered clues in language: he spoke of 'young heroes' who seek to redefine physiology; he frequently used the expression 'mastery' to indicate effective acquisition of the new technical skills; but above all his paper reported numerous and detailed stories of men's interactions with men whether as fathers or colleagues. The gendered murmuring of the material was unheard. Women were in consequence implicitly constructed as empty Galtonic vessels through which the male scientific line transmits itself.

But the clearest bridge to a feminist analysis was offered by Merriley Borell's exploration of the laboratory as the arbiter of medical knowledge. She described the move from demonstration and occasional 'hands-on' training in the 1870s to a situation at the turn of the century in which training focused on a systematic series of exercises which aimed to transmit both manual and reasoning skills. Above all, she identified a new labour process – the new 'hands-on' approach was to provide mental training and through this empower its practitioners. The entry of the new equipment of measurement into medicine with its attendant new labour process was as dramatic as the machine entering industry before it. It was not by chance that the new teaching laboratories which trained large numbers of students looked more than a little like factories. As the market entered medicine as the provider of the new equipment it also provided strong support for the advance of the new scientific medicine. Borell concluded by inviting critical reflexion on the nature and the limitations of the scientific medicine that this process gave birth to and on the different kind of medicine currently being admitted – namely the understanding of the importance of lifestyle and the environment for the production of health and disease – which scientific and reductionist medicine excluded.

The feminist critique of science, which would be voiced in our utopian conference in Mattapoisett or Whileaway, would continue this process of critical reflection. How far was this much vaunted 'new way of seeing', the social project of a specific gender and class, empowered by its relationship to capital? Was its triumph, the domination of nature, achieved through not only the claimed unity of manual and mental reasoning but also the unclaimed alliance of capital and patriarchy, creating and occupying new social organisations and occupations – the research laboratories and indeed scientific medicine itself? Was the exclusion of women healers, above all the midwives, a necessity for the successful domination of the body – by a masculinised and scientised medicine? What part did a far from neutral state play in regulating medicine in the interests of a patriarchical elite and the equipment (and later drug) industry? And above all was the unity of manual and reasoning skills nothing less than an expression of the masculinist epistemology which underpins the project of modern experimental science?

Yet there are difficulties, at least for those of us influenced by Marxist theorising, for only the manual skills of specific strata are acknowledged within scientific production. Thus although the left-wing scientific trade union of the 1930s was called the Association of Scientific Workers, technicians were not eligible for membership. Rather like housewives (and there are parallels in the labour process), what technicians did was not 'work'. Only what scientists did was scientific work. (Witness the standard expression even today in the research papers: 'other workers have shown'.) It was left to the New Left and its theoreticians, particularly Sohn-Rethel,[28] to insist that scientific knowledge was peculiarly abstract and alienated and that the social origins of this abstraction lay in the profound division of mental and manual labour characteristic of capitalist production – including capitalist scientific production. The project of the radical science movement – like the New Left, despite its inclusive rhetoric and the presence of women and black people, in actuality a movement of white men – was to transcend the division of Hand and Brain. Overcoming this division of labour could offer a new transformative science which would no longer dominate nature, including our own human nature, but live pacifically and ecologically as part of nature. Like New Left politics as a whole, the attempt was nothing less than to remake ourselves and the knowledges we produced. I write 'we',

[28] Alfred Sohn-Rethel, *Intellectual and Manual Labour: A Critique of Epistemology* (London, 1978).

for as part of that movement it was a long time before I fully understood that that 'we' did not include women, whether we were women of colour or white, middle or working class. The universal project of the radical science movement, while it was very clear about the class relations, was, like the universal project of science it opposed, profoundly gendered, sexualised and 'raced'.

But the point is that both the radical science movement and the new social studies of science only address knowledge derived from a production system which itself is organised through a profoundly gendered division of labour and a highly segmented labour market in which black people, above all black women, are forced to the worst positions, either as the lowest fraction of the working class or as an underclass. To overcome the division of labour within the production system, either generally or specifically within science, was to overcome the division of labour between men while leaving untouched that between men and women. It is for that reason that the project embodied in the work and writing of the philosopher Sohn-Rethel or the trade union leader Mike Cooley,[29] or in its vast societal expression, the Cultural Revolution itself, can at best be a story of partial progress.

Elsewhere I have argued that this attempt to unite the knowledges of Hand and Brain[30] is incomplete in that it leaves out the practices and the knowledges which derive from women's sensuous engagement, their practice in and with the world. While not wanting to reconstruct a Universal Woman, or enter into some naturalised conception of the separate spheres, it is important to insist that the lives of women are different from those of men. Certain forms of labour associated with reproduction, whether within or between the generations, are, except in some very exceptional households, still very much the preserve of women. This caring labour (often but not always a labour of love) develops relational ways of seeing and thinking which are not shared by those who have historically refused such labour. The knowledges, like the labour of the Heart, have been long dismissed as natural and therefore trivial. While it has been a

[29] Mike Cooley, *Architect or Bee? The Human/Technology Relationship*, (Slough, 1980).

[30] Hilary Rose, 'Hand, Brain and Heart: a feminist epistemology for the natural sciences', *Signs: Journal of Women in Culture and Society*, 9 (1983–4), pp. 73–90, republished in Harding and O'Barr (eds.), *Sex and Scientific Inquiry*, pp. 265–82; Hilary Rose, 'Women's work: women's knowledge', in Juliet Mitchell and Ann Oakley (eds.), *What is Feminism?* (Oxford, 1986), pp. 161–83. For a very similar argument see also Nancy Hartsock, 'The feminist standpoint', in Sandra Harding and Merril Hintikka (eds.), *Discovering Reality* (Dordrecht, 1986).

major feminist achievement that housework and child care are acknowledged as work, the task of convincing people that there are distinctive ways of seeing associated with relational labour is harder. There are parallels with the development of the laboratory in medicine and the claims of the 'hands-on' approach to bring the civilising influence of science to medical practice. Indeed, relational skills developed through the practice of caring would seem to offer rather more securely founded claims than those of the physiology laboratory to 'civilise' medicine. It is not difficult to share something of the rage felt by the animal rights movement at the cruelty of much experimental research (not least, but not only, that of the drug houses) compounded by the arrogance of a science which persists in maintaining that what it does is *sui generis* above criticism,[31] but few would argue that the contribution of the laboratory to medicine – even of Dr Hyde – is nil. The argument here is not that the knowledges developed by the masculinist laboratory are to be abandoned but that they are to be located – and hence changed – within a wider concept of rationality. As against the abstract rationality of science, or the practical rationality of manual labour, this relational labour offers a rationality of caring. To bring about this transformation of rationality requires changes not just in concepts but in our practices of daily life which open the possibility to men as well as women of acquiring 'loving reasoning'.

Lastly I took it as axiomatic that the utopian conference which looked back at today and our past would happen. My personal hopes are that it will be located in the post-gendered society of Mattapoisett, but I think we must be entirely clear that it is now up to the efforts of men to change themselves and their knowledges, otherwise the only place for such a symposium would be Whileaway. The remaining alternative – Manland – is too bleak a distopia to consider.[32]

[31] As a very recent example of arrogance, see the letters debate around Colin Blakemore's defence of animal experimentation, *Nature*, 6 July 1989.

[32] Manland is Russ's distopic alternative to Whileaway, no fit place for any post-sexist knowledge.

Index

Printed in the United States
By Bookmasters